D1275212

Charles F. McKhann, M.D., is a Professor of Surgery at Yale University with a special interest in cancer surgery. He has served on Advisory Councils to the American Cancer Society and the National Cancer Institute.

a guide for patients, family, and friends

The Facts About Cancer

CHARLES F. McKHANN, M.D.

A SPECTRUM BOOK

Prentice-Hall, Inc., Englewood Cliffs, N.J. 07632

Library of Congress Cataloging in Publication Data

McKhann, Charles F.
   The facts about cancer.

   (A Spectrum Book)
   Includes index.
     1. Cancer.   I. Title.   [DNLM: 1. Neoplasms—
Popular works. QZ 201 M478f]
RC262.M38   616.99′4   81-8487
ISBN 0-13-299503-4   AACR2
ISBN 0-13-299495-X (pbk.)

This Spectrum Book is available to businesses and organizations at a special discount when ordered in large quantities. For information, contact Prentice-Hall, Inc., General Book Marketing, Special Sales Division, Englewood Cliffs, N.J. 07632.

Editorial/production supervision
and interior design by Kimberly Mazur
Manufacturing buyer: Barbara Frick

Excerpt from letter by Thomas McCann published by permission of Candace M. McGuire.
All art courtesy of Robert Olson, Susan A. Hopp, and Susan Lasley.

Prentice-Hall International, Inc., *London*
Prentice-Hall of Australia Pty. Limited, *Sydney*
Prentice-Hall of Canada, Ltd., *Toronto*
Prentice-Hall of India Private Limited, *New Delhi*
Prentice-Hall of Japan, Inc., *Tokyo*
Prentice-Hall of Southeast Asia Pte. Ltd., *Singapore*
Whitehall Books Limited, *Wellington, New Zealand*

To my patients and their families

Contents

Common Cancers

Preface

This book is written primarily for you who have cancer, and for your families and friends, to help you understand the disease and your reactions to it. We will look at what cancer is, what it does to you, both physically and psychologically, and its treatment. The main purpose of the book is to respond to some of the many concerns and questions raised by my patients and their families. As a surgeon concerned mostly with the care of people with cancer, I have seen these questions take on enormous depth and complexity in the last few years. As recently as twenty years ago they were limited to what *must* be done, rarely questioning the need for treatment, choice of treatment, or the risks or disability it might produce. The word *cancer* was almost never used in questions or answers. If people knew the nature of their illness and its implications, they certainly did not find out from their doctors. If the initial treatment of surgery or radiation failed, there was nothing more to offer and the exact diagnosis did not seem very important. Prolonged illness, dying, and death were not subjects for polite conversation.

The change has been dramatic. Every aspect of this disease is now questioned daily. Alternative forms of treatment and difficult medical controversies are weighed in popular magazines. Too much treatment carries the same stigma that no treatment at all did previously. Some insist on their right to die, rejecting any treatment; others insist on their right to try any treatment, no matter how controversial, such as Laetrile. Chemotherapy has added years of comfort and productivity to the lives of those who cannot be cured.

A second reason for writing the book is concern about the way questions are answered. Several years ago a patient who was near death asked me some very difficult questions: "What is it like to die?" "Why does it take so long?" "What *really* happens after we die?" Perhaps as the wife of a minister she was better equipped to deal with these problems than I. When my attempts to be distracting and cheerful failed, I fled. At that time she was unique among patients, but I was in no way unique among doctors. Eventually I spent hours talking to her and learning from her. I realized that if people are able to ask hard questions, the least they deserve is their doctor's willingness and ability to give reasonable answers.

The final and most important purpose of the book is to encourage you to participate actively in your own care. You must have facts in order to share in making decisions. There is no way that one volume can answer all the questions related to cancer. Indeed, progress in treatment is too rapid. Instead I have tried to provide enough information to help you ask the right questions and understand the answers.

This book is based on conversations with my own patients over many years and extensive interviews with about sixty patients and families. Their words were often better than mine, and I have quoted them freely. In that sense much of the information in the first part of the book is relayed directly to you from people who have cancer and from their families. I am only the middleman. The information in other sections of the book comes from medical and scientific literature that I have attempted to translate into plain English. In these chapters I am an interpreter.

Cancer is a common disease. It will afflict one out of four Americans and affect two-thirds of our families. Fear of this disease has obscured the fact that almost half of the people with cancer can be cured, and proper treatment of those who cannot be cured can add years of comfortable and productive life. There is no reasonable alternative to getting the best care you can and joining your doctor in treating your disease.

Acknowledgments

Many people helped to make this book possible. First and foremost are the numerous patients who allowed me to probe into their lives and illnesses and who shared their concerns and advice so candidly. I also thank my colleagues, particularly Dr. Theodor Grage, for allowing me to interview their patients. I give special thanks to Paul Hamilton, M.D., Lynn Ringer, Irene Paulin, R.N., Mary Margaret Goodrich, and many volunteers from the CanSurmount Program in Denver, Colorado for their encouragement and long hours of interviews. The gentle side of care was taught to me by Ida Martinson, R.N., Ph.D., Sue Sauer, R.N., Judy Beck, R.N., and many of our staff nurses.

I am grateful to my colleagues for reviewing specific chapters that are outside my own area of expertise. They include Norma Ramsey, M.D., Seymour Levitt, M.D., Arndt Duval, M.D., Athanasios Theologides, M.D., Shelley Chou, M.D., Elwin Fraley, M.D., Theodor Grage, M.D., Thomas Jones, M.D., Robert Howe, M.D., Leon Adcock, M.D., and Arnold Leonard, M.D.

A sabbatical leave from the University of Minnesota made it possible for me to do much of my writing in idyllic surroundings, at the Institute for Experimental Cancer Research, Lausanne, Switzerland. I am indebted to the Josiah Macy Foundation and the Minnesota Division of the Veterans of Foreign Wars for support, and to Theodore Brunner, M.D., my host for that year.

Bob Olson, Susan Lasley, and Susan A. Hopp provided illustrations that saved hundreds of words. Karen Klein and Mary Ellen Gerth know this writing better than I do, having typed each chapter through an average of three revisions without losing any of the cheerfulness that makes them so delightful to work with. They were helped by Kathy Folven and Beverly Schmidt. Finally, a special word of thanks to Susan Stuart-Otto for her patience in editing the manuscript.

The Impact
of Cancer

What Cancer Does To You

As anyone who has cancer knows, it is no accident that many people look upon their disease as the enemy and speak of their battle against it. But battles can be confusing and it is easy to lose your way when everything around you appears to be collapsing, and the difference between advance and retreat is not clear. If often seems safer just to hide. The purpose of this chapter, and indeed of much of the book, is to help you understand your own war against cancer so you can be in command and assume the responsibility that is rightly yours. Most of the decisions are yours to make and most of the credit for every victory, large or small, belongs to you.

Your confrontation with cancer will require that you fight many battles. You will win some, but you must also expect to lose a few. For cancer is a tough opponent, worthy of the best in you. From each encounter you must walk away a stronger and better person. From the numbness of "finding out" comes the resolve that leads to good treatment. From the isolation caused by fear comes an expanded meaning of friendship. From thoughts of death comes awareness of life. Shadows of guilt are replaced with the light of understanding, of your illness, yourself, and the people around you.

To understand what is required, you must study your enemy. This means learning how cancer attacks your body, but more important, how it attacks your person, the *real* you.

I know what cancer is —cells that have gone berserk and are trying to take me over. The bad cells are crowding out the good ones.

WHAT IS CANCER?

Cancer usually originates from a single normal cell, one of the billions that represent the bricks and mortar of the body. The cell must be one that divides, and in dividing it begins to make mistakes. The original mistake is probably a spontaneous change (mutation), with no known cause, or it may be caused by a virus, or by chemical or radiation injury.

In successive divisions it continues to pile up more mistakes. A few early errors may be harmless and go unnoticed, or at worst be "premalignant". More errors, however, may give the new cells an advantage over normal cells, allowing them to grow faster and more aggressively. The most important changes in cancer cells are in their behavior, including escape from normal growth controls, ability to invade neighboring tissues and to spread or metastasize to other parts of the body. For example, a cancer that begins in a single cell in the lining of the bowel becomes several cells, still confined to the lining of the bowel. Later it penetrates into and eventually through the bowel wall, passing successively through layers of muscular tissue on the way. At some time tumor cells may escape into the lymphatic circulation where they go to the lymph nodes near the bowel and from there eventually into the bloodstream. Other cells may go directly into small blood vessels and be carried to the liver or the lungs.

Not only do cancer cells undergo some very basic changes that allow them to escape from normal growth controls, but they continue to undergo more changes so they become progressively more malignant. While most normal cells of any given tissue resemble one another almost exactly, tumor cells evolve into very mixed populations as they make new mistakes or mutations. Eventually some of them acquire a selective advantage, not only over normal cells but even over other cells of the same tumor. As this process is repeated, the tumor may gradually progress from a low level of malignancy, with cells that closely resemble the original normal cells or tissue, to a higher level of malignancy with more abnormal cells. With this comes an increased capacity to invade other tissues and spread to other parts of the body and to develop resistance to treatment.

HOW CANCERS HARM YOU   The disability caused by cancer can be local or general. A tumor may be disfiguring if it is near the surface of the body. A lump may enlarge until it is noticeable, it may cause a breakdown of the skin or ulceration, or it may impair motion if it is in a muscle or near a joint. A growing tumor can obstruct any hollow organ or tube within the body. Obstruction of the esophagus makes it difficult to swallow. Obstruction of the bowel causes pain and vomiting. Obstruction of the ureter causes pain in the blocked kidney whereas obstruction of the urethra, by cancer of the prostate, prevents urination. Obstruction of the bronchus from cancer of the lung causes pneumonia, and obstruction of the common bile duct, as in cancer of the pancreas, causes backing up of bile, producing yellowing of the skin (jaundice). Finally, local growth of the tumor may cause pressure and pain in nearby nerves. In the brain or spinal cord, even small tumors can cause paralysis or loss of sensation.

General effects of cancers include anemia, infection, and weight loss. Anemia is very common and results from bleeding from the tumor, as in cancer of the colon, inadequate production of blood cells if the bone marrow is replaced by tumor, or by increased breakdown of blood cells in some leukemias. Infection occurs when a bronchus is blocked by cancer of the lung, when the bladder is completely obstructed and cannot be emptied, or when the bone marrow or lymphoid systems are involved with the tumor, as in leukemias and lymphomas, and cannot produce enough normal white blood cells. Fever is usually caused by infection but a few tumors cause fever directly, particularly when the liver is involved.

Finally, cancer is very frequently associated with weight loss. Many explanations have been given for this, including the possibility that the cancer demands and gets more than its share of nutrition. At the present time we do not understand very much about the cause of this weight loss.

PERSONAL REACTIONS TO CANCER

Shock

Shock is the best word to describe the immediate reaction to learning that you have cancer. It is that brief period when the mind "blanks out" and seals itself off from all sensations and activity. It has been described as "a wave going over your head," when you can neither see nor hear nor comprehend what is going on and may not even be aware of where you are. This complete shutting off of sensation may not occur at all or may last only a very few seconds or a few minutes.

Denial

As normal sensation returns it is frequently associated with strong revulsion against the very insult that caused shock in the first place. In its simplest form this is expressed as *disbelief,* "Oh no, not me", "This can't be happening to me!"

Even though he used the word malignant and told me that I would probably have to have surgery, I did not understand that it was cancer. It went right by me. I did not understand until late that evening when I was talking to my wife and it dawned on me. She realized before I did what the problem was because I told her the words that had been spoken to me even though I had not yet had time to fully understand them.

Denial must be recognized for what it is, a very important normal and healthy defense mechanism against life-threatening situations or information. It has been described as the "morphine of the soul" and is the way we reject thoughts too painful to endure. We actually buy time to gather up our emotional strength to face reality, often letting reality come in slowly so it will not overwhelm us. By this gradual process many people go through a phase where they can accept the fact of cancer while continuing to deny the seriousness of the illness.

Denial may last minutes, hours, days, or even weeks, but most people cannot maintain it for very long. The person who denies the existence and threat of his cancer has the difficult task of swimming upstream against the current of reality, not to mention the demands of everyday life.

While denial is an important and normal defense mechanism, it can be carried to harmful extremes. Intense and prolonged denial can prevent you from seeking early medical attention or cause you to reject medical advice and treatment by failing to accept the diagnosis. People have been known to "forget" to tell their doctor of a suspicious sign or symptom, feeling that if the doctor did not find it, it could not be very important.

Denial may also be experienced by members of your family so that it becomes your responsibility to help others accept your illness.

Fear Shock and denial are replaced with more active reactions to the threat of cancer. Fear is one of the most basic of all emotions and when you realize you have cancer you also realize that you are frightened of many things. These include the threat of death, pain, loss of body functions, losing your position of responsibility in your family or at work, becoming dependent or abandoned by your friends, family, and even doctors. Perhaps most distressing is fear of the unknown and uncertainty of what lies ahead. Like denial, fear is a normal feeling experienced at some time by everyone who has cancer. When it borders on panic, fear can be harmful, causing you to flee from treatment or to seek help from "quacks". Part of our revulsion against cancer may be that we do not think of it as the result of aging and "wearing out", but rather as our own bodies turned against us. It is hideous to think that a few cells have turned traitor and are systematically trying to destroy an otherwise intact person. We associate cancer with a slow death, etched with pain and drawn out with hopelessness, but this does not convey an accurate picture of cancer today. Almost half of the people with cancer can be cured. When it cannot be cured, cancer can often be controlled, much as high blood pressure or diabetes, with treatment providing additional years of comfortable and productive life. This is not true of stroke victims, 50 percent of whom die within a year of the stroke, nor of heart attack victims, 35 percent of whom die within a month of their first attack. Heart disease and stroke kill many more people than cancer each year.

Anger is a more open form of rebellion against cancer, a cry of rage that *anything* could be so threatening and make you so afraid. If fear is hard to express, anger is not. It may be a silent gritting of teeth or it may be weeping, shouting, screaming, or actually lashing out at objects or people. The target of anger may be yourself, your family, God, fate, doctors, nurses, the hospital or the disease itself.

Anger

After the doctor told me and my parents that I had leukemia, I went into the bathroom and screamed. I yelled at God that I was being short-changed in life and that it wasn't fair to me or my family.

We tend to get angry at the nice people in our lives, particularly members of our families. Most of us are much more reluctant to turn on our doctors than on nurses or family members. This is probably out of fear that the doctor may leave or reject us if we show too much hostility.

I hated one doctor so much that the idea of failing and being angry in front of his eyes was more than I could bear. When I came back from surgery I was a real bitch and I took it out mostly on my mother. I said nasty things to her because that's what people do with their mothers when they're upset. Fortunately she was terrific and let whatever came out come out.

In fact doctors, nurses, and other professionals who have experience with serious illness are very appropriate targets for this kind of anger. They have seen it before and should be able to take it in stride. Anger is not without value, particularly when it can be directed against the disease itself. It brings out the fighter in you, and people who are angry at their disease are frequently aggressive about getting treatment.

In a milder form, anger shows up as resentment. This may be directed at the need to change your way of life, your work, having to become more dependent on your parents, children, or spouse, or at the possible loss of years of active and exciting life.

Anxiety includes worry about pain, love, job security, bills, financial future of your family, and your general ability to cope with the stress

Anxiety

that the illness is placing upon you. Cancer magnifies all the small problems encountered in daily life, and compromises your ability to cope with new problems that come up. Anxiety also comes from the uncertainty and frustration of living with cancer. You know that having cancer will probably change your life but do not know in what way or how much. There is a continuing sense of frustration and uncertainty concerning the treatment of cancer, the necessity of taking a different role at work and within your family, and the possibility of being a burden on those you love. Surprisingly, going home from the hospital can be a "scary time". After having everyone take care of you, you suddenly wonder whether you will be able to take care of yourself. All of these factors can add up to a lot of anxiety.

Guilt Guilt is an unfortunate but common response to illness. Some people with cancer seem to go out of their way to blame themselves for things over which they have no control. Guilt can arise over everyday problems such as inability to do your housework or cooking, meeting the demands of children, or responding to the sexual desires of your spouse. Men often feel guilty because they are not able to work and support their families and have to rely on their wives. Guilt may be the feeling you are letting your doctor or family down when you are not doing well on treatment. You will find it much more comfortable to *regret* that you cannot do something rather than feeling guilty about it.

Guilt can be very destructive. The heaviest burden of guilt falls on people who feel that cancer is a form of punishment for their sins. I do not know of any religion that sees God as being that wicked. Some doctors permit or even encourage people to think that they caused their own cancers. With the single exception of smoking, there is no evidence that what you do or think or say can bring on cancer. No thought process, personality type, or anxiety level has been proven to be related to cancer. To assume guilt in any of these areas is to assume a harmful and totally unnecessary burden.

I don't think that it is constructive to convey to someone that they have done this to themselves. It hits you when you are down and vulnerable and does a guilt number on you that is unnecessary.

People or influences that make you feel guilty should be avoided. They cannot help you.

Loss of Many people with cancer experience a loss of self esteem, particularly
Self-Esteem in the hospital. The lack of privacy may have devastating effects, including feelings of shame, worthlessness, defectiveness, loss of willpower and autonomy, self-rejection, and even humiliation and

defeat. All of these are caused by loss of control over yourself and your own fate. Your illness forces you to be uncomfortably dependent on others for treatments that you do not like, for an illness you do not understand.

The fact that I had leukemia meant that I was dependent on doctors and nurses. When you are in the hospital and people are doing things for you to keep you alive it is very clear that you are dependent on them. I felt controlled by it, as if I had given myself away to other people.

One thing that I have gotten out of all my treatments is an extreme dislike for having things done to my body. But doing things to the body is what medicine is all about. It is the outside coming in and there is no way that you can get away from it. I really disliked having my skin marked when I was going to get radiation. That sort of thing has nothing to do with me. *I don't like that kind of manipulation anymore.*

Depression is the common result of all these experiences and feelings. Everyone experiences depression from time to time and can recognize disappointment, sadness, gloom, and discouragement.

Depression

I was depressed when I had doubts if I was going to make it. I was depressed not so much because of my illness but because I couldn't do the things that I had always done. I was used to being a busy person. To get out of bed and get dressed and ready to do something and then find that you were too tired and have to go back to bed—that was depressing.

When you are depressed there is a tendency to withdraw from other people and be silent or moody. Often it is hard to eat, sleep, or concentrate on your work. Extreme stages of depression include feelings of helplessness and despair. Although some degree of depression is encountered from time to time by everyone with cancer, complete resignation and "loss of will to live" can increase the seriousness of the illness and even shorten one's life. Fortunately this is rare and such people can be helped. Despair and suicide are uncommon in people with cancer.

Unpleasant as they are, all these strong reactions are perfectly normal. Shock, fear, denial, anger, anxiety, depression, and even guilt are common reactions to *any* dangerous situation, including cancer. They represent responses *to* the disease and *are not* part of the disease itself. Moreover, because the illness and reactions to it are separate, treatment of the disease and control of psychological aspects are also separate. Once you understand the negative reactions to cancer, you can begin to overcome them!

Normal Reactions

two
Learning To Live With Cancer

When the shock of discovering you have a serious disease wears off, whether it is a matter of minutes or days, your sensations and thoughts reassemble themselves. Despair and fear of impending death fade as you begin to think about the good things you would *like* to do and what life *still* means to you. From there it is only a short step to looking ahead and making plans for tomorrow, the next day, and even as far as next week. You gradually realize that you have a future, that the world is still there and you are an important part of it.

"I HAVE CANCER" The sooner you admit to yourself that you have cancer—before you have a chance to build much resistance—the easier it is. One way is to look in the mirror and say to yourself "I have cancer". If saying this brings tears to your eyes or makes you angry—fine—weep or swear or beat your pillow, but repeat it again and again until you accept it as fact. Until you can say it to yourself, you will not be able to say it to anyone else and that, as we will see, is also very important.

Your conversation with the mirror should not end there. The sentence needs to be complete. "I have cancer BUT the rest of me is okay". The rest of you really is okay. Cancer is like injuring your hand; only the hand is hurt. Moreover, without the rest of you, the hand cannot get better. Finally, let the mirror really hear from you, "I have cancer, *but* the rest of me is okay *and* I am important!" You are at least as good a person as you were before, and perhaps already a little better.

Plans and Priorities *Realizing that I had leukemia required a major decision—was I going to try to live as though I was going to die quickly or was I going to try to live as though I was going to live a fairly normal life? The question was pretty much decided when I got braces for my teeth!*

A common philosophic question among college students is "what would you do if you only had six months to live?" Even at that optimistic age, most would change very little in their lives. Although actually having cancer poses a much more direct threat, most people come up with the same answer, "There is no point in dying before your time". If you are living a happy life and are feeling content with yourself and doing what you want there is no need to change your life just because you are sick.

I'm 73 years old and I can't expect to live 50 more years, but I may have another 10. I do everything I want to. I ride a bicycle, work in the garden, cut the grass, drive the car, just about anything that a man my age can do. A lot of my friends are sitting around in rocking chairs and not having nearly as much fun as I am.

Obviously living with cancer requires some compromises. The most common limiting factor following surgery, radiation, or chemotherapy is tiredness. You do not have the energy to do everything you did before. This forces you to establish some *priorities* and even to re-schedule your everyday life.

You have to put your energy to good use—doing things that you like.
When life can no longer be measured in terms of quantity, quality becomes the objective.

The limitations imposed by illness and treatment mean that some goals must be immediate, whereas others may seem almost visionary. The immediate goals may actually affect your well-being and even your survival. These may include obtaining good nutrition and sufficient rest to help your body conserve strength and maintain and repair itself. This is the equivalent of putting money into your personal energy bank account. The bills that must be paid from this account include energy to sustain you through your illness and treatment.

Beyond survival there are goals and tasks that make even the most confining days enjoyable. Reading, writing letters or a diary, telephoning or seeing friends are among them. It helps to make a list of books you would like to read, letters you would like to write or friends you would like to see or communicate with. You can then check off the items as they are accomplished, adding new ones as they come to your attention. These are not just ways of filling your time. They are steps from inactivity to full activity.

Next is to set goals that are even further in the future. Most of these should be attainable and worth working for. Goals that cannot be reached are just as discouraging for a person who is ill as for anyone else. It is also important to be flexible. If you cannot do exactly what you want, when you want, put it off for another time or try something else.

I tried three times to go back to work, to different jobs, and three times I failed. It was very depressing. Finally, with a lot of outside help, I realized that I had set my sights too high and just could not expect so much. Now I am taking some vocational tests to find out what my limitations really are.

So far as returning to activities is concerned, you should do as much as you can and give up nothing that you do not have to. Any retreat from normal activities for therapy or illness should be considered temporary until you are convinced that they cannot be resumed. This applies particularly to your work or occupation which was the focal point of your daily life.

One of the most exciting things in life is making plans. They may be short range plans for tomorrow or the next day, or they may be long range plans such as taking a trip, painting a room, building a porch, planting a garden, doing a research project, writing a paper or even a book, studying a language, or seeing a relative or friend whom you have not seen for a long time. Plans represent the future, with you in it.

Finally, there is no reason not to consider moving ahead with the big things in your life. Getting married, having a child, or changing occupations all require considerable thought but need not be swept aside because of illness.

He told me in many different ways "I'll see it through with you. I'm here and I will always be here". We had already decided and we went ahead and got married in April. (A 25-year old woman with recurrent melanoma.)

We had not thought very much about having a child but now we do. I would like to leave someone of my own on Earth.

DEVELOPING A POSITIVE ATTITUDE

My feeling was this is my crisis and my chance to deal capably with it in a manner that I will be proud of.

If I didn't have a colostomy to worry about I wouldn't be around to have anything to worry about.

No one walks away from cancer completely unaffected by their encounter. On the other hand, it does no good to feel like a helpless victim. The fight against cancer requires complete mobilization, and self-pity saps energy you could better use to combat your disease. You can do a great deal to help yourself and there is even evidence that a strong emotional stand against the disease may actually increase the effectiveness of medical treatment, if for no other reason than making it easier to accept vigorous therapy. Building your strength through good nutrition, adequate rest, and reasonable exercise are things that only you can do. Even anger can be turned against the illness to good effect.

I had a sense of being violated, that these little critters had come into my body uninvited. This idea got me out of my depression and into a frame of mind that, "God damn it, I'm not going to die of this."

One of the greatest assets a person can have is a sense of humor. People who can laugh at themselves are very fortunate. Even the black humor that surrounds medicine, war, death, and personal tragedy has its rewards.

Look at that thigh, doc! I've caught fish that were bigger around than that!

Everyone needs a good laugh once in a while. In fact what the medical profession could use is a good giggle pill. The best healer is inside yourself and a good laugh would help a lot to bring it out.

At the end of a day of worrying I have to laugh about my problems. I can't afford to stay awake nights worrying; I need my rest so that I can worry the next day.

The best thing that happened to me was the weight I lost. Before chemotherapy my life was a continuous diet, but those drugs really work. Every fat man should have some.

My real disappointment was that I never lost much weight. To go through all that hell and not lose any weight is very upsetting.

My wife took care of everything. She even told me which of her friends I should marry if she died.

I finally went from the thought "Hey, I'm dying", to realizing "Hey, I'm living". That was a very nice turn around.

Living with Uncertainty

Fear of recurrence is uppermost in the minds of most people for the first year or two. The use of adjuvant chemotherapy following surgery and the need for long-term followup are continuous reminders and may give the impression of "living from appointment to appointment". The search for recurrence with chest x–rays and liver scans and other studies seem like proof that "it could come back". Minor aches and pains of everyday life start new waves of fear and anxiety. The interval between having a chest x–ray and receiving the "OK" note from the doctor can be cruelly long.

It's on my mind. I don't really worry about it but it would be much more pleasant if I didn't have to think that there is a chance of it coming back.

Knowledge is the best weapon against uncertainty and the unknown. The examinations and tests done during followup visits are part of a search for recurrence, or for measuring recurrence if it has taken place. Your doctor can explain these tests and interpret them for you. As a person with cancer you are also subject to all of the *same* aches and pains as anyone else. Rather than worrying about each new suspicious symptom that comes up over a weekend you may ask your doctor what the signs of recurrence of your tumor are most likely to be.

Fear of recurrence fades with time as the pressures and interests of everyday life push such unpleasant thoughts to the back of your mind. Ultimately the key to living with uncertainty is *living*. Survival without meaning is not really living at all. Whether the time remaining is limited or not, the way to get as much as possible out of it is to get back into life.

I know there is a possibility that it will come back. One thing that I have learned from my cancer is how to live every day to the fullest.

Another source of uncertainty is the limitations of our medical knowledge. Many find it very frustrating to be unable to get answers to important and seemingly simple questions, not through avoidance but because the answers are not known. We do not know the cause of most human cancers. It is very difficult to predict who will have a recurrence and who will not and it is impossible to predict who will respond well to treatment and who will not. We do not know how long a person may have a tumor before it is found, or why some cancers can lie dormant for years after treatment and then show up again.

Even the knowledge that you are "home free", cured of your tumor, may be tempered with some reservations. The common definition of "cured" is the passage of five years, or for some cancers ten years, after treatment *without* signs of recurrence. As a survivor you are still not the same person you were before. You will remember that you had a close call and you will feel vulnerable to this disease. Some people seize on the concept of being cured to put cancer out of their minds. Others do not use the word "cured" but speak of "remission" or "control", perhaps avoiding a term that seems too optimistic and may bring bad luck. Such remissions may last forever.

Recurrence
Some people accept the possibility of recurrence and handle it almost as if they expect it. Others experience so much anxiety and fear that they seem relieved when it actually appears and they can receive

treatment and "do something about it." For most, however, recurrence is a difficult experience which indicates that the first attempt at treatment has failed, that more treatment is necessary and that the chances of cure and indefinite survival are decreased. At this time it is not uncommon to experience many of the reactions you had when the tumor was originally diagnosed. The disappointment may not be easy to handle alone and this is a good time to use your support system.

I had already expected from my readings that metastases would eventually appear, but even then it was very disappointing when they did.

I am not so depressed about things as they are as I am about the possibility of not seeing some things in the future. For instance my daughter is now 4 years old and I realize that I will probably not see her grow up or go to high school. This is very uncomfortable.

Recurrence does not mean that you will be gone tomorrow anymore than getting cancer in the first place did. Thirty or forty years ago recurrence could not be treated but now much can be done. Some recurrent tumors can be cured and many can be slowed down so that years of comfortable life lie ahead. The steps are similar to what you have already been through. They require a new outlook, new plans, and new treatment.

Now that my tumor has recurred I know that I have only a few years ahead of me. This is not a very happy thought but it is much less frightening than not knowing what lies ahead. Furthermore, even the estimate that I make from what I have read of three or four years is not a realistic figure. Medicine is changing and chemotherapy may prolong things considerably.

Another source of disappointment is when treatment fails and must be changed. When treatment works well you gain hope but when treatment fails you lose hope and are pushed down a little further. These cycles can be exhausting but somehow hope usually wins.

They told me that my drug wasn't working and they wanted to change the chemotherapy. Sometimes you find out things you don't want to know, but you don't always have much choice.

Treatment failure is not a personal failure nor a failing of your doctor. There is far too much variation between people and tumors to be able to say with certainty that a particular treatment will work. The treatment selected is the one that has worked best for your type of cancer in the past. If it does not work for you, alternatives are available.

It is easier to talk about it with someone than to think about it alone.

Fear of Death   Living with cancer requires dealing with fear, and for most people this includes fear of death. Death can be a painful subject to even think about, no less discuss with a loved one. However the seriousness of this threat makes it important to think about and discuss as early as possible. When you can face the possibility of death from your disease, most other threats seem smaller. It is in the front of your mind in the few days or weeks after cancer is diagnosed. The opportunity is there and the pressure to discuss it strong. Later, when you are doing well, it is hard to think about dying. Still later when death may no longer be an abstract possibility but a reality to be confronted, it may be impossible to talk about anything associated with it. If anything, early acknowledgement of the possibility of death gives you *more* freedom to enjoy life. It also makes it easier to deal with it again later if you want to. Once this door has been opened, no matter how long ago, it is more easily opened again.

It was very hard to talk to her about anything serious, knowing how ill she was and pretending that she would get over it. One day, two months before she died, she said, "I know I'm going to die." I said, "Mom, don't talk like that." She insisted that we talk about it and we had one of the most beautiful times I ever had in my life. She told me that God had been good to her, that He had let her see her children grow up and that she was now ready to let go of life. It was a very beautiful time.

Death is a topic that you should bring up yourself. Hopefully someone close to you will listen and talk about it, but you should realize that he or she is unlikely to initiate the conversation. A common misunderstanding is that talking about death means giving up hope. The two are entirely separate and many people can prepare themselves and their families thoroughly for death without giving up a particle of hope. It takes courage to talk about death but the long intervals between diagnosis and recurrence, and recurrence and death provide many opportunities.

Frank talked a lot about dying. It was much more difficult for me. He frequently brought it up and answered lots of questions regarding our property, the business, and so on. It got easier for me after a while but I couldn't have brought it up myself at first. It took six months until I was able to talk about it without crying, but I'm glad that we did.

There are practical ways to approach the possibility of death without having to face the emotional issue all at one time. These include discussing your financial situation, or children's education, explaining your life insurance structure, or writing a will. All of these help to lead up to a more direct confrontation which should be an open discussion with the person closest to you.

There are so many things that you need to clear up. We talked about everything and it was very satisfying to get all those little details taken care of so they were out of the way. Now if it comes, I know I can go on living my life.

Probably the single most important requirement for living with cancer is hope. The desire for life is a powerful stimulus and hope is one if its basic responses. Your first hope is for a quick and complete cure; get rid of the tumor and all will be well. Even if the chances of completely eliminating the tumor are poor most people consider themselves to be in the favorable 5 or 10 percent and establish a foundation of hope on that basis. If the tumor recurs, hope is transferred to controling the disease and eventual cure. With more progressive disease, hope may shrink a little further but it rarely disappears altogether.

With cancer you always have hope. I'm still waiting for someone to walk through that door with a miracle drug.

Hope is a beautiful experience and comes from many sources. Usually it comes from yourself, with no obvious outside influences. It is a vital life force expressing itself, like a crocus appearing in the spring when there is still snow on the ground. Another source of hope is the people close to you. Care and love, and the feeling that you are important to someone else transfers hope in both directions. Your loved ones generate hope for your comfort and for recovery, so that they can have you longer. You, in turn, have a similar hope to enjoy life with them. Doctors and nurses are important sources of hope for many people.

Many people turn to religion as a source of hope in the belief that God loves and cares for you, that He shares in your life in times of happiness and distress, that He will not give you a burden you cannot endure, and that He will be with you for all time.

Each person finds hope in his or her own way, through self-understanding, through love given to and received from others, and through faith. Regardless of where it comes from, hope is one of the most mysterious and sustaining values in life.

It is remarkable how many feel that their experience with cancer made them "better people". Cancer changes your concept of life in a way that has far reaching consequences. It is probably the threat of dying that so greatly increases the value of living. It begins with a

Hope

Coming Out Ahead

change in your attitude about yourself, with a greater level of self-awareness, acceptance, and love. You are forced to mature and examine yourself more than you ever did before. Although you may be more self reliant in many ways, you are also more aware of your need for others and of their need for you.

Relationships with other people may improve dramatically. Husbands and wives may be brought closer together by the common threat and need for mutual support. The words "Hi, mom", acquire new meaning. Childless couples think about having children. Attitudes toward friends change as they rally and provide help and support. Many people find that they become more gentle and friendly with their associates and friends, seeking out old friends and mending fences. You may become more tolerant of other people and find it easier to get along as you realize there is nothing to lose by being as open as you want.

I feel much more at ease with other people. I am less afraid to be frank and loving and giving because there is really nothing to lose.

Everyday I remind myself, "Have I said I love you lately?". "Have I said I'm sorry lately?". You shouldn't have to get sick to remember those things.

I found out how much more meaningful life is and how much more we should be getting out of it. I didn't realize what fun it could be to be a nice guy to everyone.

Your appreciation of the world around you may change. The freshness of every day, the smell of rain, the whiteness of snow, the flowers in the garden all acquire a new meaning.

When I left the hospital I experienced the most beautiful Fall I have ever seen. The colors of the leaves and the whole world around me were new and different. I realized that I wanted to stay in it and live in it.

The future may take on a different meaning. If you are a person totally absorbed in every day activities you may find yourself making more plans for the future. On the other hand if you constantly worry about tomorrow and next month and next year, you may find that you now get more pleasure out of today. You learn to live one day at a time.

It certainly has changed my life, but beautifully. It brought our family very close together. Before we used to plan ahead and lived very much for the future. Now we live for the freshness of every day.

Priorities change. Worries about minor aspects of work seem trivial.

Things in daily life that were irritating are now petty and easier to ignore. Material things become less important and the value of money often decreases.

I'm doing a lot more traveling. I don't want to leave money for inheritance tax.

We were maintaining a big home and I had collected many antiques and nice things, but we didn't have time to go any place or to share good times together. We sold the house and got an apartment and gave many of our things to the children. It occurred to us that we may not have next year and we had better enjoy this year.

Time becomes important. There are projects to be finished and projects to be discarded.

With time running out, I don't put things off like I used to. There are so many things I want to do that I resent having to put any of them aside, even for a little while.

I feel more responsible to the fact that if I can do something that other people cannot do, I should do it. One of them is writing a book for graduate students in my field of interest. I kept putting it off but still want to do it. Now I am aware of the fact that if I'm going to do it at all I'd better do it now.

It is easier to relax and just enjoy life.

I used to be uptight about everything but now if the leaves aren't raked—let them be.

Everyday is a beautiful day—sun, rain, sleet, snow. It's just good to be here.

three

Fighting Back:Coping And Asserting

Short-term Psychological Defenses to Reduce Tension
1. Denial—trying to forget or even refusing to admit there is a problem.

2. Anger and blaming someone else (to externalize or project, in basic psychology terminology).

3. Guilt, blaming yourself, "I deserve it" (over-responsibility).

The first three mechanisms—denial, anger, and guilt—can be considered emergency measures. They help us to avoid contact with the stress and tension that we feel, but they should not be expected to work for very long. We have already seen that denial protects us from having to recognize that the problem exists at all, while anger and guilt allow us to express our fears and frustration openly and even violently. These mechanisms provide emotional first aid but when used for too long can be harmful.

Deferral and Distraction
4. Defer thinking about the problem until you have to (suppression).

5. Diversion—turning your attention to things you like such as working or playing harder or reading more (displacement).

6. Taking on something new (redirection).

7. Relaxing with alcohol or drugs (escape, sublimation).

8. Doing something unreasonable or reckless (impulsive acting out).

Included here are some of the most common and successful coping mechanisms of all, as well as two of the most dangerous. They assume that you recognize that you have problems but serve to take your mind off of them. They are psychological vacations to a sunnier, more comfortable climate.

The next step beyond learning to live with cancer is to prepare yourself to assume a major share of the responsibility for your own care. Rather than be a helpless victim, you can join your doctors and nurses in treating your disease. This starts with learning how to cope with the many daily problems that come up and extends to learning as much as you can about your illness. The ultimate goal, however, is to be able to assert yourself and share in the important decisions that affect you.

I can cope if I know what I have to cope with.

I felt helpless many times. That is very bad in my case because I like to believe that if I understand what is going on I can do something to correct it, to change it, or improve it.

COPING WITH CANCER

Coping with cancer can seem like an impossible task. Your illness may well be the biggest problem you have ever had to face, and certainly one of the most threatening. Beyond that, it seems to make every other problem assume incredible size and complexity, all at a time when a large portion of your energy for coping is being consumed. As the days go by, however, you begin to have glimpses of strength that you did not realize you possessed. You are much tougher than you thought. The fact that you have taken your medical problem to a doctor should be recognized as a major step in coping. You no longer have to live alone with fear and uncertainty. There is more, however, to be learned about the process of coping that can help you understand yourself and enable you to solve your problems better.

Difficulties often seem to come in clusters that can appear overwhelming. It helps to identify and select single problems that you can deal with effectively. Larger problems that appear to be one "mountain of difficulty" can usually be broken down to smaller bite-size pieces. Getting rid of cancer is a staggering undertaking. However, loss of appetite and nausea are more specific and can be solved by looking for correct foods and finding out where, when, and how to eat them. Finding ways to get out of the house, to get more exercise, or to do a little work are all examples of the same thing.

We have many ways of dealing with problems and coping with adversity. Some of the most common coping mechanisms are described here. Everyone uses most of these mechanisms at one time or another and eventually, by trial and error, each of us establishes our own pattern. Our tendency is to continue to use those mechanisms that have served us best in the past. However, it is easy to see that some may be more helpful in coping with cancer than others. Indeed, exclusive use of any one coping mechanism may not be helpful. Even such a good one as "seeking more information and better understanding" (number 16) can be carried to an extreme that is so intellectual that the disease becomes a remote object rather than a personal illness. Recognizing that you have a choice and then consciously selecting coping mechanisms that will help you are two of the most important steps in fighting back.

While these are commonly used mechanisms, you should recognize that they only provide escape and do not contribute to directly solving problems. Indeed, the use of alcohol or drugs or the undertaking of some reckless action such as a hasty marriage or divorce, however exciting or distracting it may be, may be very destructive, creating serious new problems.

Deferral is when you become tired of thinking about your illness and "put it on the shelf" for a while, much as you set aside your work to go fishing for a weekend. In deferral one accepts the knowledge of cancer but puts it aside most of the time to make room for thoughts and activities that are more enjoyable. These may include work, sports, friends, and a variety of diversions that represent the good side of life.

I thought about all the long range worries and finally made an agreement with myself that I wouldn't worry about them until they happened. I just was not about to drive myself crazy.

Having cancer does not eliminate all other problems. It only adds to them. Jobs must be found, work must go on, homes must be cleaned, meals cooked, and children cared for. Major moves, birthdays, weddings, illnesses, and other joys and sorrows occur in the homes of people who have cancer, just as in any other home. All require some degree of deferring if obligations are to be met and life is to go on.

Obviously there are limitations to deferral and there are days that cannot be put off. Visits to the doctor's office are times when acceptance is forced upon you. However there is no reason not to defer thinking about cancer again until the next appointment. Deferral, more than any other mechanism, allows people to resume normal lives, to continue to pursue their career goals, and even initiate new projects while living with a serious illness.

Denial implies blocking out and rejecting the existence of the illness and therefore relieves you of the responsibilities of having to deal with it at all. Complete acceptance, on the other hand, implies passive resignation and many people are unwilling to abandon themselves totally to other people or to fate. In the past, too much emphasis has been placed on eventual acceptance of the disease and even of impending death from cancer and not enough on the sustaining value of healthy deferral.

Making the Problem Seem Smaller
9. Accepting the inevitable, "It is my Fate", "It is God's will" (passive acceptance).
10. Making a joke of it, laughing it off (affect reversal).
11. Looking for a silver lining, "There must be some good in it" (redefine, revise).

Accepting your disease as inevitable, making a joke of disability, or looking for a silver lining have this in common: they make a problem seem smaller and less threatening. If you can joke about it, it cannot be *too* bad. If you can find some good in it, it cannot be *all* bad. Even blaming fate makes problems smaller because it incorporates them into a much larger system, perhaps so large that both you and your problems may seem insignificant. Again, these are important and useful coping mechanisms but they too offer relief from problems rather than attacking them.

Getting Help
12. Sharing the problem with others, talking about it (mutuality).
13. Praying and asking for spiritual guidance.
14. Turning your problem over to someone else who will direct you and solve it for you (cooperative compliance).

The mechanisms listed in this group all involve getting outside help. These are constructive coping mechanisms through which you recruit people to help you attack your disease and the psychological effects of it. Sharing your problem with others is such an important mechanism that an entire chapter is devoted to it.

Personal Involvement
15. Seeking privacy to "think it out" (disengagement).
16. Seeking more information and better understanding (rational inquiry).
17. Considering alternatives (analytical).
18. Attacking the problem directly by doing whatever seems necessary (confrontation).

Finally seeking privacy to "think out" your problem, seeking more information and better understanding of your illness, considering alternatives, and attacking it directly on the basis of what you know, are expressions of your personal involvement in dealing directly with your illness. These are very positive and rewarding mechanisms. They do not replace seeking outside help but enable you to assume a significant level of responsibility and control over what takes place. Indeed, directly attacking the problem almost invariably includes getting good medical care and using all other available sources of help. Proper use of these latter coping mechanisms is the main theme of this book.

ASSERTING YOURSELF

It is essential to establish a relationship of complete confidence and trust in your doctor with the common goal of getting the best treatment possible. In order to do this you must understand and communicate with each other. The first step is for *you* to decide what kind of relationship you want to have. For some, this means giving the doctor full responsibility, turning the entire problem over to him on the understanding that he will keep you informed whenever something comes up that you should know about. If you want this kind of relationship, in which you hear no more than absolutely necessary, by all means say so. It will help your doctor avoid upsetting you unnecessarily. There is nothing wrong with this and many people feel very secure with it. You can always change your mind and ask for more information when you want it.

This time honored dependent relationship, is not sufficient for many people who wish to know more about their disease and take an active role in its treatment. To do this you will have to reach an understanding with your doctor. The responsibility usually starts with you. Your doctor has a great deal of information about your illness but, unless he already knows you well, he will have no idea how much you really want to know. He is in a difficult position and until he knows what you expect he may hold back and be careful what he discloses. He knows that what he tells you may be painful to hear, difficult to understand, and hard to accept. He may not be used to talking openly with patients and may even find your questions painful himself. Physicians who have real experience with cancer, however, will usually be glad to share their responsibility with you, but only *after* you take the initiative. A few examples of how other people have handled this are as follows:

I know he will answer anything I ask, but I also know that I have to ask. My doctor was shaking his head and looking down and finally I had to wrench it out of him. I mean, I made him say something. He's a very sweet man and he brightened up after that.

Damn it doc, you got something to say? Say it!

I've never had that problem but if I thought he wasn't telling me the truth I would put it to him, "Are you giving me the straight goods?"

I just ask questions and I expect answers. We understand each other.

Other factors may contribute to a physician's attitude. Although he may be able to help a lot, he knows that his overall success in curing cancer is less than 50 percent. He must live with the knowledge that often he cannot do as much as he would like. The fact that he cannot work miracles may make him feel helpless and his frustration is increased when the news he must share is not good. Cancer is full of unknowns and some doctors retreat when they do not have quick answers to what seem to be simple questions. Many people want their doctors to have God-like qualities; some physicians enjoy this role and the amount of authority and control that go with it. As father-figures they also try to protect your peace of mind. If you want information and your doctor says, "Leave all that to me, I'll do the worrying for you," he is not helping *you* cope with your disease.

Some doctors find it difficult to be open and honest with cancer patients and many people complain that their doctors will not answer their questions. Examples of poor communication are far too common and a few examples will be enough to show you that things can be better.

Poor Communication

If you don't get your questions answered in the doctor's office, after you get home you are a wreck. Furthermore, you are mad at yourself.

When you really want to know what's going on, the obvious person to ask is your doctor. It's a sad day when you can't get a clear answer.

A resident doctor said to me, "You know, if you were not an intelligent person you wouldn't even know about these choices". Many times doctors simply tell a patient what to do and leave because they figure the patient has absolutely no idea of what is going on, and they like to have it that way.

I really had no choice about the operation. They said it had to be done and they explained nothing. They just went ahead and did it. (A woman with cancer of the lung).

I asked him what caused an embolism and what can be expected of it. He said that there are basically three types of embolisms, small, medium, and large ones. They had me on two drugs, coumarin and heparin, to thin my blood. I wondered whether it was somewhat dangerous to be on both drugs at the same time. He looked at me, "Well, no. You see heparin works this way", and he waved his one hand in one direction, "while coumarin works in this way", waving with the other hand in the other direction. That was the entire explanation. Rather primitive. (A professor of mathematics being treated for a blood clot in his lungs)

The surgeon just abandoned him. We saw him seeing patients across the hall but he never came in to see us. I could never get to him, he was always in too much of a hurry.

Doctors are detached. They have got to be. They couldn't take it if they weren't.

At first my doctors were really helpful and seemed sympathetic. Now they're withdrawing. The more serious your case gets, the harder it is to get hold of one, even a sympathetic one.

The Whole Truth

In order to make decisions you should understand the advantages and disadvantages of the treatment being recommended and the alternatives. Unfortunately some doctors neglect to mention alternatives or undesirable side effects of their proposed treatment, presumably because they are afraid that their treatment would be turned down.

What made me very mad was that after my radiation treatment they told me that I would not be able to bear children. I think that is dereliction of duty not to have told me before. It probably wouldn't have made any difference, but I should have known.

I asked what he thought the probabilities of complete cure were. He said that this was not a scientific subject and that he could not give any exactness. I explained that I was only asking for probabilities based on similar cases in literature. He said that it was a little better than 75 percent. In going back in the literature myself later, I found out that it is nowhere near that. It is less than 5%. After five or six years the tumor always appears in the lungs. There was no hope at that time to stop it from spreading and the operation they did was unnecessarily aggressive.

I think the surgeon should have told me before surgery that the operation would make me impotent.

Time as a Form of Pressure

There are very few emergencies in cancer and you should not submit to unreasonable pressure. Treatment, particularly surgery, may be urged on you as if a day is the difference between life and death. This is very rarely the case and it is often reassuring to have a second opinion. It also may help to find out what is involved from someone who has had the same type of operation and your doctor can usually find another patient for you to talk to.

If you have the right doctor he should make you feel as though you are his only patient for the time that you need to get your questions answered. One obvious problem is that doctors are busy and good explanations take time. Many people are afraid to risk their relationship by being too pushy. In the long run however, you will be better off if you are assertive when necessary. Your doctor will not leave you because you are angry or depressed or ask too many questions.

Sometimes you just have to push and not worry too much about what your doctor thinks. "I know that you are busy but I am important too. I'm sitting right here until you answer my questions."

I like my doctor very much but he is always in such a hurry. The other day he stopped in my room for just two or three minutes. He said he had to run off and pick up his daughter at swimming. I felt like saying, "Let her drown!" I had a lot of questions—and it is always so hard to get him to stop.

Getting What You Want

If your doctor appears to be sidestepping your questions or shutting them off, try asking him why he is not more open with you. If you tell him that you really want answers but still get nothing, you have several alternatives. Your family doctor will usually be kept completely up-to-date on your care. He may not only be able to explain your illness to you but may also convince the specialists caring for you that you are serious about understanding more. Most hospitals have an elected chief of staff whom you may ask to see. He is usually a senior member of the staff and a word from him may encourage your doctor to be more open with you. Finally, there is always the possibility of asking to have your care taken over by another doctor.

A PARTNERSHIP WITH YOUR DOCTOR

Our doctor is very kind and gentle, and he explained things at our own level. He always has time to answer all our questions. He is never in a hurry. I don't know what he does in the O.R. —and I don't care! His ability to communicate makes him a great doctor.

The first stop in learning about your disease is to find out the exact diagnosis. This information must come from your own doctor. Ideally it should come directly to you but may be shared with a person close to you at the same time.

The doctor spoke to my husband alone in his office first and I just sat there quaking and wondering what he was telling him.

After surgery your surgeon must disclose what he found to your family in the waiting room long before you wake up. My practice is to tell the family *exactly* what was found and inform them that I will give my patient the same information later in the day or the next day. I also tell them to feel free to discuss it and if questions are asked that I will explain it in more detail to everybody over the next few days. Some families feel that they can break the news better themselves, and frequently they can, but eventually it is your doctor's responsibility to explain your illness to you and your family in terms you can understand. This is when trust and confidence are built.

Understanding Your Illness

The next step is to find out all you can about your disease. Usually the desire for detailed information comes shortly after the diagnosis, when you want to get a better idea of what the problem really is. Again, the obvious source is your doctor. In general the more you know and understand about your disease, the *easier* it is for your doctor to talk to you and take care of you.

In addition to explaining your disease your doctor can provide you with articles to read that deal specifically with your type of cancer. These may require some explanation on his part but will give you as complete and up to date a picture as possible. Medical articles are objective and factual and can be frightening. They deal with statistics derived from the treatment of large numbers of people. However, even bad statistics are beatable. Moreover, because of earlier diagnosis and better treatment the figures change from year to year. You will also find that a great deal is published on cancer in magazines and newspapers. Unfortunately some of it is premature or not proven and you should always check the accuracy with your doctor.

I read all I could find. I don't remember it all now, which is probably just as well, but I had to find out.

I like statistics—they are not me.

The average lifetime for my tumor is reported as seven years, but there are reports of people who lived 18 to 20 years—that's quite a difference.

If you wish to see documents that pertain directly to you, ask to see the pathology report which identifies your cancer in medical terms and the operative note which the surgeon dictated after your operation. This is a description of the operation. Both are filed in your hospital record and can be made available but will require help to understand them.

It helps to learn the language of your disease. You do not need to be an M.D. to understand a reasonable amount of medical terminology. Later chapters, and the glossary in this book, will provide a start for some of the more common cancers.

I wanted to know all about Hodgkin's disease. When I was told that I was a II-A it didn't mean a thing to me. Now I know all about it.

Many articles, particularly those written by physicians, advise you not to compare your treatment with someone else's. This is hard to do if you are alert to what is going on and interested in getting the best available care. Although there are many different tumors and treatments, you have every right to know why yours is being treated the way it is.

A final reason for learning what you can about your disease is that it helps you ask questions. It is difficult to ask intelligent questions or interpret the answers unless you have some idea of what to expect. Also, the more real information you have the greater will be your resistance to misinformation.

Asserting yourself means not only collecting information about your disease but also using this information to make decisions which concern your future. You need not accept treatment blindly but should feel that you can share in any major decisions. Doctors cannot give you orders, they may only suggest. While your doctor may recommend a course of treatment, it is you who must decide whether or not to accept it. The optimum level of personal control is sharing the responsibility for your own treatment.

Being Responsible for Your Treatment

Goals of Treatment. The purpose of treatment may be to try to cure the cancer, to prolong your life, to keep you actively at work or able to care for your home, or to relieve pain or discomfort without necessarily prolonging your life. Whatever the goals of treatment are, you should understand them if you are going to participate in the planning.

Doctors commonly speak about "controlling" cancer while one of the first questions that their patients ask concern "curing" cancer. Some cancers are more easily cured than others and your doctor can tell you about your particular disease. The tests and examinations determine whether or not your cancer is still in the place where it began, making cure more likely, or has spread elsewhere, making cure less likely.

One of the most common questions after surgery for cancer is "Did you get it all?" There are only two truthful answers to this question, "No. There was cancer that we could not remove which may need additional treatment", or "We removed all the cancer we could find, *but* I cannot be sure that it has not spread somewhere else that we cannot see." The surgeon cannot assure you that he has cured your cancer because he has no way of knowing if a few cancer cells may have spread beyond the range of his operation and will show up months or years later.

Some Important Decisions.   Modern medicine has added years to the lives of people with cancer using several forms of treatment during that time. There is a series of choices and options; the final choice is yours, if you wish to exercise it. However, in order to make intelligent choices you must have all the information and facts that are available. The first choice, following the diagnosis, may be between no operation, a small operation or a big operation. For example, a woman may elect to have a partial mastectomy for cancer of the breast. In doing so she should know that she *may* be undertaking an unnecessary risk, but if that is her choice, she is entitled to the smaller operation.

Another time the choice may be between different forms of chemotherapy. The difference may be small, or it may be large, with one treatment requiring hospitalization each month while the other may be carried out at home and in the office. Other factors include not only the drugs themselves, their side effects, and their chances of influencing your tumor, but also relative costs, hospitalization, and inconvenience.

Occasionally a decision must be made about whether to discontinue treatment. To make such a decision, you must have evidence to show whether or not the drugs are really helping you. These may include x–rays and other measurements of changes in your tumor during the past several months, as well as your own feelings of comfort or discomfort. Even when there is no evidence that chemotherapy is helping, the drugs may be continued at low doses for psychological reasons. Many people take comfort in the knowledge that *something* is being done. Most important is to realize that the likelihood of success of any form of treatment does not *necessarily* out-weigh the side effects of the treatment. Surgery, radiation, and chemotherapy all have their limitations.

Many people take great comfort in turning all responsibility for their care over to their doctors. Most doctors are used to this relationship and like it. However, expectations and medical practices are changing rapidly and this may not be the best relationship for you. If you are intelligent and take the time to find out all you can about your disease, you can be confident that you will make the right decision. More often than not it will be the decision that was recommended, but now it is *your* decision. It may not be the same decision that someone else would have made because you are not someone else. Your decision is personal property, suited to your own needs—and that is what really counts.

four

You Are Not Alone:
Using Your Support System

Cancer is too big to deal with alone. Support from other people is essential for coping with this disease. It is hard to understand how sharing one's concerns and fears lessens them so significantly, but the fact remains that it does. The sure knowledge that other people understand and will not abandon you is the reward for communication and few can do without it.

What needs to be talked about? Anything and everything! Fond memories of experiences together, plans for the future, the trials and tribulations of parenthood, appreciation of love and friendship, anger, worries, fears, death, finances, personal problems, all of the problems associated with or made larger by illness.

Some people have shared their problems with others throughout their lives and are so candid and open that they almost *have to* communicate. Others, unfortunately, are exactly the opposite and are unable to share their troubles with anyone else. Most of us are between these extremes and have found from experience that sharing helps, that support is essential, but that it can be difficult to bring ourselves to ask for it.

Secrecy and Silence.   Lack of communication often results in a conspiracy of secrecy and silence created by the families of a person with cancer. Some people with cancer isolate themselves from their loved ones.

The single most frightening thing is thinking that other people know things about you that you don't know. They are not giving you the credit that you deserve as a human being if they don't recognize that fact.

On many occasions I have been asked by families not to tell a person that he has cancer on the grounds that he "couldn't stand to know"

With rare exceptions I have refused. If a person really wants to know, it is my obligation to tell the truth. Requests for secrecy are much less common than they used to be.

The conspiracy of silence, which forces people into isolation and loneliness, is a cruel game doomed to failure. People who have lived together for years and love each other are unable to protect each other from bad news. They communicate their distress and fears just as surely through their actions, expressions, and moods as they do through words. The only thing missing is mutual acknowledgement and information about what the problem really is. From this silence, however, comes the miserable game of hiding from each other, with both sides *knowing* what is really going on but literally spending their last days together talking about the weather because they are unable to consider the one subject uppermost in their minds. When this game of hide and seek can be stopped in the middle, and communication re-established, it is remarkable to see the enormous relief and the feeling of warmth that everyone experiences.

Before trying to embark on a conspiracy of secrecy, ask yourself whom you are sparing, the other person or yourself. It is usually yourself. There is only one kind of advice that I could possibly give: do not do this to your family and do not let your family do it to you. If possible, decide in advance that you want to know what is going on and insist that they know too.

Lack of Support.   It can be very distressing to turn to a person for support and find they are unable to respond. This may be a wife who cannot talk about cancer, a husband who will not touch his wife after her mastectomy, or a parent who cannot accept the illness of a child. Rejection by a friend is bad enough but when it comes from a close family member it can be very painful.

My sister didn't visit for a year. When I called her about it she said, "I just couldn't cope with the fact that I thought you were dying. I didn't want to come over and see you die". To me that was a cop-out. When you truly care for someone you have to share bad things with them.

My mother was completely unable to deal with it. So far as she was concerned there was nothing there, even when she could see there was something wrong.

I was most concerned about my 21-year-old son. He couldn't accept it at all and just ran away from himself, from me, and everybody else. I finally realized that I would have to do something about it. Here I am with a malignancy trying to console him.

I was convinced that I could lick it. She was convinced that I would die. She was not at all supportive for me and didn't even want me to have treatment. (This young man with a brain tumor divorced his first wife and remarried someone who was much more supportive.)

I came early one day when he did not expect me and I saw him sitting at the end of the hall. He looked like a little lost puppy. That's when I made up my mind to come down and stay with him. I realized how lonesome it was not to have anyone to sit with.

In dealing with this type of rejection you should understand that the other person usually cannot help the way he feels. Family members who have shared a good relationship do not reject each other on purpose. Your illness is too threatening. It may help to discuss it with them and find the reason for their rejection. This is when a third person can be very helpful. Your doctor, nurse, minister, or a professional psychologist or social worker can frequently help rebuild the relationship that previously existed. This is particularly important if your illness is threatening your marriage or another important relationship. Finally, it may be necessary to turn to some other person for your main source of support, another member of your family, or a close friend. It is natural to be resentful, disappointed, and even angry about lack of support. Although it usually does little good to express it continuously to the person involved, it can help a great deal to discuss it with someone else.

YOUR SUPPORT SYSTEM

While you may turn to one person for most of your support, if you stop to think about it you will realize that you actually have a whole system of support to use when you need it. Visualize yourself as sitting at the head of a conference table with several empty chairs in which you will seat members of your support system, much as the president seats his advisors. Now place names over each chair to identify the people whom you would include in your personal support system. These may include your spouse, a close friend, your children, your parents, your minister, priest or rabbi, your doctor or nurse, a professional counselor, friends in general, and other patients.

While you are doing this, bear in mind that some chairs are closer to you at the head of the table than others. Give some consideration to who occupies these more important chairs, and why. They are usually the people who are closest to you and to whom you turn most frequently for help. There may be times when you will wish to bring together different combinations of people such as your family and your doctor. There may even be times when you would like to encourage certain members of your support system to meet without you (your spouse and your doctor, or your children and your clergyman), knowing that this will help everyone.

Support is needed in times of stress. In cancer some of these times are predictable: when the diagnosis is first made, around the time of surgery, when starting new treatment such as chemotherapy or radiation, when meeting with a new doctor, when recurrence has been discovered or therapy has failed. A good support system should be available for emergency meetings at any time of the night or day.

A few people appear to turn entirely to themselves for support. They give the impression of being very self sufficient and some of them are. Others have good support systems which they use but are embarrassed to acknowledge. An unfortunate few are reclusive and lonely and in desperate need of help. Most of us, however, have support systems which we use and appreciate. It is worth taking a close look at the people in your support system.

You.   You are very important in your own support system. You decide who is in it, where they sit, and what role they play. It is you who set the tone and mood for your relationships with the various members. A genuine appeal for love, understanding, and help is met with love, understanding and help. On the other hand, self rejection encourages rejection. You will find that there is much that you can do to influence your own moods and in so doing also influence the response of others around you.

You will not have to tell people close to you that you want help. They know that they are undertaking love and care for you and are willing to stand by you. On the other hand, in order to fulfill their obligations it is essential that they know a lot about your illness, and it is up to you to be sure that they do.

Husband, Wife, or Close Friend.   Your husband, wife or a close friend may be the person to occupy the seat nearest you. This is usually the person who loves you, knows you best, and is the one you turn to for help. A serious illness can create a feeling of sharing in a new adventure that can bring people close together. This is often a seesaw arrangement with each supporting the other in turn.

There were days when I was up and my husband was down. Then I would try to cheer him up. The next day it could be the other way around.

Your spouse knows your moods and is most apt to recognize changes. Moreover, your spouse has learned to live with these moods and is best equipped to help you deal with them.

I can tell when he is depressed. I ask him what he is thinking about and he says "nothing". Then I just start talking to him and try to get his mind off whatever he is thinking about. I talk about things that won't worry him, such as our grandson's birthday or a trip that we are planning.
I realized that he was so depressed in the hospital that his treatment wasn't going to have a chance to work while he was in that state of mind. My work and

the money were not as important as having him around and so I just cut back on the work to be with him in the hospital.

There are many ways of helping but the most important is just being there at the right time. This is particularly important after surgery and during hospitalizations when you are away from home or any time when bad news is expected. Communicating love and affection does not require words.

It helps to have my wife just sitting here holding my hand. After she leaves I often wake up at night and feel she is still here. It's not so helpful if she asks too many questions. Sometimes I don't like to go into how I feel, particularly when it's not good. It's hard to tell her that.

Children. Some older couples drift far enough apart that the major support comes from a grown child rather than the spouse. Grown children, often with families of their own, are usually capable of dealing lovingly, sympathetically, and realistically with illness of their parents, but within the limitations of their obligations to their own families.

Parents. The role that parents can play in the life of a person who has cancer depends on their respective ages and ongoing relationship. The parent is enormously important to the young child and this is covered in a separate chapter. It is usually difficult for an adult who has cancer to keep the information from elderly parents if they have been at all close in other respects. If the parents are in good health there is no reason why they cannot assume a place in your support system if they have continued to be close to you in other aspects of your life.

Religion. Religion is an important source of support for many people. This may be on a private basis through prayer, or it may be through ministrations from the clergy and members of the church.

If you have been a church-goer it can be very distressing to be forgotten by your clergy. The most direct approach is to ask a friend to arrange for a visit from your minister or someone representing the church.

If you have not had strong religious beliefs throughout life you are unlikely to turn in this direction for support, and may resent any intrusion or attempt to force religion into your life at this time. Friends who would like to pray at your bedside may not be very helpful and should be gently but firmly kept away.

Doctors and Nurses. Doctors and nurses can be in your support system if you wish. It is a great help to have a doctor in whom you have complete trust. That relationship alone may place the doctor high in your support system.

I have all the faith in the world in my doctor. I have always said that as long as my doctor is beside me I can carry on.

He popped in and out every time he was on the floor. At that point I wanted to be his most important patient and this made me feel that I was.

There seemed to be a lot of people in my room all the time. Nurses would come in and tell me their problems and listen to my problems and I got to know some of them quite well.

If you want to know your doctor or nurse better and to include them in your support system, try to talk to them alone. If they are busy ask them to come back when they have more time. Then offer a chair or move over and made a place on the edge of the bed. It is an invitation that is hard to refuse.

Professional Help.   Help is available to work with you directly or to help you establish your own support system. The skills of psychologists and social workers trained in this area should not be underestimated. They can be of enormous value and are available in many hospitals.

Friends.   Most of us have a circle of friends ranging from those who are very close to mere acquaintances and associates. There is often a desire to see old friends and renew old relationships but it is hard to predict how other people will react to your illness. This is one of the most clear-cut situations where your own attitude can have a huge influence on others. A truthful and candid approach makes it easier for everyone. If you are open and confident, must of your friends will acquire the same attitude, although initially they may be tentative and need help.

At first she couldn't believe that I have —and everyone hesitates to say that word, so I said it for her—"cancer".

At the periphery of your circle of friends may be acquaintances and associates from work whom you do not want to have to deal with directly. One approach is to ask a close friend to let others know what is going on and that you are feeling better and will be back soon. This will get you over the hurdle of wondering who knows and who does not when you go back to work. If you find it difficult to say that you have cancer you can always say that you had an operation or are being treated for a digestive disorder or whatever you feel is appropriate.

Most people I work with know I have cancer. I see no point in lying about it. Besides I have to take a certain amount of time off for my treatments and I would rather have them know why so they won't think that I am just loafing. My friends know too but I don't bring it up with just social acquaintances. I tell them I had a problem with lymph nodes and stay away from words that might scare them.

I found that it helped me to talk about my illness and I soon realized that it also helped my friends. They were surprised to find that leukemia is not necessarily "Love Story".

Most friends will respond well to your illness if you encourage them. A common opening is for friends to offer to help in any way they can. If you need help with shopping, or cleaning, or driving, say yes. Some may be overly protective and try to do everything for you. This can be turned aside by gently explaining why it is important for you to do as much as you can for yourself.

Some friends may avoid you because they do not know what to do or say. It is clear that they are interested in you because they ask others about you. You might initiate contact by asking a close friend to tell the person that you are feeling well and hope to hear from them.

Well-meaning friends may offer medical advice in the form of newspaper or magazine clippings, telephone calls, or letters about others who had similar illnesses.

I got opinions from all sorts of friends. People with knowledge, people without knowledge, telling me to go to this place or that place and get this treatment or that treatment. A person could lose their mind if they listened to everything.

This barrage of information is part of friendship. Unfortunately much of the information is new and untried, appropriate for some tumors but not yours, or just plain untrue. The best approach is to take their suggestions to your doctor for his comments. Most cancer doctors keep up to date with what is going on in their field.

Occasionally friends say the wrong thing by mistake, usually because they are embarrassed but feel that they must say something. Although these thoughtless comments can be painful, it helps to maintain a charitable attitude. They do not know what they are saying.

He said, "Don't worry, God only gives this to people who are strong." My hope was that perhaps God had made a mistake and I'm not strong after all and he will take it away.

She came in the room when I had tears on my cheeks and had obviously been crying. When I told her I was depressed she said that she had never been depressed a day in her life. I wasn't ready to hear that, and anyway it wasn't true. I think she was scared. She had cancer of the breast too.

We were at a staff meeting, in front of other people no less, when he said,

"Well, Nancy, you know everybody has to die sometime. It just looks like you may go before the rest of us." It freaked me out!

One way to avoid uncomfortable social situations is to get control of the conversation yourself. If someone asks how you are doing say, "Fine, how are *you* doing?" By taking charge of the conversation you can put off questions you don't want to hear.

Unfortunately a few people are so threatened by cancer they will back away and reject you rather than deal with your illness. Although there is absolutely no evidence for it, some are convinced that cancer is contagious. They may avoid you altogether or may talk to you but avoid physical contact, even with objects you have touched. These people are to be pitied but often cannot be helped. Their beliefs are frequently unshakable. One lovely patient of mine of about seventy was very depressed because her family would hardly touch her, either in the hospital or at home. I began kissing her soundly on both cheeks in front of the family every time I entered her room and within a week she brightened up and began to receive the affection from her family that she badly needed. Others may avoid you because they are afraid you are going to die, and they cannot deal with your death or their own.

Other People with Cancer

I've talked to quite a few people who have cancer and feel sorry for themselves. They walk around with long faces and say that they have cancer. I say, "So what — join the club! I've got it too!"

People with serious illness have much in common that they can share. Someone who has already undergone treatment, particularly for your type of cancer, can be of enormous help. Above all, they can show you that someone with *your disease* can do well and live a normal life. This takes away a lot of fear and helps you to see yourself well again. They can share your worries and fears and answer many questions. It is often easier to talk to an objective and sympathetic new friend than to a close family member or to a doctor or nurse. You do not have to be guarded in what you say. You can get used to talking openly about your disease before facing friends who may not be so comfortable.

In the hospital you live next door to other people, some of whom have cancer. Various treatment areas, particularly radiation therapy, are good places to meet other patients. Your doctor can also help you to meet someone and you should not hesitate to ask him to do so. Most people feel as lonely and isolated in a hospital as you. Conversations based on "How do you feel?", "How is your treatment going?", or

"Are you having any problems with it?", can lead to lasting friendships.

Trained Volunteers. This approach to the problems associated with cancer has been so successful that many hospitals and communities have developed organizations of trained volunteers who are cancer patients and have taken training in counseling. There are many such programs now similar to the CanSurmount Program in Colorado with which I have had close contact. Started in 1973 by a doctor and one of his patients in Denver, this program has now trained more than 300 volunteers. It was adopted by the Colorado Division of the American Cancer Society in 1976 and by the Service and Rehabilitation Program of the National American Cancer Society in 1978. The volunteers are people with all types of cancer who are in the middle of, or have completed, treatment. They are all people who have adjusted well to their illness and who are interested in helping others. They undergo about eight hours of formal training by a doctor, nurse, and two people with cancer who were founders of the program. The new volunteers are trained in small groups and part of their training is to tell their own stories, much as they will later exchange information with people they meet. The training emphasizes listening and understanding and provides the volunteers with a great deal of information to answer questions.

Volunteers are usually assigned to people who have the same kind of cancer and have undergone similar experiences. They visit you first in the hospital and are free to see you as often as they are able. Sometimes these visits continue at home and lead to close friendships. The volunteers can see someone only after the physician has requested such a visit. Helping other people also has enormous rewards for the volunteers.

It gives you a piece of immortality. When I am gone I can only live in the thoughts of other people. If I'm able to help them just a little bit, that makes my life just that much better.

There is no way people with cancer can manage by themselves. They might be able to manage without me, but not without all the me's.

In addition to the help they give other people, volunteers in these programs obtain a great deal of support from each other. The mutual experience of getting to know a few other cancer patients well provides a foundation of understanding and friendship that goes far beyond the duties of a volunteer. Indeed, it is not surprising that as cancer patient volunteers who have busy professional or personal lives get further away from their own illness, many of them stop their counseling activities but continue to maintain contact with their volunteer group.

The CanSurmount Program in Colorado is just one example. Others include the TOUCH Program at the University of Alabama, Reach to Recovery, Ostomy Clubs, Laryngectomy Clubs, and Make Today Count. There are so many services available now, both local and national, and they vary so much from one community to another that there is no way to catalog all of them. The best place to find out what is available in your community in the way of established support groups, volunteer programs, or professional services is through your local chapter of the American Cancer Society.

Cancer Support Groups. The simplest and most effective method of interaction between cancer patients are the cancer support groups. No special training is required, and anyone can belong. Groups can be formed in small communities or single hospitals as easily as in large cities. They can meet once a month or more. Members may come or go and may include not only people with cancer but also family members, close friends, and even children.

Some groups hold special meetings for their children at the same time that the adults are meeting. The children are taken to see different parts of the hospital, and learn from a doctor or nurse what tumors are and why mom or dad is not feeling well all the time. They have an opportunity to exchange their own ideas on what it is like to live with someone sick in the house.

Support groups can call upon the entire community for information, including doctors, nurses, social service workers, clergy, psychologists, and many others. They can learn about the different forms of treatment they are receiving or new treatments they have heard or read about, and encourage each other to continue treatment and follow-up and avoid unproven methods and quacks. In these groups you can get answers to questions concerning insurance, employment, community resources, and financial problems. You can share experiences of family and sexual problems arising from the illness, of how to occupy your time when you are not able to work, and how to deal with children when there is illness in the home. You can obtain information about the side effects of chemotherapy, loss of appetite, altered looks, and changes in sexual activity. There is the enormous value of experiencing together hope and joy, as well as loss and grief.

Support groups can be very small with six or eight people and a nurse, social service worker, or psychologist to help. If you are interested, ask around and see if there is one that you can join, either through your own hospital or through some other hospital in your community. If there is not, you can easily start one yourself.

five

For Family and Friends

This chapter is primarily for the family and close friends of someone who has cancer. You must face many of the same problems as the patient, and find your own solutions. At the same time you are obviously the core of the support system and you will have many demands placed upon you. Throughout this chapter I am reluctantly going to refer to "the patient" for simplicity, rather than "the person in your family who has cancer". Families are complex structures of two or more people, each of whom reacts in his or her own way to illness. The apparent unity of the family does not in any way lessen the importance of each member. It must also be recognized that some families are much closer than others. Some husbands and wives are not really friends. People who have not communicated well in the past are not likely to start when one has cancer. The following ideas and suggestions are to help you—whatever your relationship to the patient—give the support that is needed.

WHAT CANCER DOES TO A FAMILY

Cancer affects the entire family but particularly those who are closest to the patient. The age of the patient and his or her role in the family are important factors. Illness of a young child, a breadwinning father, a mother of small children, an elderly parent, or a distant relative each have a different impact. The changes that cancer brings into a family include the need to care for and provide support for a person who is seriously ill, increased financial obligations, the need to assume new duties and even different roles in the family, and fear of loss of one of its important members. Moreover, serious illness does not simplify life by eclipsing other problems; it adds one more large one to those that are already there.

Being stuck at home is a great loss for a man. For thirty years I had a husband who went to work at 8:00 a.m. every morning and came home at 6:00 p.m. every evening. Now he is home all the time. When I am doing the laundry, cooking, and cleaning, there he is. I think he is enjoying it. My problem is that you can't get mad at him and I have an Irish temper. If I even look cross I get back a black look as if to say "Don't worry, I won't be around much longer". I would like to blow up just once but I know that if I do I will feel guilty for the rest of my life so I just don't.

The reactions of family members to cancer are very similar to those of the patient and may include shock, denial, fear, anger, anxiety, guilt and depression. Not everyone experiences all of these, and no two people react at the same rate or at the same time. Indeed, one of the problems that families must face is the need to adjust to each other, particularly when one person's reactions seem inappropriate or out of phase with the rest. Although many of your responses to cancer are similar to those of the person who is sick, the reasons for them are often quite different. As you will see, some of these conflicting reasons are not comfortable to live with.

Denial. Every member of a cancer family who is old enough to appreciate the problem experiences denial. The rate at which different members of a family begin to accept the realities of illness may be quite different. Most adults with major responsibilities, including raising small children, cannot afford to deny the illness for very long, even if the patient does. Family members who have come to grips with reality find it hard to understand others who have not. This is a dangerous situation because when an individual is made to feel weak and nonsupportive for not being able to accept the illness, denial turns to guilt. Such a person needs help and understanding.

Fear. As a member of a cancer family, you experience many fears and anxieties, and not all of them are for the patient. We each have our own private fears. Foremost among these are the fear of loss, including loss of a loved one, of financial security, of emotional security, of physical affection and sexual activity. Another fear is that you may not be able to cope with a long and stressful illness. Finally, there is the unfounded but common fear that cancer is contagious and that you may catch it through physical contact. All of these fears have one thing in common. They could be considered *selfish,* placing your own concerns ahead of the person who is sick. Again, the result of such thinking is guilt. However, fear of being abandoned by someone you love is normal, and anxiety about your ability to cope expresses concern about your own self-preservation. Even the guilt that you feel when such feelings clash is normal. Eventually you will realize that you can feel concern for the person who has cancer *and* for yourself and the rest of your family at the same time.

Guilt. Guilt is the unfortunate result of many emotional con-
flicts. When you cannot be in two places or do two things at the same
time, and they are both important to you, guilt is frequently the
product.

*When I'm here at the hospital I feel I should be home with the children, and
when I'm home with the children I feel that I should be here with Dan in the
hospital.*

*Our daughter lives out of town and feels bad because she is late in her
pregnancy and cannot be with her father. He pointed out to her that his
children and his grandchildren are his only real legacy and she is performing a
very real service to him by having a grandchild in the first place, even if it
prevents her from being with him.*

Guilt results when you have thoughts or feelings that you think good
people should not have. You may be angry at the sick person because
she is a burden on you and unable to do her share. You may even find
yourself hoping that the person will die sooner rather than later so
that you can get on with your own life. You may be worried about
money but feel guilty because you should not at a time like this. You
may feel guilty because your are enjoying some things in life (a movie
or a ball game) when your loved one is so sick. You may be experiencing strong sexual desires when you know that your mate is not capable
of responding to them. It is the guilt these thoughts produce that is
harmful, not the thoughts themselves.

People do not give other people cancer but they often feel that
they have. Grandparents feel that they have caused their children and
grandchildren to inherit their cancers. Husbands or wives may feel
they have given it to the other person. More complicated is the
problem of young children who understand little about the disease
and think back over the things that they have said or done that may
have harmed their mother or father.

As if self-generated guilt is not enough, we may even encourage
other people to feel guilty. Families may make a patient feel guilty out
of frustration and helplessness. Similarly, an angry patient may say,
"Well, I'm not going to be around much longer so you won't have to
put up with me".

*After his tumor was discovered I realized that I had to move on my own. Before
that my job was just a pastime. Since then I have gone ahead to get better
positions and better pay and taken the attitude that I cannot goof off anymore.*

**Role
Changes:
Doing Others'
Work, Too**

Inability to carry out your normal work usually places an extra burden on someone else. Both parties are upset, because they cannot do
what they want to do and, in fact must do more. If a man is unable to

work, his wife, who is already a fulltime homemaker and mother, may have to become the breadwinner for the entire family. This may be a difficult transition if she has not worked before. Similarly, if you are a working man and your wife has cancer, you may be faced with the added responsibility of shopping, taking care of the house, cooking, and being a mother as well as a father to your children. Although your roles are not really reversed, your responsibilities may be enormously increased and resented. Distress caused by changing roles can be decreased by sharing your feelings with each other.

Sure, I mind doing housework, just as much as you did. But it's not that *bad. (Husband to wife)*

When she was working I'd come home and there was no supper and I was too nauseated to make it myself. Anyway kids are the way kids are. They eat different. I just got more and more nervous and upset. (Husband undergoing chemotherapy)

With my new job we were getting leveled off financially a little bit but at home I could see that Frank was getting depressed. He was down in the dumps and just didn't feel well. I decided that maybe I shouldn't work so much and I explained to them that I would only work three days a week and that I wanted at least one weekend day off. That did the trick, he felt better. It wasn't really the sickness that was getting to us, it was the fact that it was wrecking our family. (Wife of same patient)

Another approach is to make a list of all the things that need to be done, and divide up the duties so everyone in the family, including the children, does what he or she can. In this way everyone has a useful role and each person is needed for the smooth operation of the family unit. The husband who can no longer work can supervise the household, handle the finances, make repairs around the house, plan the meals, and even learn to cook. The wife, who can no longer cook or manage the house, can handle the finances, choose the menu, making shopping lists, read to the children, and supervise the household from her chair or bed. Children can prepare meals, fix the yard, wash dishes, make their beds, and clean the house.

Children One of the most difficult decisions for parents is what to tell young children when someone in the family has cancer. Everyone finds this difficult and many react strongly against it, feeling they can spare the child unnecessary fear and sadness, and spare themselves the distress of having to tell the child. Some parents even ship the children off to live with relatives or friends. Your children are already worried because their lives are being upset. Security is important to children and the closer you can come to maintaining your normal home the better. They also want one person to be in control, to pick up the pieces when life seems to fall apart, to love and hold them and take them into bed at night and tell them that everything will be all right.

Why Children Should Know What Is Going On. There is no way that children can be shielded from the disruption and pain of a serious illness in the family. They are under stress, too, and they handle it better if they know what is going on. Children should be told as much as they can understand. You can not hide from them the fact that something serious is wrong, only exactly what it is. The illness will affect their lives even more if you do not talk about it. Young children are quick to assume guilt and to feel that they *caused* the illness by something that they said or did that was unkind. By knowing something factual about the disease they are less likely to imagine that they contributed to it. Older children have concerns and even guilts of their own that they would like to talk about but cannot until the door has been opened for them.

Children look for information wherever they can find it: an older brother or sister or a friend who lost a parent, but rarely from adults outside of the family. They naturally look to one or both of their parents as the main source of reliable information, if that avenue is open. This may require several explanations to children of different ages and the children are certain to compare notes and explain things to each other. By understanding the nature of the illness, children are less apt to resent the special attention required by a sick sibling.

My sister always gets more attention. I understand why but I don't like it. When Dad comes home he always asks where Christine is. He never asks for me. If we ask Mom how Dad is, she tells us, and I ask her quite often.
I asked my mom why she had to have her hair cut—"Because I have a tumor". What is a tumor?—"It is something that is growing in my head that is not supposed to be there." I didn't understand that at first because I was only in the first grade, but now I understand. I'm kind of scared that something will happen. I asked my older sister and she helped to explain things.

Knowing in advance what to expect helps children accept the changes they see. The side effects of chemotherapy, irritability, unexplained anger, and the cycles of good days and bad days are less confusing if the child can be told, "It is not your fault. Mommy still loves you and doesn't mean to be upset".

Dad began to fly off the handle and get mad at us for nothing at all. I didn't know what it was all about and got angry at him right back. Later I became upset because I was angry. We didn't know at that time that he was getting sick.

Even with advanced warning some outward aspects of treatment cannot be hidden and are embarrassing for children. Hair loss is one of these.

It bothered me when Dad didn't have any hair. At first everybody stared at him and it was really cruel. Some of my friends didn't like to look at him at all. Then everybody asked and I told them and now they're used to seeing him and they don't ask anymore, but I still wish it would grow back in.

Children who are kept informed and share their parents' confidence are often more willing to share in other areas. They may welcome an opportunity to help care for the sick person by preparing meals, reading out loud, washing clothing, or just playing nurse and providing entertainment.

Reactions of Children. In addition to being understanding and supportive, children may go a long way to protect their parents. They try not to show their distress because they are afraid to make their parents cry. It is a rare child who does not begin to cry when he sees his parents crying.

Children often try to escape from the tension created by illness. If they are old enough, they get away by spending more time in homes of their friends. Another form of escape is the child's capacity to live in dreams.

Many children have responses that adults find difficult to understand or accept. Nonconcern, callous or unsympathetic attitudes, selfishness in maintaining their own lives with as little disturbance as possible, even resentfulness of the illness are not only common, but are perfectly normal. "They should be more sad then they are" or "They never want to help out" are common complaints. In fact, each of these is an expression of the normal psychological energy with which the child forces his way towards adulthood. A child who did not want to wash dishes before and still does not, in spite of the fact that his mother is sick, is not abnormal.

It doesn't affect my life much now. I don't think about it anymore. I go my own way and do my own things unless something brings it back.

If you have difficulty understanding why your child seems unconcerned, selfish, resentful or jealous, there is a pretty good chance that the child does too. Children are often confused about the contradictions they experience in their own feelings and behavior. You can help them sort out their feelings and give them *permission* to feel angry and upset and resentful and selfish.

How am I supposed to feel? I think I have some right feelings and some wrong ones and I don't know which they are.

Every child expects his or her share of attention. Sometimes a child may acquire some of the physical symptoms of the illness, such as loss of appetite, nausea, or headache. Problems in school, nervousness, and depression are all part of this picture. Signs of real distress are regression to childish or abnormal behavior, such as stealing, unusual violence, temper tantrums, fighting in school, or bedwetting. If there were behavior problems before the illness, they are apt to return and be more severe. A little regression is normal but a lot is a distinct call for help.

The most important thing that you can do is provide love, care, and support, the normal products of a close relationship. As a provider of support for a person with cancer, you have an awesome responsibility as well as unique opportunity. Whether you are a husband, wife, parent, child, or dear friend, you are being asked to help someone who really needs you. To do this you should learn what you can about the illness, particularly if you are the one closest person. Understanding the symptoms, the medical procedures, the alternatives, and the decisions that are made will enable you to share the burden. As you learn about the disease you will realize that a little preparation for what may lie ahead is much better than none at all. It is often said that no one can really understand disability without experiencing it. However, I know families and friends who do understand the meaning of a mastectomy, of impotence, of a colostomy, or of life without a normal voice. They are the people who really help.

PROVIDING SUPPORT

It is also important to recognize the emotional threat that cancer in a relative or friend poses to you. You have your own feelings and fears to deal with. Fear of loss, of added responsibilities, of financial or emotional security, and of your ability to cope with the demands that may be placed upon you, are personal fears that you must live with and understand. It is impossible to provide real support at the same time that you deny the existence of the illness or what it means to you.

The main pillars of support are love and hope. "I love you", "I am with you", "We are in this together, no matter how it turns out", can be expressed in hundreds of different ways. When words fail, just being there can be enough. Hope cannot be forced on a person, but it can be taken away. The challenge is to support whatever hope is expressed without losing your credibility by pushing an illusion of your own. When the patient recognizes that there is little hope for and accepts that, you can accept it too.

If love and hope are the pillars of support, communication is the mortar that binds them together. The more you talk, the better you feel. Open discussion of the anxieties and fears that come up can make your family a closer unit, responsive to each other, and helpful to the patient. The following are a few areas that are of particular concern to families.

Recurrence and Treatment. It is natural to be concerned about the possibility of recurrence or progression of the disease and about the medical treatment being given. The significance of new symptoms or side effects of treatment as well as where treatment should be given, who should give it, and even the choice of treatment itself are problems that most people want to share, and you will have your own ideas. It is impossible to close your eyes to the many articles you will see in papers and magazines or which will be passed on to you by other relatives and friends. You should ask your doctor to help you interpret them in light of your own situation.

A Place at the Table. The person who has had to give up many normal duties wants to retain his or her place in the family and be included in its activities. The key is to feel needed. Meals should be eaten together and family discussions should include everybody. Children should share their school experiences and the working people in the family, their work experiences. Elderly parents have a great deal to offer. One patient of mine was the repository of an enormous amount of family history which was taped while he talked to his grandchildren. He left behind more information about the roots of the family than they could ever get from any other source, and in his own voice.

Contact with the outside world helps maintain your place in it. Television can bring in world and local news, and friends can bring in a different kind of news. You can also help the patient get out into the world. Special activities such as trips, camping, travel, building something, visiting children in other cities, attending weddings or graduations mean a great deal to a person who has been shut up in the house. In short, if there is something you want to do as a family, do it *together*.

Fear of Being Dependent. Serious illness makes a person feel very dependent on others, particularly in the hospital. This frustrating situation can be made worse by the family and loving relatives who foster dependence without meaning to do so. Most people with cancer feel their need for independence very strongly and do not want to be protected or treated as a sick person more than necessary. They prefer to do things on their own without always having others jump up to help them.

Occasionally adult children take over responsibilities that are not theirs and are actually pleased with the power they now exercise. The parent may have ceased to be a parent years ago but he should not be further reduced to the status of a child. Overly protective parents can be just as hard on their grown children.

Parents can treat you as if you were six years old and slightly retarded. While their intentions are the finest, they are the most impossible people to have around. They love you and they want to help, but their idea of what you need is completely wrong. It's just impossible to live under suffocating conditions.

Patients can encourage over-protectiveness, too. Terminating employment unnecessarily, pushing other members of the family to do all the housework and cooking, resisting sex, or making it conditional are all ways of manipulating people. The tendency to regress in this way to demanding, dependent, and childish behavior is common in serious illness but has more time to be expressed in cancer. Eventually manipulation and demands lead to resentment on everyone's part.

The best way to avoid unnecessary dependence, be it real or imagined, is to encourage the patient to maintain and *control* as many areas of his life as possible. Most people do not want to impose upon their children to take them to the doctor each week, or to take them into their homes permanently. Grown children, on the other hand, may not feel that they are being imposed upon and may like being able to help in some way. Or they may feel badly because they have all that they can deal with in their own families so that they can offer very little help. Only open discussion between the people involved can solve these problems.

Finances. A separate chapter is devoted to the many financial problems that cancer can pose for a family. These problems are sources of real concern and should be discussed. They may include loss of the usual sources of income and the need to find a job, as well as sharing and transfer of financial responsibilities. The person who must take over and who is going to be the survivor if the disease is fatal must know what money is available in the forms of savings and insurance, and what bills and income to expect. If you are the person who will eventually have to handle these matters and you have not done so in the past, you should insist that you learn while you can do so with help and guidance.

Changes in Sexual Expression. Sexual activity can be affected by any kind of cancer. Occasionally, as when some hormones are used, sexual desire is increased. More often it is decreased, temporarily or permanently. The range of sexual adaptation is enormous and the results are *frequently* influenced by attitudes of the people involved. Impaired sexual function may be caused by physical damage from the tumor or its treatment. The impairment may directly prevent normal intercourse, or it may involve a loss of sexual urge, or cause emotional barriers. In the acute stage of any serious illness, when life is truly threatened, priorities change at a basic level. Life and recovery are obviously more important than sex. This withdrawal of sexual interest is not a sign of weakness nor a cause for shame, it is just a matter of first things first. In general, however, if you had a normal sex life before your illness, and there are no new physical or medical limitations, you should be able to get back to where you were after treatment is completed.

Your doctor can tell you what to expect in the way of sexual impairment during and following treatment. You should ask if there is any reason that you will not be able to resume normal sexual activity. It is very important for partners to find out *in advance* what sexual impairment may result from surgery or medical treatment.

Treatment of a few tumors may make normal intercourse impossible. Amputation of the penis or removal of the vagina are obvious examples, but both are very rare. Removal of the prostate or the rectum causes impotence in men. Removal of one testicle has no effect on sexual activity and does not cause sterility. However, removal of both testicles causes sterility but may not affect sexual activity. Removal of the uterus or radiation for cancer of the cervix may shorten the vagina enough to require some modification of sexual practices. Loss of sexual urge or interest may be experienced during chemotherapy or radiation but usually returns to normal after treatment has been completed. Some hormones can also suppress the sexual urge, as when cancer of the prostate is treated with female hormones. Some operations have a very profound effect on a person's sexuality even though they do not impair sexual function directly at all. Colostomy and removal of the breast are both examples. The sexual impairment, which may be negligible or profound, is entirely emotional and can be greatly influenced by attitudes, support and, if necessary, professional help. The major problem is fear of loss of desirability and the answer is an understanding and supportive partner.

Finally, there is a general sexual impairment that is experienced by many people with cancer. It, too, has an emotional basis and comes from the damage that being treated for cancer does to the picture of yourself as a whole and healthy person. Since sexuality is an important part of your self-image, it is not surprising that it is hurt in the process.

Just as the sexual roles of men and women differ, so do their fears and anxieties. Men fear sexual failure. Inability to perform brings on feelings of shame and fear of ridicule and rejection. For many men it is safer not to try at all than not to perform well. This in turn leads to guilt about not being able to fulfill one's expected role. The woman who understands this and is able to take the lead when necessary, and reassure her partner if he is indeed unable to perform can do much to rebuild a normal sexual relationship. The woman whose sexual urge is decreased feels guilty because she knows that she can accommodate her partner but does not feel like it. There are other sources of guilt. Wanting sex when your partner is unable to perform, or not wanting sex when your partner is able to perform, are both common. Finally, there is the completely unfounded fear that cancer can be transmitted between husband and wife by sexual intercourse or other physical contact.

Partners can help each other in many ways but none is more critical than the re-establishing of a normal sexual relationship. If you work together to accept and understand the original illness you will be better able to overcome sexual limitations. Even physical defects can be shared. The husband who can look at and touch his wife's mastectomy scar soon realizes that it is living flesh, her living flesh. It may be more or less sensitive than normal, but it is essentially skin that has healed. Similarly helping to care for a colostomy is one way of sharing the distress of having one. Reaffirming the attractiveness of your partner as a person creates confidence and helps re-establish the normal male or female outlook that will lead to sexual responsiveness.

Physical and psychological recovery require patience with yourself and your partner, and returning to a completely satisfactory sexual relationship is no exception. Understanding and patience are the key to overcoming the frustration of early attempts. Premature ejaculation, trouble with erection, or failure to achieve orgasm are problems only if you *let* them threaten you. Privacy, comfort, a warm and relaxed atmosphere all contribute to good sex. Anxiety, stress, and fatigue interfere. Depression almost always includes depressed sexuality too. Give yourself every chance by picking a time when you are in a good mood, you are feeling well in general, and when desire is real. Use little things that helped you in the past: perfume, lights on or lights off, bathing together.

Changes in sexual expression may be necessary. These may require experimentation with new positions, manual, oral, anal, or inter-thigh intercourse. You can provide sexual gratification for your partner without being able or wanting to receive it yourself. These are not causes for feelings of inadequacy, or shame. They are not aberrations but rather adaptations to your own situation. They indicate your willingness to try something new in order to regain the sexual companionship that you need. If both partners understand and accept any limitations that exist, whether they are temporary or permanent, sexual expression can continue to convey its message of love. Sex is a language of communication in which there are many different forms of expression. These include not only intercourse but lying together, petting, touching each other, holding hands, or just being together. Our desire for affection comes into our lives long before our desire for sex, and when fullscale sex can no longer be accomplished, the desire for affection is still there and can be easily gratified.

Sexual companionship plays an important role in the lives of people of *any* age. Recovery in this area is important for itself and for its contribution to emotional and psychological recovery in general. If your own attempts at re-establishing sexual bonds are failing, professional help is available.

FAMILY
AND
DOCTOR

Members of the patient's family often need to have their own relationship with the doctor. Ideally, close family members should receive the same information from the doctor as the patient, even if it cannot be given at the same time. This avoids unnecessary concerns that the doctor may have told a different story. It also helps improve communication within the family and avoids unreasonable denial. Family members tend to leave the hospital room when the doctor comes in. While this may be necessary at the time of actual examination, it is much better to remain or return for any discussion that follows. On the other hand, it is possible to intrude too much on the patient's relationship with the doctor. Some people like to be accompanied to the doctor's office for moral support. Others, however, resent this as an intrusion on their independence. Both of these are normal reactions and should be respected.

It is common for family members to wish to get some information from the doctor separately, even if it is exactly the same information that the patient received. This is often information of a very practical nature concerning care, side effects of chemotherapy, what to eat, when to be up and around. It may also include a very real desire to know "how long". It is important for family members to discuss their feelings and their hopes that death may come soon to relieve unnecessary suffering. This type of conversation is usually too painful to be carried out in the presence of the patient. In addition to giving support, almost every family member *needs* support and establishes his or her own system. Some cope with their problems alone, others turn to each other, and still others go outside to classmates or close friends. Even the person who is ill may be the main source of support for one or more members of the family.

I was asked to talk to a family of a mother and her three grown daughters because they seemed to the nursing and resident staff to be very weepy. We talked together about the father who was quite ill and soon out came the handkerchieves. It was clear, however, that they understood and accepted his illness completely and were handling the situation very well. When I mentioned the concern of the staff about their weeping they said, "Oh, tell them not to worry about us, we always cry together when we're in trouble".

You and your family still have needs of your own which should not be neglected because one member is sick. These include employment, education, money, sex, vacations, and entertainment. Early in the illness you think mostly about the patient and not about your own needs. But the illness can last a long time, with many ups and downs. To completely neglect your own life is to risk building up resentment against the person you are trying to support. It is important to get away and do things on your own without feeling guilty. You should have some time and place to express your own feelings, particularly your "selfish" feelings which are not really selfish but which can easily make you unhappy. Families can also get a great deal of help from others facing the same problems, either in the hospital or as organized groups. Most groups include the family as a unit, including children over the age of ten or twelve. The patient may or may not be included, depending on how the group functions. Some are oriented towards improving communication with patients while others are primarily outlets for expressing thoughts and concerns which would not be expressed if the patient were present. The common bond of experience, both triumph and tragedy, is more than enough to bring families from widely different backgrounds together in a spirit of sharing.

FOR FRIENDS

Thank you for brightening my day. One of the hardest things about being confined is the peace and quiet. As you know, I am not a loner. I miss my friends. So a word, a thought, or a prayer means more than you know. (Hubert H. Humphrey)

As friends of a person with cancer, it is easier for us to turn away from a friend who is sick, depressed, or whose appearance has changed, than it is for a family member. Our acceptance and understanding are not obligatory, but voluntary, and therefore both mean a great deal. We can provide vital contact with life outside of the hospital or home, with life as it was before, and as it may be again someday. Finally, there may be things that are more easily discussed with friends than with family. We are further away and less involved so that expressions of anger, sorrow, or disappointment, are less painful.

Visiting someone who is seriously ill can be a strained and frightening experience, at least for the first few minutes. Indeed, apprehension and fear are what keep so many friends from visiting at all. Be sure to set aside plenty of time for your visit so you can both relax. To feel comfortable, you must be comfortable. This means sitting where you can see your friend easily, preferably close enough that you can touch each other if you want to. Some people like to be touched, others do not. Look into your friend's eyes when you talk. If his appearance has changed since you last saw him, he is not as aware of it as you are. He thinks of himself as being the same person and indeed he is. Looking directly and continuously at him tells him that although he may have changed a little, you realize he is still the same. Remember that your voice and expressions speak for you just as plainly as your words.

It is not so much what you say but what you hear that counts, and worrying too much about what you should say only distracts you from listening. Let your friend take the lead and talk about what he wants to talk about. You can show your interest by paying attention and asking helpful questions. Above all do not change the subject until it has been exhausted. If the mood is light, do not make it heavy, or if it is heavy, do not try to be funny. The mood of the conversation should reflect your friend's feelings and not yours. You will have plenty of time to absorb your own after you leave. In discussing a problem or decision that must be made, try to put yourself in your friend's place and see it through his eyes.

One of the most important aspects of supportive friendship is to show understanding and sympathy for the situation as it is. If your friend is upset, angry, or depressed, agree with him, at least at first. This shows that you understand and care. Acknowledge that you would probably feel the same way. Confrontations, argument, and outright rejection of another person's feelings do not constitute support. Later, if you disagree, you can add things that may help change his mind or mood, but only after you have accepted him as he wants to present himself.

Cancer patients do not always want to talk about their disease. Even the very ill have sunshine in their lives, things they enjoy, and often even a sense of humor and perspective about their situation. Some like to recall old times, and the things that brought you together as friends. Children growing up, fishing trips, and work done together are a part of this. Visiting with someone who is sick does not require continuous, high pressure conversation. Silence can say a great deal, too, and should not make you uncomfortable.

Little things count, too. Your visit may be an important event so you should dress nicely and be cheerful. A small gift from home such as food or a book stay as a reminder after your visit. More important is your role as a contact with the outside world. Write down in advance a list of things you want to remember to tell your friend: news of the community, what others have said or are doing. Also make a note during your visit of anything that is needed, and others who should be encouraged to visit.

If you are a frequent visitor you can do things together, such as reading, card games, chess, or, if your friend is able to go out, shopping or a trip to the movies. Many of the things that you used to do that were fun will still be fun.

After you leave you may reflect on your own feelings and fears. You will quickly see that the comfort and pleasure you have given outweighs your own fears or discomfort. That, after all, is what friends are for.

six

Doctors, Nurses, and Hospitals

Modern medicine presents a bewildering array of specialists, nurses, technicians, hospitals, and clinics. Understanding our health care system and the roles of the different people involved will help you get the best care available.

DOCTORS

Who Are the Cancer Specialists? Most people first face the possibility that they may have cancer with their family doctor. It may be your family practitioner, an internist, pediatrician, or an obstetrician-gynecologist. Beyond them are a confusing variety of medical specialists with extensive experience in the treatment of cancer. It is important for you to know who these people are and what they can offer.

Medical Oncology. A medical oncologist is a doctor who specializes in treating cancer with drugs. In the past his training was often in the treatment of blood diseases (hematology), particularly leukemia and lymphoma, since these were the first tumors to be treated with drugs. Some hematologists expanded their experience to treat other types of cancer. More recently a new medical specialty of medical oncology has been developed which trains doctors exclusively in the use of drugs for treating cancer. Good treatment can now be obtained from a medical oncologist or a hematologist who has taken a special interest in cancer. A pediatric oncologist limits his practice to children with cancer. Specialists in oncology should have passed appropriate examinations and be certified by the American Board of Internal Medicine, The American Board of Pediatrics, or The American Board of Medical Oncology.

Radiation Therapy. The treatment of cancer by radiation may be called radiation therapy, therapeutic radiology, x–ray therapy, or cobalt therapy. The physician who practices this specialty is a radiation therapist, an x–ray therapist, or a therapeutic radiologist. He should not be confused with a radiologist, whose specialty is the making and reading of x–rays for detection of disease. Qualified therapeutic radiologists should have passed the appropriate examinations and be certified by the American Board of Therapeutic Radiology.

Surgery. The treatment of cancer by surgery is divided into even more specialties. While medical oncologists and radiation therapists deal exclusively with cancer patients, most surgeons do not. Their practices may include a variety of diseases. This means a surgeon may have a great deal of experience with cancer surgery or may have very little. For this reason the choice of a good cancer surgeon requires more investigation than one would expect. The very minimum that one should look for in a surgeon is that he be certified by the American Board of Surgeons or by one of its subspecialty Boards such as Neurosurgery, Obstetrics and Gynecology, Orthopedic Surgery, or Urologic Surgery. Some surgeons have special training and limit their practices to the surgery of cancer. Although there is no certification to indicate such training, it is important to find out what a surgeon's interest and experience are. Surgery for cancer of the head and neck, for example, should only be done by surgeons who have developed skill in this area. Qualified surgeons can usually be recommended by other doctors in the community, particularly those in medical oncology or radiation therapy who have previously shared in the care of their patients. It should also be realized that people with very rare tumors, such as sarcomas of bones, can receive the best treatment in only a few centers where significant numbers of people with similar tumors have been treated.

In addition to general surgery there are other surgical specialties for treating cancers of particular parts of the body. The chest surgeon (thoracic or cardiothoracic surgeon) is best qualified to treat cancer of the lung, esophagus, or other more rare tumors of the chest. In many medical centers, a plastic surgeon is best qualified to operate for cancer of the head and neck. In others, this surgery is done by surgeons trained in otolaryngology or by general surgeons with special interest in this area. Tumors of the limbs involving bones, joints, muscle, and other connective tissues are frequently treated by orthopedic surgeons, or by a general surgeon with special interest in cancer surgery. Urologic surgeons treat cancers of the urinary system, and gynecologists treat cancers of the female genital organs. Brain tumors and malignancies of the nervous system are treated by neurosurgeons, and in some medical centers tumors of the bowel or rectum are treated by surgeons who have special training in colorectal surgery.

Choosing a Doctor The person with cancer has a very special relationship with his doctor. It is a long-term association that should sustain you through good and bad, through the uncertainties of the disease, the triumphs of success, or the disappointment of unsuccessful treatment, possibly to the very end of life. A doctor in whom you have real confidence can make everything more tolerable. Your doctor should be compassionate, understanding, and interested in you as a person as well as a patient. If honesty is important to you, insist that you discuss your disease and its treatment openly. For many, however, it is more important to know that lines of communication are open and that your questions will be answered than to ask actual questions at the time. While it is not essential for good care, it helps a lot to have a doctor whom you really like.

Once doctors realize that I really want to know what is going on, it is okay. Even if the situation is pretty grim, we can be friends and share our laughs. Our relationship changed very quickly one Sunday morning. He spent half an hour telling me about his childhood, his schooling in Germany, leaving home at thirteen, and his own family and children. After that he was much more than just my doctor.

The best time to form an opinion of a doctor is during your first visit. Do not be afraid to trust your opinion. These simple steps will help you judge his professional competence. The questioning and examination should be thorough and suggestions concerning further studies or treatment should make sense to you. He should have time for you and not make you feel rushed or confused. He should be knowledgeable and flexible enough to discuss all available forms of treatment for your disease, including any suggestions you may have. If there are several hospitals in your area, ask which one he is affiliated with. There is an advantage to being treated in a larger hospital where doctors from different specialties can be called upon to help with your care. If money is a problem, be sure to discuss it. Cancer can be a very expensive disease and your doctor may be able to help you find resources of which you were not aware. Question the priorities of a surgeon who asks for "one third down" and wants you to sign a contract before he will agree to operate.

For many people, their association with a surgeon is brief, with additional treatment carried out by a medical oncologist or radiation therapist. While surgical competence is obviously the most important single factor, larger communities have many surgeons. There is no reason not to find one who understands your own needs.

After your first visit, ask yourself whether your questions were answered fully and whether the suggestions make sense. Ask yourself if this is a person whom you would like to know, and whom you are comfortable talking to as a friend.

Finding a Doctor

Once the diagnosis of cancer has been made, it is to your advantage to find the best cancer specialist available. If you live in a large city there is obviously more choice than in a smaller community and it is well worth taking a little extra time to find the right doctor.

Most people are referred to a surgeon, radiation therapist, or medical oncologist by their family doctor, and this usually works out well. However if your are not satisfied, the correct thing to do is tell your family doctor why you are unhappy and ask him to suggest someone else. If you are concerned about the possibility of cancer but have no family doctor, there are ways you can find one without great expense in time or money. Friends usually have suggestions. A more direct route is to go to the emergency room of a nearby hospital, explain your problem, and ask them to help you find a doctor. An alternative is to write or phone the director of the hospital of your choice. He is usually not an M.D. but will know the members of his staff well enough to get you to the right person. If you are located near a medical school, a call to the office of the department of surgery, department of medicine, or the department of radiation therapy will provide you with the names of the people on their faculty who see patients. If you live near one of the comprehensive cancer centers in the United States, a telephone call to the administrative office will provide you with the information you need. In most cities the American Cancer Society cannot provide you with the names of cancer specialists because they do not keep such lists. However, many communities have Cancer Information Lines, usually developed through the cooperation of the local medical society, which will either provide you with the names of several physicians or will suggest how best to find a cancer specialist in the community.

Getting a Second Opinion

There are several reasons for wanting to get a second opinion from another qualified physician. Foremost is reassurance that the first opinion is right. A second opinion may also be wanted when surgery has been recommended, when you question the evaluation made by your first doctor, when you think the doctor is underestimating the seriousness of your illness ("nervous stomach"), when he seems unable to find out what is wrong with you, when he says you have a very rare disease requiring a long and complicated treatment but will not tell you what it is, or when you think there may be another better form of treatment. If you really think that there is something wrong with your doctor's advice, you owe it to yourself to get a second opinion and even to change doctors if necessary. Do not be afraid to do this, it is common practice.

Changing Doctors

More difficult than asking for a second opinion is telling your doctor that you would prefer to go to someone else, yet this may be the most important step you can take. If you are not satisfied with your relationship with your doctor you have every right to shop around. The most common reasons for changing doctors are a personality conflict, loss of confidence in his ability to help you, or the feeling that your doctor is not interested in you as a person. Feelings of anger and frustration will not help you get better, and it is certainly in your own best interest to end an unhappy relationship. You should not be afraid to discuss your concerns with your doctor. No doctor likes to hear this but *every* doctor has experienced it in the past. A way of softening this conversation is to thank your doctor for what he has done, indicating your appreciation, and assure him that his evaluation is probably right but that you would prefer to try to find another doctor who is more suitable for your own particular needs. Your doctor is morally and legally obliged to help you find someone else and to provide your new doctor with any existing records, x–rays and test results.

I just didn't have the confidence I wanted. I asked real questions and I got run–around answers. Finally I told him I wanted to change, that we just didn't have a relationship that would be beneficial to me. He was very cooperative and I think he probably felt the same way.

Your Interactions with Your Doctor

It is remarkable how your attitude can influence your physician's attitude. Every doctor responds to a patient who is warm, friendly, and grateful. A relationship based on friendship and trust, with open discussion of even the hardest and most sensitive questions, also makes it much easier for your doctor to help you. Fear of your disease is the natural barrier which makes communication difficult. It helps to recognize fear and to come right out and express it. One of the most frightening questions is "Could it be cancer?" Having asked it, however, you will find that most other questions are easier. Above all, treat your doctor like a person, not a god. "M.D." does not stand for "Medical Diety". If you are angry or upset or you disagree with your doctor about something, say so.

In general it is best to let your physician guide the initial conversation by asking you questions that will give him the information he needs. He is trying to put together a pattern that will accurately establish the nature and extent of your disease and lead him to the best treatment. You should answer his questions honestly and fully, giving as much detail as he wants. Do not make him dig for information. On the other hand, if he appears to be passing over something that worries you, be sure to mention it.

It is important not to deny or hide any signs or fears you have that something is wrong. Putting on a good front for your doctor when you really feel ill or frightened will not help you in the long run. Your doctor wants you to feel well and would like to think he has helped. His own behavior may encourage you to pretend to feel better than you really do just to avoid disappointing him. It is clearly in your better interest to present yourself as you really are rather than as you think he would like you to be. If you feel well, tell him. If you do not, tell him. It may help your physician to get to know *you* by discussing your family, your work, your religious views, and hobbies. The better he knows you, the easier it will be to treat you as a person as well as a patient.

Memory often fails when we talk to doctors. A good trick is to write down your questions, even if they look like a shopping list and, if you have trouble remembering the answers, write them down too.

What Your Doctor Should Tell You

At your initial visit and examination your doctor should be able to tell you what may be going on ("Yes, the lump you found in your breast may be cancer, but it is probably just a cyst.") and what studies should be done. If the exact diagnosis is already known, and it frequently is by the time you have been referred to a cancer specialist, she should be able to explain it to you in detail, giving you some idea of the implications of your disease, and what the treatment should be. In discussing her recommended treatment, she should explain the potential benefits as well as the dangers or side effects. She should be able to tell you about other forms of treatment and give you some idea of what may be expected if you have no treatment at all or if treatment is delayed. You should discuss the chances of the treatment not working and what other treatment can then be given. If money is a factor, and it frequently is if full insurance coverage is not available, you should not hesitate to discuss treatment costs. Your doctor can usually tell you whether the treatment she proposes will be covered by your insurance, if you will have to be in the hospital, and for how long. Some time early in the course of your disease your doctor should be able to outline a long-term program for you, including other forms of treatment that will be used, and other doctors who will take part in your care.

You should understand the answers and explanations your doctor gives you. Doctors have a language of their own it took them years to learn and you cannot expect to pick it all up in a few days. Unfortunately the answers that doctors supply are often over simplified or too obscure to really qualify as answers at all. The opposite can also happen. It never pays to try to bluff your doctor and sit there nodding as if you understand when you do not.

Hard Questions

Cancer can bring up difficult questions: Is it cancer? Has it come back? Can it be cured? How long? How will it end? You must choose what you want to hear. Your doctor is unlikely to force information on you that you have not requested and are not prepared to deal with. The doctor should wait for you to ask. When such questions do come up, your emotional state can make it difficult to understand the answer the first time, and you may find yourself asking several times. It helps at these times to have a member of your family present who can go over what was said with you later. If your family is not available, a close friend or one of your favorite nurses can do the same thing.

I want the straight news. I may not like it at the time but I can get used to it.

NURSES

The nurse has a very special role in caring for a person with cancer. In the office, the hospital, or in your home, she is much more than just an extension of your doctor. Nurses can do some things better than doctors. The nurse who sees you before the doctor, after the doctor, and even without the doctor, often has more time to answer your questions and help you. She provides a different point of view which may be more compassionate and understanding. She also has a different type of responsibility. Her training allows her to provide practical answers to practical questions that are part of your everyday life. It is your nurse who can teach you and your family to take care of dressings for unhealed wounds, to get around better when you are still not very stable on your feet after an operation, to take the medications that are necessary to avoid nausea or vomiting, to care for your skin or your mouth during radiation and chemotherapy. The nurse is usually an expert on the various medications that can be used to control pain. She will teach you to use them properly so you can take care of yourself at home.

In many hospitals nurses have training in particular areas related to cancer. The specialized art of teaching people how to care for a colostomy and other similar surgical procedures is greatly improved by having someone available who is really expert. The same special type of help is often available for people who have had laryngec-tomies, mastectomies, or major amputations.

In addition to direct care, your nurse can be an excellent sound-ing board for your worries and fears. Most nurses who take care of people with cancer know a great deal about the disease and can answer many questions. They can explain tests and studies, including what they are for, how they are done, and what the different results mean. Your nurse can help you understand and accept your treat-ment and even to choose between alternative forms of treatment. She is able to explain to you the side-effects of chemotherapy or radiation, to tell you what to expect before surgery and help you to a speedy recovery afterwards. If there are things you would like to say but do not feel like telling your doctor or your family, your nurse may be just the person. If you wish, she can relay your concerns to your doctor or handle any complaints you may have about your hospital care.

Your nurse can help you understand your family and your family to understand you. At the same time she can serve as a buffer between you and your family and friends during periods of unusual strain or adjustment. For example, she can remove your phone from your room during the evening or when you wish to rest so that you will not be disturbed by incoming calls. She can insist that all visitors go to the desk and then she can check with you so that you have only those visitors you want to see and when you want to see them.

Many people notice that it is easier to become angry with their nurse than their doctor because the nurse's contact is more direct and personal. People are often afraid to get angry at their doctors, but not at their nurses. It helps to express your feelings of anger and frustra-tion to someone. Your nurse should understand this and not be offended. However, it does help to apologize when you are feeling better, recognizing that these feelings are usually not directed to-wards your nurse personally but toward the situation in general. If you have some complaint about the general nursing care you are receiving or what appears to be a personality conflict with one par-ticular nurse, you should bring this to the attention of your doctor or to the head nurse on your floor.

When you are in the hospital you will notice that different nurses appear at different times from day to day. They usually have rotating schedules so no one works just days or at night. If there is one nurse whom you particularly look forward to seeing, you can ask her what her schedule is so you will know when to expect her. After you leave the hospital it is very gratifying to the nurses who took care of you if you to drop in from time to time and just say hello. They like to maintain contact with their patients but often are not able to do so on their own time.

HOSPITALS   The best medical care can usually be obtained in a hospital. As much as most of us dislike the idea (and expense!), this is where the most highly trained people and modern equipment are brought together. Hospitals differ in their capacity to treat certain diseases. There are now several large comprehensive cancer centers in the United States which specialize completely in diagnosis, treatment, and research in all types of cancer. Most of them are associated with medical schools and all of them offer the best treatment available. University hospitals, also associated with medical schools, are staffed by highly skilled people brought together for treatment, teaching, and research of many diseases, including cancer. Next is a broad range of teaching hospitals many of which have affiliations with medical schools. They share with university hospitals responsibility for training young doctors (residents) in the medical specialties. Members of the hospital medical staff who undertake this teaching are usually highly qualified. Many private hospitals do little or no teaching and are not closely tied to the local medical shool but have excellent staffs, with expertise in all areas of cancer treatment. The way to identify a private hospital that can care for most cancers is to find out if it has a department of radiation therapy, one or more surgeons who specialize in cancer surgery *and* one or more specialists in medical oncology.

There are many excellent smaller hospitals in cities as well as suburban and rural communities. Because they are nearby, particularly in smaller communities, these hospitals may be the best place to have initial diagnostic tests and biopsies done, and later some forms of treatment. In general, however, once a cancer has been identified it is usually to your advantage to be seen in a large hospital or cancer center where more expertise is available. On the other hand, it is frequently possible to have some treatment, particularly chemotherapy, in your local hospital or in your own doctor's office under the supervision of a specialist in a larger center. The larger centers work very closely with their referring physicians to give you the best possible care.

Who Are All the People?   The most bewildering aspect of a large hospital is the number of people with whom you come in contact, each with his or her own special job to do.

Many Doctors.   In the hospital you may see many doctors besides your own. All hospitals have physicians who are on their permanent staffs, including doctors in family practice, surgery, internal medicine, and radiation therapy. University or teaching hospitals also have younger doctors or residents who are in training in various specialties. These residents spend from one to six or seven years learning their specialties from the staff physicians who are their teachers. University hospitals closely associated with medical shools usually have medical students. Most of them are nearing the end of medical school and can relate to you in a professional way. While they are not responsible for decisions concerning your studies or treatment, they can usually help you understand them.

Your own doctor is a member of the staff of the hospital and is the person responsible for your care. However, he has plenty of available help. In a large hospital he may call upon colleagues in his own or other specialties for advice. These consultants can include a radiologist who does the x–ray studies and reads the x–ray films, a heart specialist (cardiologist) who reads the electrocardiogram and may examine and treat you if necessary, a pathologist who examines the microscope slides of the biopsy to determine whether you have a cancer, and anesthesiologist who may put you to sleep for surgery, rehabilitation specialist, and many more. All of these people help in your care even though you do not meet them.

Nurses.   Most of your day to day care in the hospital is carried out by nurses. Their duties are determined by the type and amount of training they have. The registered nurse (R.N.) takes instructions directly from the doctor and has a great deal of responsibility, including giving medicines. The licensed practical nurse (L.P.N.) and the nurse's aid have much less responsibility and work under the supervision of an R.N. Many hospitals have teaching programs for student nurses.

The nurses in most hospitals work eight hour shifts. The day shift, from 7:00 a.m. to 3:00 p.m., is the busiest and has the largest nursing staff. Most of the work of the day, including bathing, exercise, and changing dressings is done during these hours. The evening shift, from 3:00 p.m. to 11:00 p.m. requires fewer nurses. The amount of individual attention they can give may be somewhat less, depending on the number of patients for whom they are responsible. The night shift, from 11:00 p.m. to 7:00 a.m., involves still fewer nurses, so their time is occupied mostly with people who need close supervision and special help.

Technicians.   Many departments employ individuals trained in the techniques used in that department. X–ray studies are often performed by technicians, but then looked at and evaluated by the radiologist who is a doctor. Day to day treatment in radiation therapy is usually given by a technician under the supervision of a doctor. Laboratory studies, including those that require drawing blood, are done by technicians.

Social Workers.   Serious illness and hospitalization brings up a variety of problems that are not purely medical but have a great deal to do with your ability to recover quickly. Some of these problems include finances, care of children or family members, where you will go and what help you will need after you leave the hospital, and psychological problems. Many hospitals also have psychologists who can help with emotional problems of cancer patients and their families.

Chaplain.   Spiritual needs often increase in time of illness and most hospitals have one or more chaplains available to see you and your family. The chaplain will usually introduce himself within a day or two of your admission, to let you know that he is available. If you want to see the chaplain, your nurse can notify him. However, while some people want to see a chaplain, others do not and he will not know what his role with you may be until you tell him.

The hospital chaplain's experience makes him a unique person. In addition to the ministerial function of prayer and sacrement, he is usually a patient and compassionate person who has time to listen. Since he is not directly connected with your medical care you may feel that you can turn to him with problems, concerns, anger, guilt, fear, or even joy, that you would not share with anyone else. He is apt to be someone who understands feelings and who is truly interested in you.

Dieticians.   Nutrition is a very important component of the treatment of cancer. The simple act of consuming enough food can be a real problem for a person who is nauseated from chemotherapy or has difficulty swallowing from radiation. The dietician's job is to help you get the best meals that are compatible with your illness. You should not hesitate to talk to her while in the hospital and, if necessary, have her help you plan for after you go home.

Respiratory Therapists.   If you have a lung problem or are going to have a chest operation you may be seen by a respiratory therapist whose job is to teach and help you cough correctly to clear your lungs and windpipe of secretions, and to supervise giving oxygen, if you need it.

Physical Therapists.   If your tumor, or its treatment, causes you to lose some important body function, such as the use of an arm or leg, a physical therapist will help you regain the lost function.

Occupational Therapy.   Prolonged hospitalization can become boring, particularly if you do not feel sick. An occupational therapist can teach you crafts and skills ranging from woodworking and weaving to knitting and leather work. Many people take their new skills home and enjoy them long after leaving the hospital.

Orderlies.   Orderlies help patients get from one place to another in the hospital. While they need no special training in medicine, they are frequently students interested in careers related to medicine. You will find that they can be very friendly and understanding.

Other Patients. The most enjoyable and helpful people you can meet in the hospital are often other patients. They are either going through experiences similar to yours, so that you can share with them, or they may be ahead of you in their treatment and can tell you what to expect. Friendships that begin in the hospital are frequently close and longlasting.

Entering the hospital can be a confusing and frightening experience. Your feelings may range from hope that you are entering a place of expert care and modern scientific machines to the fear that you are in a cold, efficient institution which is incredibly expensive.

What Happens in the Hospital?

Going to the hospital is always stressful. Either you are sick and need treatment, or you are going in to find out what is wrong (and it may be serious), or you are going to have an operation. Suddenly you are surrounded by doctors and nurses in an unfamiliar environment, along with many people who appear to be even more sick than you. All of this is frightening. Nobody wants to be in the hospital and it is not surprising that most people are upset when they first arrive. Most hospitals try to make you feel comfortable as quickly as possible and these feelings usually disappear in a short time.

When the decision and arrangements have been made, your doctor will notify you of the day and time you should go to the hospital. On arrival, you or a member of your family should go to the admitting office to give them some basic information. This includes such general information as your name, address, phone number, marital status, age, birthdate, social security number, husband's/wife's or nearest living relative's name, address, and phone number, and the name of your referring physician and/or family physician. They will also want financial information, including your insurance company's name and address, your policy number and group number, and the subscriber's name, Medicare (if applicable), with claim number and effective date; Public Assistance (if applicable) with agency name and address, case number, and caseworker's name; your employer's name, address, and phone number; your employer's insurance company's name, address and claim number; and often the name of a guarantor or person responsible for expenses not covered by insurance and their address and phone number.

Entering the Hospital

If you do not have adequate health insurance you may be asked to provide more financial information, including number of dependents, gross income, amount of unpaid medical bills, whether you rent or own a home, the market value of your home, your savings amount including stocks and bonds, other real estate assets, and other income rather than your own. Community and welfare programs can often help if you are unable to pay your medical bills, but the hospital needs this information so they can begin to help you look for assistance as soon as it is needed.

Your room may be a single room or shared with one or more people. Some people prefer to have a room to themselves while others prefer company. You may have a choice in this matter, and if so, you should discuss it with your doctor in advance or at the admitting office when you first arrive. You should also express your preference about smoking. The first doctor to see you may be your own or a resident or medical student. She will introduce herself and explain who she is. She will sit down with you and take a detailed history of your illness and many other aspects of your life which are related to your general health. This will be followed by a thorough physical examination. In a university hospital this procedure may be repeated by another member of the team a short time later. It takes some patience on your part to answer the same questions again but you will be surprised at how different the emphasis may be between two doctors. This duplication is not only instructive for them but introduces an element of safety for you since it makes it less likely that anything important will be overlooked. Your own doctor should see you sometime during the day that you are admitted to the hospital to discuss your illness and give you some information about the studies or treatment planned. Usually you can also obtain this from the resident physician.

Informed Consent

Good medical practice requires that a person undergoing treatment be fully informed about the nature of the treatment, including the side effects and risks, as well as the expected benefits. While this information should be discussed fully with your doctor, there are several situations where some acknowledgment is required in writing. The most common of these is the operative permit that must be read and signed by you in the presence of your doctor. This document is usually a printed form with spaces filled in with the name of the operation and the doctors involved. Since the same form is used whether the operation is the removal of a wart or open heart surgery, it obviously contains no details. The real information must come from your doctor. The form does state that you had the operation explained to you, and you should not sign it until you have received such an explanation and all of your questions have been answered. A similar consent form is usually required before beginning radiation therapy.

Many hospitals, including the major cancer centers and most hospitals with university affiliations, participate in experimental clinical trials to look for better ways to treat cancer. These trials may involve the use of new anti-cancer drugs or new approaches to treatment. If you are asked to participte in such a trial you will be given a consent form to read and sign. This should be written in language you can understand and should contain a significant amount of information:

1. The exact purpose of the study.
2. What you will be asked to do or what will be done to you as part of the study.
3. The risks involved.
4. The expected benefits of the treatment.
5. Alternative procedures, if any, that may be as good as, or better than, those being studied.
6. How the information from the study will be used and disseminated. This should be done in such a way that your privacy is protected.
7. An offer to answer any questions that you have at any time.
8. A statement indicating that you may withdraw from the study at any time without prejudicing your continued medical care by the same doctors.
9. What treatment or compensation, if any, you will receive if you are unexpectedly harmed by the study.

The success of being adequately informed about your medical care rests strongly on the good will of your doctor and on your willingness to ask questions. The consent form merely indicates that such an exchange has taken place. One of the major difficulties in being adequately informed is that the information often comes at a time of great stress. The day before an operation is hardly the time to be thinking about technical details, however important they may be. You will find it helpful to have a friend or relative present when your treatment is being explained so they can go over it with you later to be sure you understand. Similarly, if the treatment is at all complicated, as in chemotherapy trials, you may ask to have a copy of the consent form to look over for a day or two before you sign it and to keep for later reference when the treatment is underway.

It is a pretty tall order to think that you can ever feel at home in a hospital, but a few small things can smooth over the transition. Having a friend or family member come with you enables you to maintain contact with your own *real* life during the confusion of the first few hours. Most of us do not like to eat alone and you may find it comforting to have a family member sit with you once or twice a day at mealtimes. Although the hospital will provide clothing, it will probably not be as nice as your own and many people prefer to wear their

Making
Yourself
at Home

own nightgowns or pajamas and robes. Bringing in a few things from home and setting up your hospital room a little are ways to make it yours while you are there.

It helps to start right in making new friends in the hospital. Your own doctor, the resident doctors, nurses, and medical students should be people who are responsive and understanding, with time to talk to you. Obviously, the more they know about your illness the more they can help you. I have had several patients develop such close relationships with medical students that they asked to be remembered to each other years later, long after the student graduated. Other patients make excellent friends and you can share a great deal with them if you are willing to open up.

One way to feel more at home in a hospital and meet other people at the same time is to be up and around. If you are not confined to your bed there is no reason to stay in your room. There is usually a lounge where you can meet with your family and other patients. Your hospital world can be still larger. The cafeteria, coffee shop, lobby, library, and chapel are all for your use. Just let a nurse or the secretary know when you are leaving the floor so they can find you, if necessary. If you are confined to bed and would like company, ask your nurse to see if she can find another patient or volunteer who can visit you. Little gets done in a hospital on Saturday and Sunday. If you are able to and would like to leave for the weekend, this can be arranged by your doctor.

Another way to become part of the hospital system is to take an interest in your own care. The first step is to find out in advance what tests are going to be done and why. Within a day or two of admission your doctor will have some idea of his long-range plans and can share these with you. She should be able to tell you in advance pretty much what lies ahead, day by day. Another good source of information is the resident physician sharing in your care. Occasionally the resident may tell you something different from what you understood from your own doctor. If this happens, ask your doctor to clarify it for you. She is the person in charge.

Your nurses can help you make good use of your time. While you are in the hospital, they can teach you about your dressings, skin care, and diet or mouth care, depending on your own needs. Before you leave the hospital they should teach you about the medication that you will be taking home with you, particularly pain medication. Do not forget to include your family in these discussions. Not only do they want to know, but they can help you remember what was said. They may be responsible for your nursing care after you leave the hospital and they need time to get used to the idea and learn what to do.

Arranging to get yourself, your family, and your doctor together at the same time may be difficult. If your family has particular
hours when they visit, let the doctor know in advance so he can plan
ahead. Late in the afternoon is often a good time. If your family
arrives unexpectedly or wishes to see your doctor in the middle of the
day, the nurse or secretary can usually find him, but it may be a while
before he can see you.

Most people feel very isolated and dependent in the hospital. Although the system was designed primarily to help you, in recent years
it has developed a life of its own. Rules, regulations, and routines of
the hospital are often more for the convenience of the staff who must
be there all the time than for you or your family. Some traditions have
waited too long and should be challenged. Fortunately this rigid
system is changing. Visiting hours are becoming more flexible as it is
realized that families must work and then frequently drive long
distances to get to the hospital. Allowing children to visit a brother,
sister, or parent in the hospital is a similar step in the right direction.
If you are asleep in the afternoon, your rest may be more important
than a routine temperature and blood pressure, and when you are
not ill there is also little reason to be awakened for these at night.
Rules against telling you your temperature or blood pressure are
completely out of place now.

> Getting
> the Best
> from Your
> Hospital

There is also a lot you can do to maintain your own identity in
the hospital and even get better care. The first is to insist to yourself
and to those caring for you that you are a real person and not just an
object to be poked, examined, and eventually repaired. Self-respect
demands respect from others. If you feel you are bumping into rules,
there is no reason not to apply a little pressure yourself. There is
nothing to gain by trying to be a "good patient" in the hospital. If
there is something you want or something you do not like, say so. If
your wishes are neglected, ask your doctors or nurses why. On the
rare occasion when there seems to be a real lack of understanding or
communication, many hospitals have a non-medical person who is a
patient advocate and whose job is to try to solve these problems.

*I had been there before and I just was not going to let the hospital get to me
again. I was quite aware of what I wanted and I was not going to let anyone
abuse me. When something wasn't the way I wanted it, I just complained.
Pretty soon everyone knew who I was and was very nice to me.*

*If people keep making me wait I'm going to start sending doctors and hospitals
bills for my time.*

Another approach to getting the best out of your hospital is to express your appreciation for good care. A word to your doctor, a note to your nurses, or a letter to the hospital administrator will find its way to the right people.

I cannot say enough for the entire nursing staff, doctors, or any of the personnel. They treated me as an individual human being. I am very grateful to all of them. On my return it was like coming home after being away.

"Thank you" sounds very feeble, but we do thank you for working so hard to save my husband's life. We are grateful that a hospital like this was available to us. The doctors and nurses were as concerned about me as they were about my husband.

For the concern, gentleness, and patience shown by all staff members during my stay, I am most grateful. God bless you all.

In all the hospitals I have been at, I have never come in contact with such nice nurses and doctors. They treated my son like one of their own children. The nurses were also very good to me too. Everything was explained to me. The atmosphere was friendly no matter how busy they were.

seven

Dying And Death

No one can look at death without experiencing some sadness and fear. We do not want things to end. We wonder how our world can go on without us, although we know it will. Spouses may remarry, children will grow up and graduate from school, perhaps with another father or mother. Money problems will be solved. But how can we *not* be a part of it? There are so many things we have not done, that we really want to do. Now they will never get done, or someone else will have to do them, but not the way you or I would. We know our own faults, including the fact that we have always started things we did not finish. Life is full of plans that are set aside.

The only way that you continue after death is in other people's minds so that you have to accomplish something in order to be remembered. I am frightened of death because I may not have accomplished everything I want to.

We wonder what will happen to us after we die. Walking in the woods, planting flowers, waiting for the words "Hi Mom", when the children come home from school are all beautiful parts of life.

We are afraid of being helpless and unable to take care of ourselves. Without people to wash and clean us, we may become dirty. We are afraid of being left alone. Some friends have already abandoned us, while others seem to be saying goodbye, and we are not ready for that yet. Beyond this is fear that we may be abandoned by those even closer to us. We realize that we are causing them pain and upsetting their lives. Finally we are afraid of all our fears. We want to talk about them but are afraid because we know it will be painful.

Am I Going To Die? Almost everyone who has cancer realizes that it could be fatal. Some take a brief glimpse at this possibility at the beginning and then block it out forever. Most, however, accept and fear the possibility of death from cancer soon after the diagnosis is made, but then try not to think about it until it is forced back into consideration by recurrence and further illness.

I know that I am quite sick but the thought of death is still very remote from my mind. I still like to think of myself as having a while to go.

In my experience "Am I dying?" is one question people do not ask if they do not want to know. It is very difficult for most people to ask and one of the hardest questions anyone can be called upon to answer. Confirmation that the illness is indeed very serious, given with love and understanding, may be the best answer that you can get.

One man, after months in the hospital, punctuated by many operations, with peaks of hope and valleys of disappointment, was finally found to have incurable cancer. His wife, who was with him almost night and day, begged everyone not to tell him. In the meanwhile he could see that the nature of his treatment and the attitude of his doctors had changed. He asked everyone, including his wife, what was going on and whether something was being kept from him. The nurses wept for him because they could not stand his questions, his doctors avoided him because they could offer no support under the circumstances. Finally in exasperation he asked his wife one night, "If you were in my situation wouldn't you want to know what's going on?" She admitted that she would insist *on knowing. To which he asked, "Well, what about me?" The next day she declined help from the doctors and said that it was her responsibility to tell him. She did so with tenderness and understanding that filled their last days with love.*

The question is a humane as well as a medical one. While some doctors are very capable, it is unfortunate that many are ill-at-ease and even inept in dealing with dying and death. Whether they have a strong fear of death themselves or whether they look upon death as a failure of their responsibility in treatment, the result may be little support from a person who should be able to provide a lot. At the present time very few medical students or doctors receive training in this area.

How Long?   This is one of the most frequently asked questions, yet one of the most difficult to answer. Most experienced doctors know better than to try to estimate the length of anyone's life. Our ability to be precise is very limited, even when death may be just a few days away. It is doubtful that anyone really wants to know in advance the exact day he can expect to die. Some people who were told they had six months have outlived the doctors who told them.

I hate their calculated, educated guesses which are just speculation. If they can be certain about what they are saying, that's fine.

There's only one person who really knows. If He meant someone else to know, He'd find a way to tell them.

I have encountered people who were given such estimates and became angry at their doctors because they did not die on schedule. One such person, with a brain tumor, decided on his own that his disease was fatal and that he would not live very long. In spite of reassurances from his doctors that he was doing very well, he has spent over a year in front of a television set waiting to die. In every other respect he is a very healthy man.

Many doctors refuse to answer this question, or turn it around, "If you can tell me how long I have to live, I will tell you how long you have to live". However, I have found that many people want and need a more helpful answer, and for very good reasons. They have more important things to do than sit round and worry about when they are going to die. For them, some realistic estimate is necessary to make decisions and plans that will affect their lives and those of their families. These may include such things as taking a long-awaited vacation, changing business plans, or moving ahead with plans that would otherwise have been put off.

We had decided to get married in July but it was obvious that I was going to have another operation so we moved it up to April. I wanted to get married while I was still able to have all my friends around, and not have them thinking "the poor thing" all the time. My husband knew what was likely to happen, that my life span would not be a normal one. We discussed it and decided that we wanted to get married anyway.

Your doctor usually can provide enough information, in the form of estimates based on his experience, to help you make important decisions. Even early in your illness he can tell you what the probability is that you may die of cancer rather than something else. If your disease was widespread when first discovered, or has recurred, he can estimate your chances of being cured and set reasonable limits on how long you may expect to live. Guesses of "six months to four years" are often better than no information at all. You may find such figures reassuring to live with, so long as you understand that they are only estimates.

I really wanted to know how much time he had. They told me between two and six weeks and it was very close to six weeks. It helped me to know because we had lots to talk over.

Some tumors are very unpredictable, particularly when chemotherapy and radiation may control the disease for long periods of time. In such cases, even the most open doctor cannot be very helpful in predicting what lies ahead.

Finally, some doctors cannot bring themselves to deal so directly with their patients under any circumstances. They are, however, legally obliged to share their knowledge with *someone* in the family.

I asked him how long I would live. He just evaded the issue and wouldn't talk about it at all. Finally, he said about five years. Later I had to find out from my son that the tumor hadn't been removed at all and that he had been told maybe six months. I'm a grown woman. He should have told me.

How Will It End?   No one can accurately predict how the end will come for any particular person. The presence of incurable cancer does not eliminate the possibility of dying from any number of other things. You may have some ideas of your own concerning how you would like to have it end and you should consider them with your doctor. At the very least your doctor should be able to assure you that he will care for you throughout your illness and that you will not suffer unnecessarily.

YOUR REACTIONS TO DEATH   The common reactions to death, first described by Elizabeth Kubler-Ross, include *shock* and *denial* ("No, not me"), *anger* ("Why me?" "Why my child?"), *bargaining* ("I'll be good"), *depression* ("Yes, me!"), and *acceptance* ("Yes, me, and I'm ready"). These may seem similar to those feelings you experienced when you first became aware of your illness. Indeed, shock, denial, and anger experienced early in illness may not be experienced again or they may be much reduced as you live with your disease. On the other hand, people who accept their disease but reject the possibility of death may encounter these strong feelings again, or even for the first time, late in their illness. In my experience, bargaining is not very common, since most people with cancer live long enough to establish realistic goals and see them achieved. When death is recognized as the eventual outcome, denial, depression, and aceptance are the most common reactions. No one necessarily goes through all of these steps or from one to another in an orderly sequence. There may be flashbacks to denial and anger. Indeed, a person who feels ready to die today may not be tomorrow. Most important, there is no right or wrong. Each person meets death in his own way.

Denial.   Many people are never able to accept the fact that they are dying. Effective coping with cancer does not necessarily mean that the person is ready to accept death. This is particularly true of men, for whom accepting death is a sign of defeat and giving up, which they are not able to do. They are fighters and they are going to fight to the end. "Show me a good loser and I'll show you a loser" and "Good guys come in last" are competitive concepts that sustain many people. A person who has had this attitude throughout life is not likely to change near the end, and forcing a discussion of death on such a person can be harmful since it breaks down important defenses.

We could not talk to our son [a college student] about dying because that would require that he admit that he was dying. That was too frustrating and made him angry.

No one should have to know something he does not want to know and it would be cruel to force unwanted information on a person who is not prepared for it. Some are able to deny effectively to the end and their right to do so should be respected. Denial is a normal and healthy form of protection. We occasionally lose sight of this and try to push our loved ones beyond the limits of their endurance.

We could not work Mother up to the acceptance stage before she died.

The best that the family and friends of such a person can do is support the denial as long as it lasts, without necessarily encouraging or augmenting it. Too much emphasis has been placed on eventual acceptance of death and not enough on the sustaining value of denial for the emotional health of many people. Families feel guilty because they think that they should be talking about dying, since so much is being said about it in the popular literature.

There is an important difference between denial and inability to talk about death. Some people who have a very close relationship cannot talk about death together. Although they have shared most things and can talk about any and everything else, this is one event that must be understood without words. These are times when both patient and spouse may seek release by speaking freely of death to doctors, nurses, close friends, or other family members, but not with each other.

Depression. Anger and depression are two clear signs that denial is beginning to recede and that some degree of acceptance is making itself felt. In cancer anger is often dissipated early in the disease, but may return in full force when the likelihood of death is recognized.

When a person close to you dies, your sense of loss may be

enormous. From this common experience you can begin to understand the loss experienced *by* a person who knows he is dying. It means leaving behind all family, all friends, and all possessions, forever. Depression, sadness, self-pity, and grief are the normal reactions to such a confrontation. Mourning your own death may begin when you first realize your illness may be fatal, or not until death is close at hand. It is a mourning for what has already been lost from your life: your job, mobility, health, income, and closeness to family, as well as for what you will lose in death.

Depression shows up as withdrawal, quietness, sadness, and loss of appetite and interests. Weeping is common. This is a time when love and the companionship of one or a few close people are needed but when attempts to console are out of place and doomed to failure. It is an important stage that must be worked through, because it is the threshold to the peace and beauty of full acceptance that many people seek.

Acceptance. Acceptance of death at an emotional and personal level usually comes as a *relief* from the phase of depression experienced first. It is not happiness or sadness but a feeling of peace. When you are not longer afraid of your own death, there is little left to fear. Pride can be set aside and pretense dropped. Barriers between people can be replaced by bonds of friendship and love. Loose ends can be gathered together and you can now say things you have long wanted to say. Goodbyes can be tender and loving, leaving beautiful memories to sustain your survivors throughout their own lives. Fears can be dissipated by talking about them. Your personal belief and faith will contribute to your peace. It makes little difference whether this is faith in your worth as an individual, in the dignity of man as an organism, or in God and afterlife.

Forgiveness and Permission

He helped us all, particularly the children. He spoke to each one alone and told them how he felt about them and what he hoped for them. It made a great difference to us.

The sorrow that surrounds death cannot be washed away but the guilt can, by the exchange of permission and forgiveness. Forgiveness is for hurting, for being so dependent and helpless, for being a burden, and finally for leaving and making your loved ones unhappy. Permission is to go on your own way without them, leaving behind all the people and things you held dear throughout life. Your loved ones want forgiveness too, for all the unkind things that were said and done throughout your lives together, for the anger and resentment, and even for having begun to mourn before you were gone. They, too, want permission to live without you, to marry again, to grow up and graduate from school and establish their own lives.

Permission and forgiveness may be granted to different people individually by simply accepting the fact of death together, absolving each other of blame, guilt and despair, and by giving permission to go on living without you in exchange for permission to die. Frequently this level of acceptance is exchanged between two people who are very close, speaking for others as well as for themselves. Permission and forgiveness may be granted without necessarily being requested. Their message may be conveyed without words, through care given with love and understanding.

Letting Go. The final phase of acceptance is letting go of the world you have known and enjoyed. This includes letting go of your plans for the future, your material goods, your favorite places and activities, your friends, and finally your family, reducing your world to the one person who is closest to you. By agreeing to let your world go on without you, *you* are given the freedom to think and feel and do as you wish, eventually to die a free and truly independent spirit.

The Many Meanings of Hope. These several reactions to death are linked together by one thread of continuity: hope. Hope changes with your illness and your expectations. It requires abandoning yesterday's concept of hope and replacing it with today's, as the situation requires. At first you hope for permanent cure. If this becomes impossible your wish is modified to a long and trouble-free remission. Later, hope may be for a return to your family and your work, for a vacation, for a few days home from the hospital, to be able to be up and walking again, for relief from pain, and eventually for peace and rest. Hope does not necessarily end there, but it may extend to a wish that your family can get along without you, that your children will complete school and do well in their own lives and that you will be missed, but not too much. Knowing that you have a fatal disease does not in any way imply that you give up all hopes. Indeed, conscious acceptance and continuing hope cushion each other and allow you to hedge your bets against wishing for too much or too little at any time.

The Right to Die. Acceptance of the possibility of death gives you a chance to express your wishes on how you want to die. This usually requires an understanding between yourself, your doctor, and the closest members of your family and can be discussed at any time. The choices are between maintaining your life at all costs or allowing you to die a natural death without prolonging your life by artificial means. The first presupposes that life is indeed sacred and that no effort should be spared to maintain and prolong life until there is no spark left. This view sees doctors as obliged to defend life with all the means available. Medicine has been accused of leaning in this direction in the past, although I have not seen much evidence of it in the treatment of cancer.

Both arms were outstretched in the bed like the cross of our Lord. They were trying to keep her alive when she was dying. I couldn't stand it and told them to leave her alone.

An alternative and more widely accepted view is that every individual should be permitted to die in peace and dignity and that no extraordinary means should be used to prolong life. This allows, or requires, your doctor to show restraint in the face of impending death. It enables him to provide the usual measures to insure your comfort but without prolonging your life. In practical terms this means that drugs, surgical procedures, medicines, intravenous fluids, tubes of various kinds, and respirators, will be avoided or discontinued unless they contribute directly to your comfort. The extent to which these measures can prolong life is variable but ranges from not at all to several days or even weeks. In cancer, with the possible exception of some brain tumors, the maximum is usually a matter of days.

At each crisis Dr. Johnson and I looked eye to eye and I asked, "Is this the time?" I made it clear that I wanted no heroics. I even asked the nurses on each shift when they came to my room to make sure that they got the message.

Living Wills.   The desire of many people to insure their right to refuse treatment and die in peace and dignity has prompted several states to consider or pass appropriate legislation. The appearance of living wills and right to die laws are the first steps in this direction. In many states living wills are not legally binding on the physician nor do they provide him with legal protection if they are subsequently challenged. At the very least, however, some form of living will provides evidence that you, your family, and your doctor have discussed your wishes in depth. In this sense the actual discussion and meeting of minds are probably more important than the document. This type of discussion and the preparation of a living will, if desired, should not be put off until death is close. It has a better moral and legal foundation if done early in the illness, when death is still a relatively remote possibility.

Euthanasia.   One other alternative not mentioned very often is the deliberate shortening of life. You should not be alarmed about thoughts you have about ending your own life. Many people with cancer consider suicide at some time but few carry it out. Many people, however, visualize circumstances under which they would like to have their lives shortened, even though they realize that they will not do it themselves. Euthanasia or mercy killing is the obvious alternative. Many think about this and a few discuss it with their doctors. Similarly, many doctors think about it but only a few are willing to discuss it and very few admit to having deliberately shortened a person's life.

I would like to die suddenly and asleep, as free of tubes and machines and drugs as possible.

I hope there will be somebody close to me who knows how I feel and will see to it that I don't go beyond that point. Call it euthanasia or whatever you want, I don't want to live beyond what I consider living.

If asked, most of us would elect to die peacefully in our sleep. Some doctors are willing to take the responsibility to insure this. The decision is based on the extent of the illness and suffering, their personal knowledge of the patient and the family, and often some expression of hope on the part of the family that the suffering will soon end. Doctors may visualize themselves or their own close relatives as being similarly ill as a criterion for determining what is enough suffering. The usual way is through gradually increasing doses of narcotic drugs over a period of a day or two. Pain is relieved, anxiety disappears, and continuous sleep is insured. Most of these drugs depress respiration and eventually breathing stops.

There is no legal basis for euthanasia and there is unlikely to be one in the near future. Accepted medical practice lags far behind the desires and needs of some people and legal sanction lags at least as far behind medical practice. Euthanasia should be discussed much more openly by cancer patients with their families and their doctors. If wishes were more openly expressed they would be met with less hesitation and guilt.

WHERE TO DIE

Choices of where to die include hospital, home, and hospice. The decision is often arrived at through experience, based on where you have been most comfortable and received most of your care. It obviously involves not only your own wishes but also the wishes and capabilities of your family. This in turn frequently hinges on the availability of outside help.

Advantages of Being in the Hospital

The hospital is the gathering place of experienced medical people who understand your illness and know what to expect at any time, where specialized help and equipment are available if needed. This is why many people feel more secure in the hospital and are able to relax and let other people take over. While younger children usually prefer to be at home, older children and adults often feel safer in the hospital where there are people around who can take care of things.

Being in the hospital is certainly less disruptive and tiring for the family than caring for a person at home, particularly if there are small children in the home to add to the burden. This must be tempered by the distance the family must travel and the amount of time they want to spend visiting in the hospital.

Visitors in the hospital, whether they are family or friends, can devote all their time and energy to providing support without having to *do* anything. With little responsibilities for providing care, parents visiting a child can say, "You do the little things; I want to spend my time loving her."

Some people protect their families from the unpleasant aspects of the illness in the hospital. Teenage children often have very adult concerns for their parents in this respect.

In the hospital you can select who may visit you and when much more easily than at home. Your privacy can be insured, if that is what you want. Finally, families who are fearful that they cannot cope with a medical crisis or with death realize that in the hospital they will have support themselves if they want it.

Disadvantages of Being in the Hospital

Being in the hospital removes you from familiar surroundings and limits your contact with your family and friends. Indeed, obsolete hospital rules may not allow you to have visits from young children or grandchildren. Moreover, many people are very afraid of the hospital even when they are just visiting. Children in particular are often intimidated by the hospital to the point of being speechless. They then go away sad because they could not say anything.

In spite of efforts to change, most hospitals are still colder and less friendly than good homes. While there are many familiar faces, there are also many strange ones. The very fact that a great deal of everyday care is done *for* you cannot help but make you feel that you have little control over what is done *to* you. Regardless of how it is paid for, hospitalization is very expensive.

Advantages of Being at Home

Many people *really* want to be at home and many families *really* want to take care of them. Home is where you live. The surroundings are warm and friendly and they are yours. You have access to the entire family and as many friends as you wish to see, any time. Children can come in and out of the room and there are no strange faces. Life is less confusing and it is easier to relax and communicate, particularly with children. The threat of being abandoned is greatly reduced because people are not saying goodbye and leaving at the end of each day. At home you have some control over what happens to you, even down to small details. You can have your favorite food when you want it.

Caring for someone who is ill can bring the family together, and the feeling of satisfaction and accomplishment can last a lifetime. The intense involvement required of home-care decreases self-criticism and feelings of guilt after death. Finally, home-care is much less expensive per day than care in the hospital.

Most families do not have previous experience caring for someone who is seriously ill. They do not know what to expect and may not understand exactly what is going on. As a result the patient feels less secure, realizing that his family may not be able to deal with everything. Many families feel that they will be unable to cope with a long illness or with the moment of death. While a certain amount of equipment or expertise can be provided at home, it obviously cannot compare with that available in a hospital.

Caring for someone at home can be very disruptive for a family, much more so than visiting in the hospital. Moreover, even with plenty of help, it can be exhausting. Small families may realize that they need outside help but may not know how to find it or may be unwilling to ask for it.

Between home and hospital is a new concept: the hospice. Initiated in England as a special facility for dying patients and their families, the hospice is now finding its counterpart here. The first model in the United States was developed in New Haven, Connecticut as a well supported home-care program, now housed in its own building. Similar programs and units are being developed through the country. They are designed to maintain the patient-family unit, but in a facility that offers more medical support than can usually be provided at home.

Whether at home or in a special facility, the hospice concept pays particular attention to control of pain, interfamily relationships, avoiding isolation and loneliness and to the needs of the family after death. Medical and nursing help are available on a 24-hour basis and are augmented by a team that includes clergy, social service, psychology, physical therapy, and family volunteers. The hospice experience will undoubtedly have a profound effect on medical attitudes towards dying patients and their families and even on our outdated public attitudes towards death.

A dying man needs to die as a sleepy man needs to sleep, and there comes a time when it is wrong as well as useless to resist. (Stewart Alsop)

Disadvantages of Being at Home

Hospice

THE END OF LIFE

The remainder of this chapter is written primarily for the family of a person dying of cancer. It is unfortunate that our society and its medical practices exclude most of us from seeing life's two most dramatic events, birth and death. Although few think of it as such, it is a privilege to be with someone who is dying. In caring for a loved one who has cancer you may have an opportunity to be present at the time of death, whether it is in the hospital or at home. The following paragraphs are intended to remove some of the mystery that surrounds the end of life by looking at the process of dying.

Consciousness. Some people are unconscious for hours or even days before death while others may be clear and alert up to the last few moments. Usually there is a gradual development of confusion and semi-consciousness over a few minutes or hours. Any pain that was experienced before usually declines. Pain is one of the first senses to decline in death, and if the person shows no signs of being in pain, it is safe to assume that he is having none. When pain has been a problem, a look of relaxation and relief may indicate that it is past. Speech may become quiet and difficult to understand and the thoughts expressed may be quite unrelated to the events or people present. Often, the semiconscious person can still hear although he is unable to respond. Your own words of endearment and support may still be understood and appreciated. Touching, caressing, holding or rocking, are all appropriate.

Fluids. Ice chips, water, or juice may be given as requested but should be stopped if there is difficulty swallowing. Since the purpose is comfort and nourishment is no longer necessary, milk and solid foods should be avoided. If the person is too weak to drink from a cup or a straw, a teaspoon may be used. Care of the mouth is important, vaseline or some other lubricant applied to the lips will prevent drying. Secretions from the mouth can be removed with the tip of a handkerchief or paper towel or by turning the person to his side.

Temperature. As the circulation of blood begins to decline the hands and feet are the first to be affected. They become cool and darker or paler than normal. Later the same changes are seen in the face. Although the skin is cold, and either dry or damp, the dying person is usually not conscious of feeling cold, and light coverings are enough.

Breathing. Breathing is usually easier with the person on his back or slightly to one side with a pillow under his head, but any position which makes breathing easier is acceptable, including sitting up with good support. A small child may find relief by being held in your arms. Whatever position is best, it should be relaxed and comfortable. Oxygen is of little value. Occasionally breathing assumes a peculiar pattern, alternating gradually between rapid and slow. Our breathing is controlled by the amount of oxygen and carbon dioxide in the body. When these two controls give conflicting signals and fail to coordinate with each other this type of respiration results. It has no particular significance and requires no treatment.

Rattling or gurgling with each breath is from secretions in the back of the throat. These are distressing to listen to but cause no discomfort.

Involuntary Movements. Occasionally involuntary or reflex movements may take place. These are rare but may involve any muscles, particularly an arm, leg, or muscles of the face. In addition, there may be a loss of control of the bladder or the bowels as these muscles relax.

When breathing and the heartbeat has stopped, the eyes become fixed in position and the pupils dilate. After death, there is no rush to do anything and you may sit with your loved one as long as you want, whether it is in the hospital or at home. Many families find this an important time to pray or talk together, and reconfirm their own love for each other as well as for the person who has passed away.

AFTER DEATH

If death takes place in the hospital a doctor will be notified and he will make a brief examination. After that, the nursing staff will know what needs to be done and will be able to help you in many ways. Telephone calls to your doctor and to the mortuary can all be done for you.

At home the responsibility is yours and someone in the family should find out *in advance* what must be done. Regulations concerning proper notifications and removal of the body differ from one community to another and your doctor or nurse can get this information for you.

When death takes place at home, after a long illness involving a doctor's care, it is almost never necessary to have the coroner or police come to the home. Your doctor can usually bypass this by notifying the medical examiner or coroner in advance that the death of a person under his care is expected to take place at home.

If your doctor or nurse is not present, one of them should be notified at the time of death. The medical examiner should be notified by a family member or the doctor and will require the following information: place of death, date, time, who was in the presence of the person who died, the next of kin, relationship, the doctor's name and phone number and probable cause of death.

The mortician should then be notified and arrangements made for removal of the body at a time convenient for you. Some families make initial arrangements with the mortician several days in advance, when there is less stress, while others put this off until after death, feeling they are not giving up hope sooner than necessary.

If the person who dies is a child, the mortician may be asked to come with a car rather than a hearse or you may prefer to transport the body to the funeral home yourself.

Autopsy Permission.   Your doctor may wish to have permission to examine the body to obtain more medical information about the illness and the cause of death. This was once routine in many hospitals but has become less so in recent years. When death is from a rare tumor or from one that has behaved in an unusual fashion, important information can be obtained that may help your doctor understand what took place and be better able to deal with it in other patients. Permission for an autopsy is usually requested by your own doctor and he can explain why he wishes to have it. Many doctors and families find it easier to bring up their questions and discuss concerns about an autopsy before death takes place, when the reasons may be more easily understood. The actual permission can usually only be given by the next of kin. If the patient requested or made known his desire to have an autopsy, or not to have one, that request is always honored. Similarly, if one member of the family is openly and unalterably opposed, most physicians comply rather than cause unnecessary distress within the family. Some families request an autopsy in the interest of science or to complete their own understanding of the illness and death. An autopsy leaves no disfigurement that can be detected on the clothed body.

The Funeral.   Funerals and mourning rites range from the Irish Wake and full-scale service with viewing of the body, to informal memorial gatherings days or weeks after burial. They all serve the same purpose, to acknowledge the death and to permit a public expression of grief. Unfortunately, even then many feel they must be under control. Funerals also require practical decisions and preparations which help family members regain contact with the realities of life. These include the decision for burial or cremation, selection of a mortuary, finding a gravesite, funeral arrangements, planning a memorial service, providing obituary information to the newspaper, finding military discharge papers required for burial in a national cemetery, and deciding whether or not to receive friends in your home after the service.

One of the most distressing tasks is the selection of a casket. A room full of satin-lined boxes is a sobering sight at any time but can be intensely painful for family members. In addition, in their acute distress, feelings of guilt, fear of public criticism, and an attitude that "the best is not too good," may inadvertently cause families to spend far more than they can comfortably afford. Ideally, this choice should be made long before death takes place, at a time when it can be done objectively with a completely clear head. At the very least, the next of kin who is making the decision should be accompanied by someone else in the family or a trusted friend who has experience with funerals and who will encourage caution and reason.

Many of the costs of the funeral are tied to the casket as a "package." These include embalming of the body which is done routinely without asking permission. In fact embalming is rarely necessary or required by law. Moreover, when the body is to be cremated, embalming is completely unnecessary and the cost of a casket can be reduced to a minimum. Immediate cremation can be obtained for about $300, while the average funeral with burial may range from $2,000 to $3,000. More grandiose funerals can go far above these figures.

Many of these decisions can be made in advance. Indeed, some people make their own arrangements to help their families by expressing their wishes, leaving instructions concerning disposal of their bodies after death.

The best time to get a cemetery lot is on a good sunny day when you are fine.

Memorial societies provide another way to avoid unnecessary funeral expenses. There are many in the United States and Canada and they help families prearrange simple and economical funerals. "A Manual of Death Education and Simple Burial" by Ernest Morgan (Celo Press, Burnsville, NC 28714) contains much useful information and the names and addresses of all of the memorial societies in the United States and Canada.

I said goodnight and thanked him again for what he had given us and went home to cook dinner for the children, just like every other night. He died after I left the hospital. At the end I walked out of the hospital alone. It was not just the end of two months of being in the hospital, it was the end of years of living together. I realized that I was on my own and had to face life alone.

GRIEF AND MOURNING

When someone close to you dies a vacancy exists in your life. You are acutely aware of the emptiness, but it does not remain empty long. All kinds of thoughts and feelings fill the void. Some are wanted, many are not. Feelings of loneliness, despair, embarrassment, anger, guilt, and resentment conflict with each other as they battle for your attention. They confuse you and exhaust you until you wish to escape from your sorrow but find that you cannot. Eventually you must confront each of these thoughts and feelings. You must sort them out and put each where it belongs. If you do this well, the emptiness gradually disappears, filled partly with old memories and disarmed grievances and partly with new people and fresh experiences. Eventually all that remains is a small hollow that has been incorporated into the new contours of your life.

This is grief. It is hard, painful, and time-consuming work. No two people grieve in exactly the same way because no two people are grieving for exactly the same thing. The child who loses his father misses someone quite different from the wife who loses her husband. You bring into your grief your own personality, your previous experiences with death, and your relationship to the person who died. Grief is intensely personal and no one should be denied the right to grieve in his own way and at his own rate.

The Elements of Grief.   In spite of its many variations, there is a pattern to grief. Several stages can be recognized, each with its own expressions and needs. These include shock and disorganization, anger, guilt, loss and loneliness, relief, and re-establishment. They are similar to the stages experienced by the person who died. Again, they are not necessarily encountered in any precise order and any one stage may be repeated or overlap with others at various times. The entire spectrum can usually be recognized if you are confronted by sudden unexpected death. In death from cancer, often after a prolonged illness, the same stages are usually experienced but some are harder to recognize because they are spread out over a longer period of time. The process of grieving may begin with the diagnosis of cancer, or at the time of recurrence, or when the disease gradually fails to respond to treatment. These are often the times for shock, disorganization, and denial. Anger and resentment may be revived briefly at the time of death but it is not unusual for them to be "used up" long before. Outsiders often do not understand this and expect more tears when there are none left.

Preparatory Grief.   In cancer, grief often begins long before death. It usually begins when you know that death is coming and often much earlier, when death is only a possibility. This mourning in anticipation is a normal reaction that protects you from the final trauma of death by spreading it over as long as possible. In periods of preparatory grief you may feel quiet, weepy, or sad. You may want to be alone or you may be restless and want to talk to other people. It is sometimes accompanied by loss of appetite and difficulty sleeping. Understanding this process is important because it also causes feelings of guilt, as when you catch yourself thinking of the other person as dying or dead when in fact he or she may be doing very well. Inside you are saying, "I am sad because I know you are dying and I know I will miss you so much that I am already beginning to miss you now". Preparatory grief cannot and should not be avoided, nor should it cause you unnecessary guilt. It will not interfere with your ability to provide love and care.

Anger. Death is an outrage and more than enough reason to be angry. You need someone to blame: God, the illness, your doctors, your hospital, other members of your family, and unfortunately, even the person who died. After all, you have been rejected and abandoned. Following the death of a parent, children often feel that they have been deliberately deserted. If you look at it closely you will probably realize that your anger goes back beyond death. Relationships within a family are complex and lives together are never all love and smooth sailing as we like to think.

Most human relationships are tempered by storms of disappointment, arguments, and even hatred, all of which come to the surface at the same time in death. Your feelings are confused and distressing. They are also perfectly normal. Unkind thoughts do not make you a bad person, uncomfortable and disloyal as they may be. They are the ghosts of darkness in your life that should be thought about and talked about until they disappear in the light of day.

Relief. Feelings of relief can come on strongly and immediately after a loved one's death from cancer. These feelings are frequently expressed as relief that a person's suffering is over. In reality this also means that your own suffering is over. With prolonged illness you may have wished that the person would die. Now that he is dead, however, your sadness is tainted with relief that borders on happiness. Death also frees you of many demands, some of which go back to your original relationship with the person, long before illness intruded: a parent who held you too close and could not let you go, the constraints of marriage, a life-style that you felt tied into. Gradually you realize that *now* you can do things differently, that you can start again and even try to have a better life for yourself. Your secret hopes begin to come up, but often too soon for comfort.

Feelings of relief can cause enormous guilt if not recognized as a normal reaction to almost intolerable stress. How can you possibly be relieved that someone has just died? It helps to express these feelings to someone who will not be judgmental. This is often *not* a close family member who may have identical thoughts but cannot bear to hear them expressed aloud.

Guilt. Preparatory grief, anger, and relief have in common their ability to bring on intense guilt. There are other causes of guilt too. If each of us could relive our lives with those close to us, there are *always* things that we might do differently. Now we are sorry that we cannot have another chance. You *could* have chosen another doctor or a different treatment, bickered and argued less, been less strict with a child or kinder to your parents.

Probably none of these would have made any difference—but they are all sources of guilt. They are the "instant replays" of our imaginary life which should be viewed briefly and then set aside forever. Fortunately, most of these sources of guilt can be talked out. Eventually, you realize that changing things would have made little or no difference.

There are steps that can be taken to lessen or avoid guilt. Open communication with your loved one before death and with family and friends after death are the best. At various times during the illness you may ask yourself what you owe your husband or wife, yourself, or your children. Usually what is best for one is best for all. If a compromise is necessary, the reasons for it may be clear. You may also ask yourself if you have done the best that you can personally, whether you obtained the best medical treatment and support services available. Care of a person with cancer requires making many decisions, some of which are difficult and painful. Each problem should be examined by itself, looking at all the possibilities and alternatives so that you are satisfied that the choice that you make is the correct one at the time. Sharing the decisions with other responsible members of the family and your doctors also helps to insure that the best choice is made.

Loneliness.   Your personal loss can be the most painful part of mourning. It builds up gradually, spurred on by constant daily reminders: a pipe on the table, letters addressed to your loved one, photos, the empty crib, or the clothes in the closet. Even the companionship of teasing and fighting are missed.

Loneliness is expressed as sadness and depression. You attempt to recall what you can of the other person, to remind yourself in many ways how good he was. In a way, loneliness feeds itself until finally it is exhausted. As painful as it is, you leave reminders such as the pipe, the pictures, and the clothes in place because they help you to remember. In this stage of grief, you turn to people who knew you both because you want to talk and remember. Understanding friends and family members are indispensible at this time. Eventually loneliness begins to abate and the memory which was larger than life resumes a human size as you enter the recovery phase of mourning.

THE DANGERS OF UNFINISHED GRIEF

Before going on it is important to examine what is accomplished in these early stages of grief. Before you can build a new life for yourself with a new relationships that are solid and safe, you must dismantle the old one piece by piece. The early phases of grief do exactly this and they should not be slighted or suppressed.

Unfinished grief mars the lives of countless numbers of people. It can frequently be avoided by understanding the reasons for grief and actively indulging in mourning. Once established, however, it may have far reaching consequences and often requires professional help. Failure to complete the grieving process can block normal emotional growth and cause unhappiness. Failure to recognize real needs have led couples to conceive or adopt a child who could not possibly fill the place of one who recently died. Others enter marriage too soon in an attempt to replace an irreplaceable spouse. There is danger in filling these voids too quickly rather than letting them fill in their own time, in being afraid of the painful hours and days that are required to truly bury the dead.

Anger should be dissipated before it becomes too consuming. This is particularly true of anger directed at the person who died, anger for leaving you, for causing you so much pain and distress, for dying without your permission. It extends to resentment for taking so much of your time, for having an illness that drained the family's financial resources, for depriving you of the possibility of a college education. Such anger is primitive and selfish. It is also real and tenacious and normal. If you really are angry you should take the time to express it and dwell on it until you are tired of it and it is gone.

The need to put on a brave front may actually be fear of expressing grief. Refusing to mourn by going back to life as usual, dry-eyed and straight-backed is not normal behavior. In adults, this frequently is the response to unresolved grief from the past. You were hurt before and you will not be hurt again, even by death. The danger of shutting something as shattering as death out of your life is that the same barrier may also shut out life as well. Such a barrier may wall off your inner self from all but superficial relationships with others, rendering you incapable of love. If you cannot bring yourself to feel real loss, you may also find that you cannot feel real love.

Prolonged grief can prevent you from resuming former relationships and establishing important new ones. Such longing for a lost relationship that cannot be regained may reflect concern that you yourself failed in some way. Fear that you did not contribute all you could to the original relationship during life may cause you to try to improve upon that relationship after death. The continued mourning of a young person for their lost spouse years after death may represent fear of facing life with a new partner, because of real or imagined inadequacies in the original marriage.

It wasn't for quite some time that I felt the full impact of his loss. Then I was depressed for a long time. The single one thing that helped me during a bad time was a Bach festival. Bach's music seems to me to have a beginning, a middle and an end. It is in harmony with nature and the mood in it made me see the rightness of death too.

RECOVERY

We are now ready to look at the final stage of mourning: recovery. This stage begins by picking up the pieces of your life, establishing your old routines, and making whatever daily decisions are required. The shadows of loneliness diminish as you accept other people into your world and step into the sunshine of life around you. In addition to re-establishing ties with your old friends, you begin to start a new life, with new friends and new experiences.

Up to this point you have glorified and magnified the person who died and even tried to see things through his eyes, making decisions and doing things as he would have done them or would have wanted them done. Now you begin to do things your own way. In this process you sort out the values of your old life that you wish to keep but gradually reassert your own values and let them guide you to full resumption of life. Finally, you must accept the fact that your life will never again be the same. There is no point in trying to hold it back or to regain what was lost. It will be a different life, with new challenges, new goals, new hopes, and new rewards. It will include new interests and, most of all, new people.

Communication.   One of the most basic properties of human grief is our need to share it. This starts with family and very close friends, often before death. It allows you to express anger and fear and guilt and helps relieve feelings of isolation and depression. In grief there is no level of feeling or subject of concern that cannot be shared with the right people. The closeness that families acquire at this time and remember for the rest of their lives comes from exactly this sharing. Gradually the need to communicate extends beyond family to friends.

When I would mention my wife at the board of the church they would all quiet down and change the subject. Some members of the board were doctors and one of them was the quickest to turn me off. Finally I said, "I want to talk about her: I need to talk about her: let me talk about her. She still lives with me". That changed everything.

Friends.   What can friends do for a family that has just experienced a death? So little and so much. You cannot really assume their loss for them even if you are very close to the person who died or have been through a similar experience yourself. On the other hand, at a time when it is really needed, a little warmth and understanding goes a very long way.

Most of us do not want to get too close to a dying person or a family in mourning because it reminds us that we too will eventually die. We would even like to run away and avoid the entire situation. These are uncomfortable feelings but they are normal and we can learn to understand and live with them. It is all right to feel uneasy about death and even to say so openly. Everyone feels the same way whether they admit it or not.

Soon after death the family often wants to talk about the illness and the circumstances of death itself. They may repeat themselves time and again until finally they have exhausted their own tolerance for the morbid details. After that they begin to think back to the good times that they had together, listing the many qualities of the person who died. Your job is much simpler than you think it is. You have only to be available and willing to listen. Your willingness to listen allows them to work on their grief in the best way possible.

Support And Counseling. Outside support and counseling are often helpful and occasionally required. Informal groups of families sharing the same experience can go far in supporting each other. The desire of many people to remain active in these groups is good evidence of the support that they received. In addition, as these families complete their mourning process they can work with other families and show them that recovery will come with time. Some communities have organizations of trained volunteers who have been through grief and mourning who serve this function. An excellent example is the Shanti Project in San Francisco. Nurses who care for terminal patients will often maintain a supportive relationship with the family until they are clearly on their feet again. Unfortunately most doctors do not provide much support for the families of their patients after death. Even notes of condolences are rare. Perhaps this will change if the medical profession begins to take a different view of its responsibility to the dying patient.

Mom asked me "Who do you think is out in the kitchen?" I said, "Linda." It was a priest and I knew what had happened. I ate breakfast while he told me that Linda had died but that I shouldn't worry because she had gone to heaven, that she was happier there and wouldn't have to go to the hospital anymore. I said, "I know. Now leave me alone. Let me eat my cereal and be by myself ". Lisa was seven. She decided she was going to be Linda. She sat in the rocker where Linda sat a lot and rocked back and forth saying that she would be Linda, but she wasn't going to learn how to sew. Judy was only five. She was hiding behind a door and kept going back there.

HOW CHILDREN SEE DEATH

Children are full-fledged members of the family and you have an obligation to help them understand death and mourning rather than excluding them from it. To do so you should understand how children see death. Your child's attitude is colored largely by his age and previous experience and what he sees to be your own attitude. Preschool children are used to being left behind, but only on the condition that the person who leaves will come back. In everyday life they always do. Since this has been the previous experience, the child of this age has no basis for thinking that death is any different. The person who died is gone for a while but *will* come back. This is an age where death carries little or no fear and that the questions that are asked are spontaneous, naive, and innocent.

In the early school years, from six to nine, the child looks upon death as an outside force that takes you away. It is often a mysterious, bad person who kills, a black angel, a Nazi, someone from outer space, or a frightening animal. Furthermore, in our television age, death is often looked upon as violent. Children of this age are definitely fearful of death and are often reluctant to talk about it. It may even mean "being put to sleep, like Tinker". They also gradually understand that separation by death is permanent. The child over the age of nine or ten understands that death eventually comes to everyone but pictures it as being far off and usually associates it with old age.

Regardless of age, the child will feel as much final loss as anyone else and should be allowed to share in the entire experience. Children need to know a lot about what is going on and this requires openness in answering their questions. It is better to explain too much than too little since the child will filter out what he can understand. Most important, the child needs freedom and security to express his own fears and feelings to other members of the family without meeting a barrier of denial or refusal to listen. The attitudes that children develop in their first experiences with death are apt to be those they carry throughout life. Explaining death to a child is never easy but the following points may help.

Explain what really happened at the time of illness and death, stressing that everything possible was done but sometimes death cannot be prevented. Some factual knowledge about the disease helps. "A brain tumor grows and causes pressure inside the head." "Leukemia replaces the bone marrow so that it does not make enough normal blood cells."

Avoid indirect or religious concepts that attempt to make death more beautiful. "She was taken to heaven by one of God's angels", may cause a child to fear heaven, God, and the angel, none of which was intended. If "Mother is happy in heaven now", the child who is thoroughly unhappy here may actually want to join her. At the very least he may resent the fact that she is happy anywhere when he is so unhappy.

Assure the child that whatever happened to the person who died will not happen to him. This is particularly true when another child, either a brother or sister or close friend, has died.

The child does not want to be abandoned any more than he

already has been. You should reassure him that you are there and well and that you will take care of him.

Children are constantly being told not to do this and not to do that. It is inevitable that they will resent this and wish that you would go away, perhaps even die, and leave them alone. When death actually takes place it is a small step for the young child to assume that indeed he did cause the death. Reassurance that nothing that the child did or said or thought had anything to do with the death is critical if you are to avoid unnecessary guilt which can be very difficult to remove later.

The child will want to know that the body will be buried or cremated, the location of the grave, or what will be done with the ashes. He should understand that the body feels no pain but that it cannot return, that the soul has left the body and is now with you in your memories or with God in heaven, or both.

The child should be told what the funeral will be like and offered the opportunity to go. However, he should not be forced, nor made to feel that by not going he is avoiding a responsibility. If the child wishes to stay home, you should be sure that he has good companionship with someone he knows and loves and he should be included in any gathering after the funeral.

It makes the child feel closer and wanted if he is included in your mourning. There is no way that you can hide your grief from your child. Saying that nothing is wrong when you have tears in your eyes will only be confusing. Children may feel protective towards their grieving parents, making them reluctant to reveal their own sadness and loneliness. Sharing grief means being sad together.

The child should be allowed to handle grief in his own way and you should not impose your behavior on him. Do not be surprised at erratic behavior that vacillates between sorrow and playfulness. Playing is a child's release from stress. Deep inside you may wish that you could do the same. The child who is self-contained and quiet and withdrawn after death is the one who needs attention.

Adults often feel that children have inappropriate reactions to death. The reason is that most normal children, particularly in the younger ages, are unable to tolerate grief for very long. Unlike their elders who grieve continuously for weeks, the child is apt to be sad and quiet for a few minutes and then go off to play with his friends, then sad and quiet again, only to want to watch television a little later. They find it too painful to stay sad for very long periods, and are easily distracted by their own interests and the need to pursue their own lives.

Returning to school can be a frightening experience for a child. His loss makes him feel like an outcast among his own friends. Taking the child to school and talking to his friends is one of the best ways of avoiding this.

I took each of the children to school the next day and discussed with their classes what death meant to us. In the eighth grade I was bombarded with all kinds of questions and spent an hour and a half discussing the symptoms, what the loss of my husband means, and what the children and I will do now. It was very matter-of-fact and very helpful.

THE MEANING OF DEATH

To the extent that we can accept death as an important part of life and free ourselves of unreasonable fear, we are able to accept the responsibility to live our own lives now. If we are to be unique and true to ourselves, we must do so during our lives because there is no way to come back. Death allows us to live more bravely, to do what we want to do and to be what we want to be *now*.

As survivors, we have a brief moment to carry on and extend the life that is gone before we too will be gone. From the tears of our sorrow we gain strength. In our anger and guilt we see ourselves, often for the first time. In our loneliness we seek others. Eventually we rise above grief and integrate our memories and heritage into more purposeful and constructive lives.

eight

When a Child Has Cancer

Having a child with cancer is one of the heaviest burdens parents can ever be asked to carry. Marriages can be strengthened or destroyed by this experience. The shock of diagnosis, severity of treatment, altered responsibilities of mother and father, frustration of remission and relapse, and the ever-present threat of loss of a child extended over months and years, require all the strength parents can muster.

WHY MY CHILD?

Parents must learn to accept this entire range of strong feelings. They often reject the diagnosis of cancer until it has been confirmed by several physicians. Anger may be directed at the physicians who make the diagnosis or provide the treatment, the nurses who care for the child in the hospital, or the hospital itself. Cursing God, fate, or life in general is almost necessary. It is a rare mother who does not at some time ask herself what she may have done that caused the illness. Diet, environment, failure to recognize symptoms early, even punishment for imagined sins have all been blamed. In fact, there is nothing that parents do that causes cancer and there is nothing that they can do to prevent it. There is no answer to the most reasonable of questions, "Why my child?"

Parents frequently wonder how much their child understands about his disease. Although this is closely related to age, the answer is usually "More than you think".

THE YOUNG CHILD

Children under five have no concept of serious illness or threat to life. They fear being alone and separation from their parents more then anything else. They quickly learn to fear doctors, nurses, and technicians, and they protest against all medical procedures with screaming and temper tantrums. They cling to their parents and demand that they be with them constantly in the hospital or clinic. At the same time, they shy away from any new people who enter their lives, particularly medical personnel.

The child who is over five or six almost invariably senses that his illness is serious. He realizes that something is very wrong when he has to go to the hospital or clinic frequently, takes medicine all the time, may be restricted in his activities, and is the subject of constant concern and attention. In the hospital he sees other children with similar illness, many of whom are older and know what they have. He hears doctors and nurses discussing his disease matter-of-factly and the exact diagnosis usually surfaces.

Between the ages of five and ten the child can better tolerate separation from parents because he knows they will come back. His major fear now is of pain and injury. He knows what hurts. On the other hand, the age of reason also begins. The more the young child understands his disease, and particularly the need for unpleasant medical procedures, the better he is able to deal with them. All treatments and procedures should be explained in advance. This is a difficult age, when information must be fed to the child as it is needed in order to accomplish the immediate goals of diagnosis and treatment. The best people to provide this information are the parents.

THE SPECIAL PROBLEMS OF TEENAGERS

Adolescents and teenagers understand serious illness and fear the possibility of death. Their need for constant association with their parents is usually gone and fear of pain and injury are replaced by hope, if the promises of long-term benefits are adequate. The goals of maturation are interrupted just when the teenager is trying to establish an identity of his own and beginning to realize the promise that life holds. A year or more of school may be lost. Getting a driver's license may be delayed, independence is limited, planning for the future is discouraging, relationships with the opposite sex seem more difficult to initiate. While some may rage over this, many are very stoic about their illness but burden themselves with enormous guilt over what they are doing to their families. They are sensitive about the fact that they have interrupted the plans of the family or that they are backing out of an area of assumed responsibility. They feel that the father who was formerly an alcoholic may become so again, that things that the family needs will not be bought because of their medical bills. Older children may feel particularly guilty for not fulfilling the hopes their parents have for them and that they have for themselves.

Many teenagers make plans that they wish to see fulfilled and adhere to them doggedly. One thirteen-year-old boy insisted on leaving the hospital in October to buy Christmas presents for his family when he knew that he could not possibly make it until Christmas. It was a piece of business that had to be taken care of. Three teenage boys who became friends in the hospital discussed plans about building a kayak when they got out. Only one survived to do this with the help of his grandfather. It was a promise that had to be fulfilled.

Physical appearance is important to all children over the age of six but particularly to the teenager. Lumps, scars, and physical disability are all deviations from normal that are hard to accept. Most common, however, is hair loss from chemotherapy or radiation. Every child who is to receive such treatment should be told about this possibility. A variety of wigs are available although they are not completely satisfactory. This should be discussed and, if desired, purchased *before* treatment begins so that it matches the normal hair as much as possible. Even if the child decides not to use the wig, the fact that it is available, perhaps for special occasions, makes it a source of comfort.

The only thing worse than *not* telling a child that his hair will fall out as a result of receiving chemotherapy is to deliberately lie. Similarly, it is better to tell children when something is going to hurt. It does not hurt any less, but truth generates respect and confidence. Most doctors and nurses who deal with children with cancer have developed very open attitudes about the disease, finding that this is the best way to build confidence and cooperation. Everything is explained completely, so that the child is well prepared for whatever must be done.

SUPPORT FOR THE CHILD

Dealing honestly with a child requires answering all questions to the best of your ability. Direct explanations are best. "You are going to receive a transfusion to help make the bleeding stop." "We are trying a new drug because we want to do everything we can to help you." The more you know and understand about the illness and its treatment the easier it will be to translate these things into words she can understand.

Painful questions may be asked with disarming openness. These range from "Why do I have to go to the hospital?" or, "Will it hurt?" to "Do I have leukemia?" or "Am I going to die?". Failure to accept this responsibility may undermine your child's relationship with you at a time when she needs you most. Questions have always been answered, and when the usual sources of information become silent or evasive, the intelligent child can only be worried that terrible things are being hidden. Imagination can make illness and treatment even worse than they are. You should ask your doctor for a list of questions that your child can be expected to ask and what he thinks are appropriate answers.

Adolescent and teenage children need adult support. It is no longer a question of just explaining the treatment but also willingness to listen and share concerns. The intensity and duration of treatment can wear down the adolescent if she does not have adequate support. She may consider her situation hopeless, seeing the treatment as worse than the disease. The teenage child does not have a backlog of achievements on which to rebuild morale and occasionally must be reminded that others care about her and that she is indeed of value to her family. Sympathy, optimism, and respect for bravery are good places to start. Acknowledgement of common fears of relapse, continued illness, and even death, can build relationships of incredible beauty and strength.

As children grow old enough to assume more responsibility for themselves, doctors usually begin to deal directly with the children as young adults. This is not to bypass the parents but to help build the child's confidence in her doctors and nurses, relieving the parents of the difficult position of being a go-between. Ideally, this is a joint effort that includes the patients, parents, and doctors, but some teenagers insist on seeing the doctor alone. This is a sign of normal growth and development and should be respected. The parents, of course, are entitled to the same information and should get it separately.

A few teenagers refuse to communicate about their illness and parents should be sensitive to any withdrawal on the child's part and encourage her to share her thoughts and fears. This may be an attempt to spare the parents unnecessary pain. By deliberately not letting them know how much she understands, the child tries to protect them.

Others exert the adult privilege of denial. They may grudgingly acknowledge their disease by name but then shut off any conversation about it, regardless of how much the parents desire more open exchange. There is little that you, as parents, can do except be receptive and available should the situation change.

Different Responsibilities. The greatest responsibility usually falls on the mother. She is in constant attendance and eventually becomes expert in child care. More than anyone else she influences the atmosphere both at home and in the hospital, and the responses of others to the illness usually reflect her response. The father has a less direct but very important role. Life cannot be allowed to stop. In addition to providing support for his wife, the father must undertake more responsibility for running the household and managing the other children while carrying on with his own work.

These different demands on husband and wife can easily cause them to drift apart. As time goes by, the mother may resent the burden of child care that is hers, and the father may feel left out. Compromise is obvious but often difficult: the father should spend more time alone with the sick child and the mother more time with her family. This greater sharing of responsibilities has several important effects. At the same time that it makes the father more sympathetic and understanding of the daily stress on his wife, it also gives her relief and time off. While it helps the father maintain closer contact with his sick child, it also reminds the other children that Mom loves them, too.

Caring for a child with cancer is a long-term project and parents should try to conserve their energy. Major changes should be considered very carefully. If marital separation is inevitable it will probably progress. However, if it appears to be a solution to problems caused *by* the illness, it may not be a good one. The divorced parent who is coping well with the illness may only add unnecessary burdens by remarrying. Moving or changing jobs are upsetting and may add unnecessary stress. Becoming pregnant is occasionally suggested as a way to prepare for the loss of a child, but a child cannot be so easily replaced.

Both Parents Together

We have a very good marriage but Susan's illness just about destroyed us. We were used to leaning on each other. In the past when one was down, the other was up, and we could always help each other. This time we were both down, and down, and more down. It never seemed to end. Sometimes we couldn't even talk to each other without getting upset or angry.

Parents who can support each other and work together with their child against the common enemy of cancer fare better. The keys to dealing with these enormous problems are love, understanding, and communication. This begins between the parents and then is extended to the sick child and her brothers and sisters. Once the parents and family members begin to talk to each other about the things that are really important, most problems become smaller and may seem to solve themselves. If parents know the facts, agree on what must be done, and are able to communicate this effectively, the child will trust their decisions about what is best. To be able to speak with one voice and avoid confusion requires constant discussion between husband and wife on every phase of management.

Parents Need Support Too.
Most parents find they need outside support. The obvious source is other parents with the same problem. The value of this is so great that it is now provided by virtually all hospitals that take care of large numbers of children with cancer. It ranges from informal group meetings arranged by the hospital staff to national organizations with local chapters. Only a

person going through the same ordeal can really understand your concerns.

As close as my husband and I have always been, we just could not talk about Tim when he was in the hospital. We would spend every minute we could by his side but on the way home we never even mentioned his name. When we attended our first meeting with other parents we were amazed to hear the others' feelings regarding our son's illness. Up to then it had been territory too frightening for us to venture into alone. But once the door was open it stayed open and we went on to deal with our own feelings together very well.

At the third meeting I finally opened up and told the group a lot of what I was feeling about my son's illness, things I had never told anybody. After that I felt like 10,000 pounds had been lifted off my shoulders.

In addition to providing much needed understanding, these groups are sources of practical information, ranging from how and what to tell the sick child, and what to expect from chemotherapy, to maintaining discipline at home and dealing with behavior problems in the other children.

Suggestions for Parents

1. Learn all you can about your child's illness.
2. Discuss all aspects of the illness, your feelings about it, the treatment, your doctors, and the hospitals, together. Include the things you agree upon and feel the same about as well as the things about which you disagree. Learn to compromise and finally to agree on all decisions.
3. Be as open with the sick child and other children in the family as their ages permit.
4. Get outside help.
5. Resolve to maintain your family unit no matter what happens. Sacrificing your marriage for a sick child will have no influence on the outcome of the illness.

How Children See Hospitals and Doctors

Treatment of childhood cancer is highly specialized and relatively few hospitals in the United States have the required experience. The best are the children's hospitals in many major cities. The advantage of which compromise her independence. Anger is the normal outlet and it is often directed at the parents. Open rejection, such as "Why entire team of helpers.

The hospital is a very frightening world for the young child. She wants her mother constantly with her and that is exactly where she should be. The older child may resent the fact that she is being manipulated. She is being *taken* or *persuaded* to go to the hospital, both of which compromise her independence. Anger is the normal outlet and it is often directed at the parents. Open rejection, such as "Why did you do this to me?" and "I hate you" are common. Modern hospitals are trying to smooth out this transition by making themselves more attractive to children. Well-equipped playrooms allow children to relax and feel at ease. Trained personnel help children get the most out of their playtime. Bringing one or two prized possessions from home also helps this transition.

The hospital provides a good opportunity to learn about various tests that must be done, particularly those that will be done routinely in the future. If you do not understand the need for a procedure, ask that it be explained again, by someone else if necessary. You do not need to consent to anything that does not have potential benefit for your child. You certainly have no obligation to do anything just to please the doctor. If you are not personally convinced of the value of a procedure you will have a hard time convincing your child.

Writing down information you receive gives you a permanent record, by date, of drugs that are started, blood counts and bone marrow results, clinic visits, changes in treatment in the clinic or at home, and any new symptoms or problems. Furthermore, if you call your doctor when he is out of his office and can remind him of what drugs your child is currently on and what the most recent blood counts were, you will be helping him with information he may not have at his fingertips.

Most adults have a great deal of respect and even affection for their doctors. This is not so of the young child who soon learns to associate the doctor with pain and discomfort. You can be an important bridge here. In addition to helping your child understand what the doctor is saying and doing, you can do a great deal to influence your child's image of the doctor. It is important to explain that you go to the doctor or to the hospital when you are sick and need help, *not* as punishment for being bad, as some children imagine. Stress to your child that the doctor is doing everything she can to help him, and that even though the tests and treatments may be painful, the doctor is very sorry they are and really loves the child. Thanking the doctor in front of your child at the end of each visit sets a good example. You should encourage the child to do the same, but do not force her. Reminding the child that she may feel more appreciative later usually brings about the same result. Regardless of how much fear must be overcome, kind and appreciative parents usually bring up kind and appreciative children.

A parent should be with the child throughout all unpleasant procedures. This provides more reassurance than almost anything else. You cannot suffer for your child but you can suffer with her. The child appreciates this. Even the mother who cries with her child can be very supportive. If for some reason it is not possible to be with your child, as during radiation therapy, she will be reassured to know that you are right outside the door. Finally it is very important to praise the child for her cooperation and bravery when the procedure is over.

TAKING CARE OF YOUR CHILD AT HOME The initial treatment of childhood cancer usually requires from two to six weeks in the hospital. After that, most of the management can be carried out in the clinic or office with the child living at home. Clinic visits often require some waiting so bringing a book or a favorite toy is helpful. The onus can be removed from the day by adding a more cheerful event such as a picnic, lunch at a restaurant, or shopping. When you leave the hospital, your doctors and nurses will give you detailed instructions on treatment that is to be continued at home and any signs that should be reported. However, experienced help is only a telephone call away. Your family physician or pediatrician will be notified that you are coming home and will know what has taken place and what is to be expected. You should also have the office and home telephone numbers of the doctors who cared for your child in the hospital and should not hesitate to call any time if you have questions. As you gain experience you will find that you know the answers to many questions yourself. In the hospital your child was confused and frightened. It is not surprising that she wants to put that memory behind her. Unpleasant memories are best dealt with directly, usually by talking about them. Young children may even deal with them by playing doctor. You will be amazed at how well a young child can understand and accept his illness when he can be the doctor and the patient is a teddybear.

Back to a Normal Life. Today the child with cancer will have many years of life and may be cured. During that time he must mature and grow in a normal fashion. The value of treatment is lost if you cannot have a good time at home. When a child leaves the hospital in remission he usually feels much better than he did a week or two before. He is usually anxious to get home and back to his *normal* life. He should be welcomed back into his *usual* place in the family. The sick child does not want to be considered different. Any favoritism is sure to be resented, eventually by everyone concerned.

Parents often disagree about how to discipline normal children and the problem is much more difficult with a sick child. Most children test their parents soon after they get home. Failure to set limits and stick by them can create a monster out of a perfectly normal child.

Healthy brothers and sisters will soon turn against a sick child who is deluged with presents or given the keys to the kingdom in behavior. For everyone's happiness, you should treat the children equally, and return to the standards that you set before the illness occured.

Protection and Overprotection. The child may be in remission but the parents often are not. Fear of recurrence of the disease or complications from treatment make it easy to be overprotective. It is hard for the child who is just getting over his own fear to deal with parents who are anxious and fearful about every little thing he does. Your doctor will inform you about any restrictions that must be imposed on your child's activities. You should make every effort not to add more of your own. The child in complete remission from leukemia, for instance, usually has almost no restrictions. If he is on maintenance therapy and receiving drugs that may suppress his resistance to infections, exposure to contagious diseases should be avoided. If the white cell count is at a normal level most infections are not a serious threat. Measles and chickenpox are exceptions and contact with other children who have these diseases should be avoided or, if exposure takes place, reported immediately to your doctor. The same precaution should be taken with the child who is on chemotherapy for a solid tumor.

When leukemia is not in remission there is a somewhat greater risk of infection, depending on the severity of the disease. These children should avoid crowds and people with colds. Infections do not reactivate the disease but recurrence of the disease or intensive treatment can reduce resistance to a variety of infections. Vaccinations or any other shots should only be given on the advice of your doctor. If an infection does develop, anticancer drugs are often discontinued for a few days or weeks to allow the normal immune resistance to come back. These brief interruptions will not interfere with the overall success of the treatment.

A low platelet count, due to suppression or replacement of bone marrow, increases the risk of bleeding. In this situation the doctor may recommend that the child's physical activities be restricted to avoid possible injury. There is no such risk or need to restrict activities if the platelet count is adequate.

Children should understand why a low white count means they cannot go to the movies and why a low platelet count means that they cannot play outdoors. Restrictions must have reasons and rewards at the other end.

School. Just as adults have their occupations and professions, so do children: going to school. The child with cancer must miss a certain amount of school because of hospitalizations and clinic visits. However, there is no reason to miss year after year of school and risk growing up to be a social and psychological cripple. When such things do happen, it is usually because the mother is unable to accept the full implications of the illness and feels she is protecting the child by having him with her at all times. The child takes advantage of a good thing, provides a few common complaints such as a headache or stomachache, that any normal child can come up with before breakfast, until the mother gives up. The mother's fear soon makes the child equally fearful of separation and the pattern becomes established. Eventually both may grow tired of it. The child resents her complete dependence on her mother and the mother resents being so tied down. By this time, however, it is very difficult to change.

This situation is much easier to avoid than to remedy. School work should be kept up as much as possible in the hospital and it should be made clear on going home that as soon as strength permits school will be resumed. Home education and other means should not be substituted for class time in the normal school system.

Most schools are very helpful. The school nurse is usually the best person to talk to. It is often helpful for a parent to go to school with a young child and spend a few minutes discussing the illness with the class. Alterations in appearance are more readily accepted if the reason is understood. Older children usually prefer to tell their own friends.

THE LAW AND LEGAL RESPONSI-BILITY

Very complicated questions have arisen over legal responsibility for the sick child. While most parents seek the best treatment available, occasionally a family will refuse treatment on religious or personal grounds. The conflict between parents who wish to avoid unnecessary suffering for their child and for themselves, and the long-term well-being of the child, is a difficult one. Several recent cases have been widely publicized where parents refused to initiate or continue medical care for children when the treatment appears to have had quite a lot to offer. Previously, most children with cancer were doomed, but now they can expect long remissions and some will be cured. In light of this the courts usually assume responsibility for these children and insist on appropriate medical care on the grounds that the parents have no right to impose beliefs on minor children that may jeopardize their health or lives. This usually requires that good medical care can provide *reasonable hope* of helping the child.

LONG TERM EFFECTS OF TREATMENT

Until a few years ago there were so few long term survivors of childhood cancer that the late effects of treatment were of little consequence. Now some long term effects of radiation and chemotherapy are beginning to be seen. Radiation of the skeleton causes problems of growth and development, particularly when it is given to children who are under the age of five or to adolescents in their growth spurt. Sexual development is usually normal after chemotherapy but about 20 percent of girls have problems, particularly if the treatment is given in early adolescence. A few children show personality changes or some impairment of intellect following chemotherapy or radiation of the brain early in life. The risk of starting a genetic disorder that will be seen in a later generation appears to be remote, but there is almost certainly a slightly increased risk of developing another type of tumor later on in life. It will be many years before the extent of these risks will be known. In the meantime all possible steps are being taken to minimize them.

Children view their own deaths very much as they view the deaths of others. With increasing age and awareness, death becomes more frightening and harder to accept.

WHEN A CHILD DIES

The dying child who is old enough almost always finds out. Usually progression of the disease allows him to figure it out for himself. Being in the hospital with other children who die of the same disease carries its own message. Children in school may pass on things heard at home. You should prepare yourself to confirm his suspicions when he asks. As a child begins to comprehend his own death he wants two assurances from his parents, "Tell me that everything will be alright" and later, "Don't leave me alone."

Children are perceptive and sensitive to fear, anxiety, a forced smile, evasion, or outright dishonesty. To a large extent, the child's handling of death depends on how much the parents reveals themselves. The mother who cried outside and goes into the child's room with red eyes forces a distance between them and the child is much more apt to be silent and reserved in her own expressions. Weeping is a demonstration of love, and the mother who cries in front of her child conveys a message that is immediately understood.

Physical intimacy in the form of touching, caressing, and holding, are extremely reassuring to children. A mother's hand under the covers on the backside of a young child may bring comfort and sleep when nothing else does. Every child knows how comforting it is to snuggle in bed with her parents when the thunder is too loud and the night is too dark, and there is no rule against lying beside your child in the bed in the hospital.

Eventually, a time may come when a cancer is no longer responding to treatment and a conscious decision must be reached about whether anything more can or should be done. Even when treatment is stopped, care goes on and the important choice must be made between keeping the child in the hospital and trying to provide comfort and care at home. The child will almost always prefer to be at home, although older children sometimes elect to stay in the hospital, feeling more confident of the care they can receive. The decision to have the child die at home requires that the child wants to be home, that the family accepts the impending death, and that all active treatment of the disease has been discontinued. It is not an irreversible decision and the child can always be readmitted to the hospital.

A Mother's Grief. Death of a child is one of the most painful experiences parents can be asked to face and mothers and fathers have different reactions to it. The major role of the mother during illness, as a source of love and virtually constant care, brings her very close to her child, and death presents her with a devastating loss. Many mothers fear they will "lose control" and even wish to die with the child when the time comes, so much of her life is taken away. Moreover, the mother is constantly reminded of her loss by things around the house. Everyday a toy, a piece of old clothing, or empty bed renews her loss and she weeps frequently. A mother tends to be less restrained in her angry questions about why she lost her child and may actually be jealous of friends who have healthy children. She can flare up or break down at stupid questions such as, "Why don't you have another baby?", knowing that the dead child cannot be replaced. At the same time that she may be preoccupied and have little interest in her family, she may also feel left out by them. The family has become more independent in her absence. A mother's grief is apt to be open and emotional, full of tears, anger, frustration and guilt.

A Father's Grief. If the mother loses flesh of her own being in the death of her child, the father is more apt to lose a companion or a potential companion whom he saw growing up. During illness, many fathers enjoyed doing things with their child and put a great deal of effort into activities and trips, and these are what he remembers. In the rearrangement of family life he may have taken much more responsibility for the children at home. As a result he may feel guilty that he did not spend enough time with the child who was ill.

Men are expected to be uncomplaining and strong, emotionally stable and reserved. Fathers often feel that they should grieve alone and silently. They feel that they should keep up a brave front, even though they do not feel very brave; they may feel that they should not break down and cry, even though they would like to. One father sat on the lawn in front of the hospital and looked at the window where his child died for an hour every day before going home and looking brave. This lasted for six months and led to serious conflict because the mother thought she was feeling everything and that the father was feeling no pain at all. Eventually, with outside help, he revealed this and the relationship immediately began to improve. Because many fathers are unable to let themselves go, they tend to grieve slower, longer, and perhaps less effectively than mothers.

Many fathers bury themselves in their work to escape their unhappiness. If the mother's open and tearful grief is too painful, the father may even begin to avoid her. Such escape is a common coping mechanism and does not in any way reflect lack of concern. While it may offer some relief for the father, it increases the burden on the mother. The father is more apt to blame the illness rather than any individual person. He may feel that his work is going poorly, that his luck had run out, or that life is against him in many areas, all of which reflect his depression and loss.

Keeping the Family Together. Illness and death can bring a family together. One of the important goals should be to reconstruct the strength of the family so that everyone gains something. The illness of the child provides a focal point, an all-consuming activity for much of the family. For that reason, the maximum period of stress is usually *after* death when everything seems to come to a stop. The incidence of serious emotional problems has been estimated as high as 80 percent and the divorce rate in such families is above average. In their anger and guilt, parents blame themselves and each other when the real problem is unbearable pain and frustration in not being able to do anything to change events or escape from them. Each parent wants to crawl into his own hole, lick his wounds, and above all, not cause more pain for the other. They often fail to realize that they *cannot* cause more pain, that the maximum level has been reached. They can only hope to reduce it. In spite of the strong tendency for parents to drift apart at this time, their best chances of preserving their home and family are in getting closer together. Sharing will dilute the misery instead of intensifying it and this can only be done by working together instead of apart.

Parents should understand that their basic patterns of grief may be quite different. By admitting their feelings to each other, they can grieve together. The father can learn to accept the mother's open mourning, showing tolerance or joining in if he can. The mother, in turn, should encourage the father to mourn more openly with her but she should not be surprised if he cannot. In recalling the illness, it helps to realize how well you did most of the time, that your great strength carried you through an experience that makes you unique in many ways.

There are about 7,000 new cancers in children under the age of fifteen each year. The most common are acute leukemia, brain tumors, sarcomas, Wilm's tumor of the kidney, and neuroblastoma. **CANCERS OF CHILDHOOD**

The first three of these are discussed elsewhere, and this chapter will conclude with a few words about Wilm's tumor and neuroblastoma, both of which are quite rare.

Wilm's Tumor of the Kidney. This tumor is seen most frequently between the ages of one and five and is rare in children over eight. It occasionally occurs in young infants. It shows up as a mass on one side of the abdomen which is usually noticed by the mother or by the doctor on a routine examination. The mass may be very large and is painless. The child is usually otherwise completely healthy and active. The diagnosis is made by x–ray studies of the kidney.

Other procedures are not necessary and a separate biopsy is not done. The large size of the tumor has no relationship to the possibility of cure and the treatment is to remove the affected kidney. Depending on the age of the child, radiation is then given to the area of the kidney, or to the entire abdomen if it appears likely that the tumor has spread within the abdomen. Chemotherapy is also given and usually includes Actinomycin D and Vincristine. The most common places for this tumor to spread are the lungs, liver, and bones.

Wilm's tumor is another childhood cancer whose outlook has greatly improved in the last few years, primarily through the use of these combined approaches to treatment. The cure rate is greater than 90 percent if the tumor is confined to the kidney, especially if the child is under one year of age and the type of tumor is favorable. Spread to the lungs and other areas still carries a cure rate of about 50 percent. Occasionally this tumor occurs in both kidneys, in which case the usual approach is to remove all of one kidney and part of the other. Even these children do surprisingly well, with a cure rate that may be as high as 30 percent.

Neuroblastoma. Neuroblastoma is a tumor of developing nerve cells which occurs in the adrenal gland near the kidney or in the chain of nerves that lie on both sides of the spine. Twenty-five percent of the children who develop this disease are less than one year of age while half of them are under two and 75 percent are under four. Occasionally the tumor is present at birth. This is an important distinction because children who are less than one year when the disease is found do much better than those who are over two years old. The signs of the disease are directly related to the tumor mass itself and are therefore extremely variable because the tumor can occur in so many different parts of the body. Moreover, about 75 percent of these tumors have already spread by the time the diagnosis is made. The most common places for the tumor to spread are the liver, the bone marrow, bones, and under the skin.

The treatment for neuroblastoma is surgical removal of as much of the tumor as possible, sometimes followed by radiation since many of these tumors cannot be completely removed. Chemotherapy is being tried in children over the age of two but has not greatly improved the results, especially when the tumor has spread. Age and extent of disease are very important in the treatment and outlook of this tumor. The results are extremely good in children who are less than one year of age. If the tumor can be completely removed by surgery, most of them can be cured of their disease. Indeed, within this age group there are a small number of children who need no immediate treatment at all, even though the tumor has spread to the bone marrow or liver. The body seems to resist the tumor, possibly by producing an immune response capable of reducing the size of the tumor. Later, when the child is older, the remaining tumor is removed. On the other hand, children over the age of two have a poor outlook unless the tumor is small and can be completely removed.

nine
The Cost of Cancer

The cost of cancer creates serious problems for many families. Treatment is expensive and often prolonged. The direct costs of medical treatment alone can range from $5,000 to more than $100,000. To this must be added the indirect or hidden costs due to time out from work, loss of employment, child care, transportation, housekeeping, lodging and meals away from home, if medical care is being given in another city. Families must continue to function in spite of the illness. At the same time that you are faced with enormous medical costs you must continue to have food, clothing, and shelter. The net result can range from postponement or cancellation of college educations, to true hardships and the accumulation of thousands of dollars in debts. The purpose of this chapter is to provide some facts and figures on the financial impact of cancer and to urge you to be realistic about how these figures fit into your own circumstances. The earlier you understand the cost, the better you can plan how to meet them.

For many families cancer is indeed a catastrophic illness, yet it is amazing with what courage people face their financial and personal problems. Spouses who were not previously employed take jobs and those who were previously employed undertake second jobs in order to hold the family together and meet their bills. It can be a heartbreaking experience for a family to run out of money in the middle of such an illness. Turning to government welfare agencies is distasteful for many and impossible for some.

DIRECT COSTS The major direct costs are hospitalization, doctors bills, and home care. Of these, hospital bills are the most staggering. In general, hospital bills can be broken down into room and board, pharmacy or

112

medications, supplies, laboratory studies, x–ray studies, operating room and anesthesia time, and oxygen and inhalational therapy. These do not include professional fees for the surgeon, medical or pediatric oncologists, radiation therapists, or other consulting physicians. All of these costs, institutional and professional, are increasing rapidly in our current inflation.

Over 95 percent of all people newly found to have cancer are admitted to the hospital for initial treatment. Only radiation therapy is usually done on an outpatient basis, through daily visits to the hospital. Hospital costs vary from one part of the country to another and even between different hospitals in the same community. In general, university teaching hospitals are more expensive than private community hospitals and these, in turn, are more expensive than city or county hospitals. The differences, however, are relatively small and the room and board rates per day are almost the same in the different hospitals in any major city.

Physician's fees vary considerably between individuals and from one community to another. Most physicians and surgeons adhere to a standard and customary fee schedule established by tradition in the community and accepted by Blue Cross and Blue Shield. Schedules are usually reviewed annually and serve as guidelines to the participating physicians and surgeons. It is customary in many teaching hospitals and in city and county hospitals to forego any professional fee if the person does not carry appropriate health insurance. On the other hand, there is no legal limit to what a physician *may* charge over and above the insurance guidelines if the patient is able and willing to pay more in order to see a particular doctor. Physicians and surgeons can tell you what their usual fees are and you should get this information before treatment begins and the bills pile up. Most physicians are willing to modify their fees or help you get financial help if this is a problem.

Home Care. There is a definite trend toward home care. The increasing desire of many people to stay out of the hospital as much as possible means that many of the expenses of home care must be considered directly related to the illness. These include drugs and supplies, laboratory tests, equipment, and special diets that would be provided in the hospital. However, they also include transportation to the doctor's office or to the hospital for checkups and treatment, visits by professional nurses to supervise and assist in home care and housekeepers to help maintain the home if the family is unable to do so. Home care expenses are of particular importance because, if adequately documented, many of them are covered by medical insurance and others can be deducted for tax purposes.

Nursing Home. Many nursing homes will not accept people

with advanced cancer because of inadequate facilities and personnel to provide the necessary high level of individual care. However, they often will accept those who are not ill enough to be in the hospital but who cannot or would prefer not to be at home. Nursing home care for such people is usually covered by health insurance.

INDIRECT COSTS

In addition to the more obvious indirect costs of cancer, there are numerous hidden costs that are dictated by the needs of each individual family. The most significant is loss of wages, particularly if the person who is ill is also the breadwinner. Second to this is the loss of wages by other working members of the family when they accompany the patient to the hospital or doctor's office or provide care at home. Families with small children must consider the cost of babysitters or any other arrangements that must be made to care for the children when both parents are away from home.

A significant factor is the location of the hospital where most of the treatment is given. Travel can be very costly since it may include lodging and meals away from home. Finally, professional counseling and psychiatric help for patients and their families is being recognized as an important but often expensive need.

SOURCES OF MONEY

The main source for paying medical bills is insurance. Over 90 percent of the people in the United States have some form of health insurance, usually through their employment. This insurance, however, often falls short of that needed to cover bills resulting from a catastrophic illness such as cancer. Additional sources of money include savings, money set aside for college educations, sale of personal belongings and jewelry, sale or mortgaging of homes, and cashing in of life insurance policies. The cost of treating cancer can be staggering and the family striken by this disease should examine its finances carefully and early in order to avoid having to sell property, use savings, or make unwise decisions that perhaps could be avoided. Your doctor and hospital social service worker can give you an idea of the long term cost of the illness and help you find out about your insurance coverage. Several government and private sources of funds are available. Some of these sources of money for medical care are Blue Cross and Blue Shield or other private insurance carriers; Medicare; Medicaid; Supplemental Security Income; Social Security Disability Insurance; General Assistance; Crippled Children's Services; Veterans Administration; and The Clinical Center of the National Institutes of Health. This listing includes only the major sources of funding that are available. Many communities have additional public and private sources of their own. They include special benefit programs for children, for workers in certain industries, for service people and their families, and for illnesses requiring prolonged hospitalization and care. The best sources of information for your community are a hospital social service worker or your local welfare office. Two additional sources of information are the American Cancer Society and the Leukemia Society of America, Inc. which have chapters in each state and many communities. The important thing is to start immediately. Many programs require extensive paper work and a lengthy waiting period before they can help you. Moreover, they may *not* pay for services or bills that you have already received. If you are applying for Medicaid, social security disability insurance, supplemental security income, or general assistance, you should be prepared to provide accurate personal and financial information. This includes name, address, social security number, citizenship, age, the amount of income of each member of the family, the amount of savings of each member of the family, cash value of life insurance, market value of stocks, bonds, and other investments, and the value of real estate, automobile, and even personal belongings. All of this information must be documented and is subject to verification by the welfare agency.

Most people value their ability to work and resent anything that interferes with their capacity to support themselves and their families. An important aspect of feeling well is to be able to resume your normal life, including work.

EMPLOYMENT

Returning to the Old Job. Most people with cancer are middle-aged or older and are able to return to their previous employment. If an employee has been loyal to his company, the company is generally loyal to him during his illness. Many are very accommodating and make special arrangements for time off for treatment, shorter work days, or job reassignments. It is better to let your employer know the nature of your illness from the beginning so he can know what to expect and make adjustments that will keep your job available for you. It is also best not to return until treatment is essentially over and you are strong enough to work at least part time. This avoids unnecessary absenteeism. Your return to work should be gradual, starting with part time and slowly increasing your hours. This enables you to regain your confidence and strength at the same time, and demonstrates your willingness and ability to work. About 80 percent of people with cancer who were previously employed are able to return to their old jobs. Most of the others do not because they elect early retirement or are too ill to return to work.

The county board was really good to me. They said I could still work and take leave without pay and that they would pay for any days that I can work. They have been very understanding about when I can't come in and said to come back when I can. I'm getting in about three weeks a month now.

Finding a New Job.   Applying for a new job, particularly for a young person without much previous work experience, may be more difficult. While a history of cancer may be a barrier to employment in some companies, many other factors are obviously involved. These include the general job market, the number of qualified people available for a particular type of work, and the economy. Some companies are reluctant to employ people who have cancer because of general fear of the disease, particularly the possibility that it may be infectious, fear of a poor work record and absenteeism, physical limitations, and inability to perform assigned duties, threat of recurrence, or increased insurance costs to the company.

Public fear of cancer and the possibility of infection are prejudices based on ignorance and are slowly being combated by public education. Companies whose senior executives and employment staffs have encountered cancer in their own families are apt to be more liberal about employing people who have a history of cancer. Fear that people with cancer will not perform their jobs well and will have a high rate of absenteeism is being dispelled by the experience of several large companies who have examined the records of their own employees. Notable among these was a study of seventy-four cancer patients hired by the Metropolitan Life Insurance Company. They ranged from twenty to fifty years of age and were followed from one to fifteen years after treatment. At the end of the study 55 percent were still working for Metropolitan Life, 42 percent had discontinued their work, mostly to take other jobs, move to other communities or retire. Three percent were disabled and 2 percent discontinued their work for health reasons not related to cancer. No individuals were discharged from work because of poor performance. The turnover was very nearly the same as the normal population and it was concluded that employment of people with cancer presented no particular risk for the company.

Physical limitations and inability to perform assigned duties are obviously concerns for any employer. Many companies screen potential employees for a variety of health problems, including heart trouble, alcoholism, diabetes, and back problems, as well as cancer. The screening is usually done before a person is hired but occasionally after hiring. Most companies ask applicants about their health and over half also require medical histories and/or physical examinations. Medical screening may relate only to the ability to perform a particular job or it may include other medical conditions not related to work. The first type of screening should not be considered discrimination since it enables the company to place the right person in the right position. For example, a woman who has undergone mastectomy may not be able to do any lifting, although she can handle many other types of work. Screening for general health problems that are not related to the job, on the other hand, may constitute a very real form of discrimination. This requirement is frequently not instigated by the employer but rather an insurance company, particularly when a physical examination is required.

Employment Benefits. Virtually every company of any size is required to provide its employees with benefits which usually include health insurance. It is at this point that your interests, and those of your employer and his insurance company may be in conflict. Many companies insure all their employees under group policies that have clauses concerning pre-existing health problems, including cancer. This may be on an individual basis so that the insurance plan, even though it is a group plan, singles you out as being a higher than average risk. The insurance plan may insist that you be temporarily or permanently ineligible for insurance or that you may be insured for *other* health problems that may occur, but *not* for cancer. Some states, such as New York, require that every employee receive full fringe benefits, including life and health insurance, if the company carries this type of coverage. If hired, a person with cancer must be included. While the original purpose of this law guaranteed employees adequate insurance coverage, the result can be the opposite, making the company reluctant to employ anyone with a history of cancer.

Some insurance companies place all the responsibility on the employer, notifiying him from one year to the next about whether his insurance record for the past year has been good or bad. If the amount of money received in premiums was more than that paid out, the record was good; if it was less than that paid out, it was bad. The employer then adjusts his employment policies to assume as much or as little risk as he wishes. Many employers fear that hiring too many people with higher than average health risks will increase the insurance rates. Until insurance companies liberalize their policies concerning pre-existing illnesses, the best approach in looking for a job is to request a waiver of insurance related to your previous cancer.

The fact that you have had cancer does not necessarily imply disability, and most employers realize this. Improving cure rates and long term remissions providing years of productive life make it very hard to predict the fate of any individual, and employers and company physicians are under strong pressure to acknowledge this and modify their practices accordingly. The Flynn Act in New York notes that the person with cancer may be a long term risk but that if "the condition does not presently interfere with the individual's ability to perform, it may not be lawfully used to bar employment".

Job Training. If illness has made it impossible for you to resume your old job but you wish to find a new type of work, help is available. The Vocational Rehabilitation Act of 1973 applies to people who have had cancer. It provides federal funds for counseling, training, financial assistance, special equipment, and speech lessons for the person who has lost the use of his normal voice. Any physical defect that interferes with your normal work can qualify you for retaining in some other area. The only requirements of these programs are a reasonable outlook for recovery combined with your ability and willingness to return to some kind of work. Information can be obtained from your state vocational and rehabilitation agency which has offices in the state capitol and usually in many other communities. Your physician can help you get into a job training program.

What You Can Do. Most people who have had cancer *are* able to obtain jobs. The most important factors are acceptance of your disease and any disability that it has brought on and a genuine desire to work. A positive attitude about yourself and your own future is hard to overlook. Being turned down for a job can be unfair and discouraging but an optimistic approach on your own part and a little help from others can usually overcome most obstacles. A person who is handicapped is often thought to be in pain and this frightens people away. If there is no pain associated with your handicap, let others know. It will make them feel more comfortable to be reassured that you are comfortable. It is also important to explain to a potential employer exactly what you can do and what you cannot do, being open and matter of fact about your limitations, but firm about your desire to work.

If you encounter difficulties either in getting back your old job or obtaining a new one there are several sources of help. Your doctor can inform your employers that you are indeed able to work and can frequently put some pressure on them to give you a job. The American Cancer Society has an ongoing campaign to encourage employers to hire people who have had cancer, and representatives from your chapter will be willing to talk to the employer. Both your doctor and the American Cancer Society can provide employers with facts and figures about different types of cancer, survival rates, and the outlook following various forms of treatment. While the American Cancer Society must deal with generalities, your doctor can provide information that directly relates to you. More and more companies are hiring people who have had cancer, and these companies are accumulating experience with job performance, absenteeism, and length of time on the job. The American Cancer Society is collecting this information and can make it available to your prospective employer. If you have held a job in the past and belong to a labor union, you may get some support there. In general, however, unions have not been very forceful in this area. Your State Department of Human Rights can provide legal advice and directly help you regain or obtain a job in your community. Another, not very subtle, way to apply pressure is to discuss your problem with the medical writer of your local newspaper. Adverse publicity, or even the threat of it, can be very persuasive.

When I wanted to go back to work they just dumped me —no job. G is a huge company where I had worked for 30 years. The cost of my illness now is already about $20,000 out of pocket, primarily because of losing the job.

The Law and Legal Steps.   Laws providing help for disabled also apply to people who have had cancer. The Federal Rehabilitation Act of 1973 has been active in this area. Whether you only carry a diagnosis of having had cancer or are obviously disabled, if you wish to find some kind of appropriate work, it is against the law to discriminate against you. Unfortunately pressure cannot be brought to bear on all companies for all kinds of jobs. However, if the company to which you are applying employs more than fifty people and sells services or materials to the federal government that exceed more than $50,000 annually in value, the Rehabilitation Act can stand behind you. The threat that it carries is the cancellation of the federal contracts the company currently has and disqualification for receiving future government contracts. The act requires that you be judged specifically in terms of the job to be performed and not against any general standard. Moreover, if the employer finds that you cannot perform the duties of the job you applied for, he is required to try to make a "reasonable accommodation" so that you can be employed. This may involve altering the work setting. Since the enactment of this law, more than half of the states have come up with similar legislation forbidding discrimination against individuals whose disabilities or handicaps are not related to the jobs they wish to perform. People in remission from cancer are covered by this law regardless of whether or not they have any obvious disability.

This law is administered through the Office of Federal Contract Compliance of the U.S. Department of Labor, Washington D.C. The official regulations can be obtained from the Employment Standards Administration, U.S. Department of Labor, Washington D.C. 20210. Complaints must be filed in writing to the Office of Federal Contract

Compliance of the U.S. Department of Labor. It is probably best to do this with the help of a legal advisor from your own community who has experience in labor law. Other sources of information include the American Cancer Society, and the American Civil Liberties Union in your own state or in Washington D.C.

To initiate action against a particular company, it is important to have some statement from them in writing concerning their refusal to hire you. This may say that you are being turned down for employment specifically because you have cancer or, more generally, for "medical reasons". In any case, you should write to the company and request a written reply stating why you are being rejected for employment. A verbal statement will not do.

INSURANCE The two forms of insurance of greatest importance to people with cancer are health insurance and life insurance. Both can pose problems. If you have been treated for cancer, a company can refuse to insure you, require a long waiting period or impose additional premiums. To understand the reasons for this one must look at the business philosophy of the insurance industry. When they offer insurance to a person who appears to be perfectly healthy they are gambling that the person will *not* get sick or will *not* die before reaching a ripe old age. By insuring large numbers of people, of whom only a few can be expected to get sick or die young, they can offer protection at reasonable cost. When someone comes along who has already had cancer, the balance is tipped. Instead of having one in several hundred chances of becoming seriously ill and even dying at an early age, the odds may be considerably higher and the risk in insuring such a person much greater. Insurance companies have several ways of dealing with this. They can refuse to insure you at all. They can make you wait several months or years before they will insure you, knowing that with each passing year your chances of having a recurrence are less. They can offer to insure your health or life with respect to *other* illnesses, but excluding your cancer, on the assumption that your chances of having a heart attack are no greater than average. Finally, they can charge you more for your insurance. Obviously there are opposing points of view and what may seem like discrimination to a person who has cancer are sound business practices for the insurance companies.

Life Insurance. In spite of these restrictions, most people who have had cancer can eventually get insurance. Exclusion clauses, increased premiums, or waiting periods are the penalties that must be paid for not taking out insurance before illness. However, there is a good deal of public pressure against companies that refuse to insure people who have had cancer. The companies are also aware of the tremendous differences between various kinds of cancer and that statistics change from year to year. They recognize that basal cell carcinoma of the skin or early cancer of the cervix of the uterus (in situ) are very low risk diseases that usually carry no penalty at all. Higher on the scale are squamous cell carcinoma of the skin, papillary carcinoma of the thyroid gland, seminoma of the testis, and low grade carcinoma of the bladder which may require one to seven years waiting period for health insurance, or increased premiums for a few years for life insurance. Cancer of the lung, colon, or breast carry still higher penalties. Finally, a few tumors such as chronic lymphatic leukemia, and cancers that have spread to lymph nodes or are known to have recurred usually cannot be insured at all. Waiting periods begin after treatment is finished and may be as short as one year, or longer than ten years. An insurance policy that requires five years of increased premiums will only require two years of higher premiums if your treatment ended three years ago when you apply for the policy.

Life insurance cannot be cancelled once it is in effect. However, if it is carried through your place of employment you may not be able to renew it if your employment ends. Most policies can be converted to individual policies but require that you do so within a limited period of time, usually one month. Furthermore, *you* must initiate the transfer to an individual policy when your employment ends. Life insurance is costly and people who have cancer and are burdened with many other bills may find it too expensive. However, many policies also have waivers of premiums in case of serious illness, on policies that are already in effect.

Health Insurance. Health insurance is often obtained through employment groups. Some insurance companies accept all members of the group together even if one has a history of cancer. Others identify each individual and can select, reject, or modify on the basis of individual health histories.

Health insurance penalties are usually more severe than those on life insurance because the amount of money that the company may have to pay is much more variable. Health insurance by Blue Cross and Blue Shield for a woman who has had breast cancer, for instance, may not be available until after five years have elapsed with no recurrence. A policy may then have a rider which excludes coverage of recurrence of that disease for another five years. After ten years of no recurrence, Blue Cross and Blue Shield will usually issue a standard policy with no rider. Penalties are not confined to people who have had cancer. Waiting periods, increased premiums, and temporary or permanent exclusions also are applied to people who have arthritis, emphysema, epilepsy, duodenal ulcer, diabetes, or coronary heart disease, among others.

Health insurance that went into effect before your tumor occurred usually cannot be cancelled or changed. The option to cancel or refuse to renew the policy must be written into the original contract and should be looked for very carefully by anyone buying health or life insurance. If your company tries to cancel or modify the policy, you have every right to a full explanation and to take legal action if necessary. The one unfortunate exception to this is when your health insurance is through your place of employment and you are unable to work, thereby losing the coverage of a group contract. Usually these policies can be converted into individual policies but occasionally this is difficult or impossible.

Some states provide special health insurance coverage for individuals who are not high risk. These policies often provide fairly comprehensive coverage for hospital and medical bills at reasonable cost. They are offered to people who have been refused health insurance, or who must pay extra costs, or have substantial restrictions put on them related to any specific disease such as cancer. These policies usually do not cover care received before they go into effect but do cover charges incurred during the first six months or one year of coverage under the policy if the illness (for example, cancer) was diagnosed or treated within ninety days immediately before applying for insurance. This type of emergency insurance for those who cannot obtain other conventional health insurance is very important for people who were previously uninsured. Unfortunately it is not available in all states.

If you are buying health insurance you will find that companies vary in their attitudes toward insuring people who have had cancer. It is very important to look at several companies. A good general insurance policy is better than a special "cancer policy". You should be sure the length of hospitalization coverage is at least sixty days, and that coverage includes outpatient or office care for chemotherapy or radiation therapy, home care by visiting nurses or homemakers, and what share of the hospital costs you will be expected to pick up. You should then weigh the value of a high deductable amount, which you must pay before coverage begins, against good long-term coverage, according to your own circumstances.

Treatment

Treatment for cancer can only begin after the tumor has been found. This is usually because *you* suspect that something is wrong and consult a doctor. Only occasionally is it the result of a routine check-up. You are your own best first line of defense.

Any unusual occurences should make you suspicious. Some are subtle while others demand prompt attention. The most frequent signs or symptoms that should be looked into include the following:

THE SIGNS OF CANCER

Bleeding: Any abnormal bleeding should be investigated. In women this includes vaginal bleeding between periods or after the menopause. Any rectal bleeding or evidence of blood in the sputum, in the urine, or the vomiting of blood is abnormal. Vomited blood may be black or like coffee grounds, rather than red.

Cough or Hoarseness: Everyone coughs occasionally, particularly in the morning. Smokers cough more than others. A change in the frequency or type of cough, in the type or amount of sputum brought up or hoarseness that lasts more than a few days is abnormal.

Lumps: Any lumps anywhere should be investigated. The most obvious lumps are in the breast, armpit, or groin but they can appear under the skin in any part of the body. They may be large and soft or small and hard, or anywhere in between. They *all* should be investigated because they could be serious. Many people have moles and freckles. It is the mole that changes that is dangerous. A change may be darkening in color, loss of color, increase in size, or ulceration and bleeding from the mole.

Bowel habits: Any change in bowel habits lasting more than a few days should be cause for concern. This may be constipation, or diarrhea, or alternating constipation and diarrhea. It is not necessary to find blood in the stool before worrying about the possibility of cancer of the colon or rectum.

Sores: Sores on any surface of the body that do not heal within the expected length of time should be checked. These include sores on the mouth, lip, tongue, genitals or anywhere on the skin.

Pain: Pain is the body's way of warning us that something is wrong. Most cancers do not cause pain early. However, pain lasting more than a few days is always a sign that something is wrong and should be investigated.

Difficulty swallowing: One would think that anything as basic as difficulty swallowing, which may be due to cancer of the foodpipe (esophagus) or the stomach, would be easily recognized. In fact, people often go from solid foods to soft foods and even to liquids before they finally admit to themselves that something *may* be wrong.

Weight loss and weakness: Less frequent as early signs of cancer are weight loss and weakness. However, when these are unexplained by diet or some other illness they are more than enough reason to see your doctor.

PHYSICAL EXAM

If you suspect something is wrong it is your doctor's job to try to find out what it is. In addition to a variety of questions related to the subjects mentioned, her physical examination should include any lumps or sores that you have noticed, your mouth, neck (for the thyroid gland), breasts, lungs, rectum, prostate gland, uterus, and examination of a stool specimen for unsuspected blood. Anemia or a low blood level requires a thorough search for hidden blood loss. The most common places for this are the stomach and the bowel. Examination of the stool for unsuspected blood can lead directly to the discovery of cancer of either of these two organs. These are the examinations that are most apt to disclose an unsuspected cancer. Obviously any abnormalities that *you* have noted should be called to your doctor's attention.

Assuming that both you and your doctor feel something is wrong and that it may be cancer, a variety of studies can be done to make the diagnosis. Each particular cancer requires its own set of examinations and studies, directed towards the area in the body that seems to be the most likely source of trouble. If the suspicious area is easily found, such as a breast lump, very few studies are required. On the other hand, if the suspicious tumor is thought to be deep inside the body, such as in the digestive tract, several studies may be required to find out exactly where the problem is.

X-ray pictures, as we ordinarily think of them, distinguish between hard and soft tissues. Bone is a hard tissue and shows up as a light area on the x-ray while normal lung, which contains a lot of air, is a very soft tissue and shows up as a dark area on the x-ray. Everything else is between these two. Most of the body is made up of relatively soft tissues. Cancers tend to be slightly harder than many normal soft tissues and therefore can be seen by x-ray. The best examples of this are cancer of the breast, where the cancer is usually harder than the normal breast, and sarcomas of the arm or leg which are harder than the surrounding soft tissues.

X-ray Dyes. Because many normal internal organs and cancers have nearly the same degree of softness or hardness when seen by x-ray, further techniques are used to outline the internal organs. Special dyes show up on x-ray, usually as white against a dark background.

In order to see the outline of the inside of the esophagus and stomach, a chalky tasting material (barium) is given to you by mouth (upper G.I. series). In a darkened x-ray room, the doctor can watch the material pass through the foodpipe and fill the stomach. He can also look for abnormalities in the wall of the foodpipe or the stomach and see if the material passes on quickly or whether there are signs of obstruction.

A similar study can be done in which the material is introduced into the rectum and large bowel after they have been cleaned by means of laxatives and water enemas (barium enema). The x-ray dye outlines the inside of the rectum and bowel, allowing the doctor to see abnormalities of the wall of these organs and to look for signs of narrowing or obstruction.

X-ray dyes are used to look for cancers in many organs including the esophagus, stomach, bowel, rectum, kidney, and bladder. In addition, certain dyes injected directly into the blood supply of internal organs so the brain, liver, pancreas or kidney, show whether the blood vessels are in their normal places or if they have been pushed aside by a tumor. This is done by inserting a needle into the arm or groin and injecting the dye directly, or by threading a tiny plastic tube (catheter) through the needle, into a particular blood vessel to be looked at. When the tube is guided into place with the help of x-ray, the dye is injected and the pictures taken.

New Techniques. A useful new x-ray technique is the CT scan (computerized tomography). This is a technique which takes pictures of cross-sections of various parts of the body. Since each organ has its own proper position in the body, these cross-sections show if some organ has been pushed aside and if abnormal tissue is present. Another new technique is the use of echograms by which an ultrasound wave is bounced off tissues within the body to identify any abnormal hard tissue that does not belong there.

Isotope
Scans

In a later chapter on radiation therapy we will see that some radioactive materials give off rays or particles that are used to treat cancer. There are similar materials which can be injected into the body in much smaller quantities, sending the radiation from inside to out, to detect cancer. The easiest of these to understand is the bone scan where the radioisotope is taken up by abnormal cancerous bone but not by normal bone. The isotope dye is injected into a vein in the arm and allowed to circulate to the bones. Within two hours a bone scan can be done. You lie quietly on a table for a few minutes while a scanning tube, which does not touch you at all, goes back and forth over your whole body looking for areas where the dye may have been taken up.

The opposite technique is used in a liver scan. The normal liver takes up the radioactive dye and gives a dark outline of the entire liver on the scan. A tumor, which does not take up the dye, will show up as a white spot against the dark background. The major organs that can be studied by scans include the brain, bone, liver, lymph nodes, and thyroid. All of these are relatively simple procedures where the dye is injected into a vein, taken up by its target organ and then looked at by the scanning machine. The only exception to this is the examination of some lymph nodes in which the dye is injected into a tiny lymphatic vessel on the foot. The next day the lymph nodes in the pelvis and the abdomen which have taken up the dye can be seen with x–ray pictures.

Medical use of x–ray for diagnosis is increasing as better equipment and studies are developed. Most of these are necessary and important for accurate diagnosis of a variety of diseases, including cancer. On the other hand too many x–rays can be harmful, and doctors may not be aware that you have had many x–rays in the past. As a result some studies are repeated more often than necessary. Of particular concern are routine examinations such as chest x–rays and mammograms. The following steps can help you avoid unnecessary medical radiation.

1. Do not repeat routine x-rays unnecessarily. If you had one a few weeks ago, ask your doctor to get the last one instead of taking another.

2. Ask your doctor if x-ray pictures will provide enough information and fluoroscopy can be avoided.

3. Avoid unnecessary dental x-rays unless you have lots of cavities

that need continuous treatment. Routine dental x-rays every six months are probably too often.

4. If you go to a new doctor or dentist transfer your old x-rays so that new ones will not have to be taken.

5. Routine chest x-rays for employment are frequently not needed. Ask if recent x-rays taken for other purposes will do.

6. If you think that you are pregnant tell your doctor. The sensitivity to radiation in children is five to ten times that of adults but the sensitivity of the fetus may be ten to 100 times that of adults. The risk of causing cancer in your unborn child is not known but usually can be avoided.

There are a variety of techniques for looking into different parts of the body without surgery, the following areas can be examined in this way:

LOOKING INSIDE WITHOUT SURGERY

Upper Digestive System. The upper digestive system consists of the esophagus or foodpipe, the stomach, the upper portion of the bowel, the pancreas, and the bile ducts. These can all be examined by a flexible instrument which is inserted into the esophagus after the throat is anesthetized with a local anesthetic to eliminate the sensation of gagging. The procedure is not uncomfortable. The examiner can see where he is moving the instrument by the lens system. He can examine the esophagus, the stomach, and the beginning of the small-bowel (duodenum). The small tubes that bring digestive juices from the liver (the bile ducts) and from the pancreas (pancreatic duct) enter the duodenum together just beyond the stomach and the examiner can frequently find this opening and put a small instrument into it. He can then obtain samples of the digestive juices produced by the liver and the pancreas to look for cancer cells. In addition he can put an x–ray dye into the bile duct or the pancreas to examine each of these systems by x–ray for evidence of cancer.

Colon and Rectum. The procedures here are called proctoscopy, sigmoidoscopy, or colonoscopy. Before any of these examinations can be done, the bowel must be cleaned out with enemas and/or laxatives. Instruments used vary from the short proctoscope to the longer sigmoidoscope to the flexible colonoscope which is capable of visualizing most of the large bowel. The procedure itself is only slightly uncomfortable and does not require anesthesia. It is carried out while you are in a somewhat undignified head-down position, kneeling on a special table that tips forward so that one's buttocks are up in the air. After the rectum is first examined by finger, the instrument is inserted and guided by the examiner through the lens system of the instrument.

The Lung.   Most lung cancers can be seen by putting a tube directly into the air passages through the mouth. This may be a rigid or flexible tube, with a light system and lenses. The procedure is called bronchoscopy because the main air passages are called bronchi. Because the tube is irritating and causes coughing, it is always necessary to anesthetize the throat and air passage with a local anesthetic or put you to sleep for this examination. The air passages have many branches and if a tumor is near the main trunk of the tree, it may be seen. Other times traces of blood from the tumor may be seen coming from a more distant branch of the tree. Cells coming from the cancer can often be collected by means of this examination.

Bladder.   The bladder can be examined easily by a tube and light system (cystoscopy). This usually requires general anesthesia for men since the passage to the bladder (urethra) is through the penis and the distance is relatively far. The same route in women is much shorter so their examination is not uncomfortable. In addition to seeing directly inside the bladder, the examiner can put dye into the tubes that carry the urine from the kidneys to the bladder (ureters) and by x-ray studies see these tubes and the central part of the kidney where urine is collected.

CANCER TISSUE DIAGNOSIS: BIOPSY

The final step required to determine if an illness is really cancer is to obtain a small piece of the suspicious tissue and have it examined by a pathologist to see if it is cancer. Although a person who has cancer rarely meets him, the pathologist is a very important figure in the medical team. He is a specialist who has learned to distinguish cancerous from normal tissues by examining them by the naked eye and by microscope. He looks for differences between normal and abnormal cells, and biopsies of tumors are often taken near the margin to include some adjacent normal tissue for comparison. Most obvious are alterations in the architecture of the tissue, with loss of the normal arrangement and orientation of the cells, or invasion or migration of cells from one layer to another (see Figure 10.1). The pathologist also sees abnormalities in the cells, with unusual variations from one cell to the next. Some are large and some are small, some have large nuclei and some small, some stain darkly while others do not. Cancer cells often have lost the characteristics of the corresponding normal tissue. Glandular cells may no longer appear glandular, muscle cells no longer like muscle.

It is important for the pathologist to distinguish between benign tumors and malignant ones. The *benign tumor* is innocent, grows slowly, and usually is limited in how large it can become. It does not invade neighboring tissues or spread to other parts of the body and it

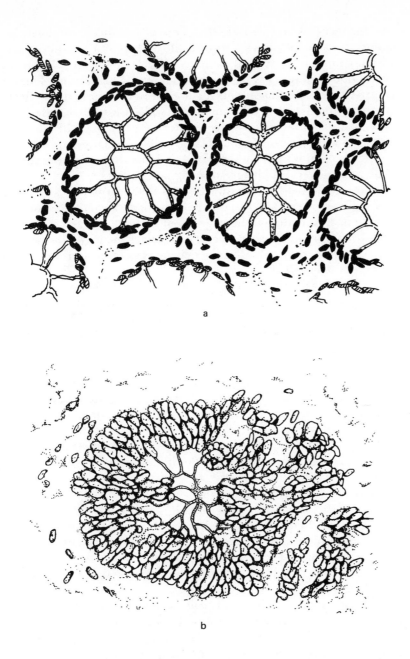

a

b

Figure 10.1 What the Pathologist Sees. (a) Normal colon showing orderly arrangement of cells into gland structures. Cells are of uniform size and shape. (b) Colon cancer showing disordered arrangment of cells. The cells vary in size and shape and form many layers but still have some resemblance to the original gland structure.

does not recur after removal. *Malignant tumors* or *cancers* have unlimited growth capabilities. They invade and spread to other tissues and tend to recur if they are not completely removed. Within the general family of cancers there are two main classifications. Tumors that arise from cells that are on surfaces or in the lining of organs or that form glands are called *carcinomas* while those that arise from connective or supportive tissues are termed *sarcomas*. In addition, there are a wide variety of tumors from highly specialized tissues, and a spectrum of tumors from the blood and blood-forming organs. In all, there are over 100 different malignant tumors.

Beyond actually determining that a tissue biopsy is cancer, the pathologist is often called upon to determine exactly what kind of cancer it is, how malignant it is (grade of malignancy, and if there is microscopic spread to other places, particularly nearby lymph nodes (stage of malignancy), all of which may be very important for choosing the best treatment.

Processing and examining the tissue take one or two days. Occasionally, when it is important to have this information very quickly, such as during surgery, the pathologist can do so by freezing and staining the tissue (frozen section). This requires about fifteen minutes.

There are a variety of ways of getting tissue. The actual taking of a small piece of tissue for the purpose of diagnosis is called a biopsy. If the suspected area can be approached through a tube (endoscopy), the biopsy can be obtained very simply at the same time that the area can be looked at directly.

Needle Biopsy. One of the quickest and simplest ways of obtaining a piece of tissue is by means of a hollow needle. The suspicious lump must be near the surface of the body where it can be felt (as in a breast tumor) or where it can be seen easily by x–ray (some carcinomas of the lung). The skin over the lump is frozen with a local anesthetic and then a special needle is pushed into the lump. A small cutting instrument that fits inside the needle is used to remove a tiny core of tissue. Since there are very few nerves underneath the skin, freezing of the skin is all that is required to make this a painless procedure.

Incision Biopsy. If the suspicious area is on the surface of the body, such as a skin tumor, or if it is near the surface of the body but not hard enough to be easily felt as a lump, it may be necessary to make a small incision through the skin to obtain a piece of the suspicious tissue. This is usually done by freezing the area with a local anesthetic, making a small cut, and obtaining a piece of the suspicious tissue. This is the method most often used for cancers of the skin and cancer of the breast, when a needle biopsy cannot be done.

If the tissue to be biopsied is deep inside the body, the biopsy usually requires that you be put to sleep for an operation. If the operation is only to obtain a sample of the tissue it may be very brief, requiring only a few minutes. On the other hand if the operation is to obtain a sample of tissue and then to remove the cancer, which is often done at the same time, it may take considerably longer.

Cancerous tissues are made up of cancer cells and sometimes these cells can be collected and examined by microscope to help make the diagnosis. The best known of these is the pap smear for cancer of the cervix which is described more fully in Chapter 21. The pap smear is done by scraping the entrance to the uterus (cervix) gently as part of a regular pelvic examination. This is a completely painless procedure. Other areas where cells can be recovered include the mouth, food-pipe, stomach, colon, lung, and bladder. In addition, some tumors that have spread to the chest or the abdominal cavity produce fluid in which tumor cells are floating. This fluid can be obtained by tapping with a needle and recovering the fluid to examine it for cells. This is done by first freezing the skin with a local anesthetic, and then inducing a hollow needle through which the fluid can be removed. Once the skin has been anesthetized, the procedure is painless. Recovery of cells from the esophagus, stomach, the colon, or the lung require looking into these areas by means of flexible tubes as described above, seeing the suspicious area that may be a tumor, and scraping or washing it with water to recover the cells.

CANCER CELL DIAGNOSIS

It has long been hoped that cancers would be found to produce some unique materials by which they can be detected early and with certainty. So far this is not the case. A few cancers do produce characteristic materials that help in their detection. These include a relatively rare type of cancer of the uterus (choriocarcinoma), tumors of the liver, bone, prostrate, bone marrow (myeloma), and neuroblastoma of childhood. Test for chemicals produced by these tumors are done on blood samples and require only a little blood from a vein in the arm.

SPECIAL TESTS AND EARLY DETECTION

Some tumors also produce substances that are normally found in the tissue and blood of human embryos. These carcinoembryonic antigens (CEA) are not specific for cancer since they are also found in the blood of people with several other diseases. Their main value has been to monitor people for early detection of recurrence. If a tumor is associated with a high level of CEA in the blood, which falls to normal after treatment, a return of CEA to a high level may indicate recurrence of the tumor. In some cases, this rise in CEA may precede any other sign of recurrence, prompting earlier treatment.

eleven
The Best Treatment for You

There are three major forms of treatment for cancer: surgery, radiation, and the use of drugs, including hormones. Each of these is discussed in detail in a separate chapter. In general, surgery is the best treatment for tumors that have not spread from the place where they began, and when they can be removed safely without causing too much disability or scarring. Examples are cancer of the colon, breast, and lung. Surgery may also be used to avoid or treat distressing symptoms, such as obstruction of the bowel, even when the tumor cannot be completely removed.

Radiation therapy is also of great value in tumors that have not spread far from where they began, particularly tumors that cannot be removed surgically because of the disability or scarring that would result. Examples include cancer of the tongue, lip, and cervix. The area that can be radiated safely is considerably larger than the area that can be removed surgically. Radiation therapy is also used after surgery when there is uncertainty about whether or not the operation was able to remove all of the tumor. Finally, radiation is of value in treating local deposits of tumor that have spread from the original cancer (metastasis) and which are causing distress, usually in the form of pain. An example is tumor of the bone that originally came from cancer of the breast.

Chemotherapy by itself is the best treatment for tumors that begin in many parts of the body at the same time, such as leukemia and some lymphomas. It is also used with surgery when the likelihood of spread from the place of the original tumor is high. An example of this is cancer of the breast when it has spread to the armpit lymph nodes. Finally, chemotherapy is of value for many people whose cancer has already spread to other parts of the body from its original location, so that further surgery or radiation therapy would be of little value.

134

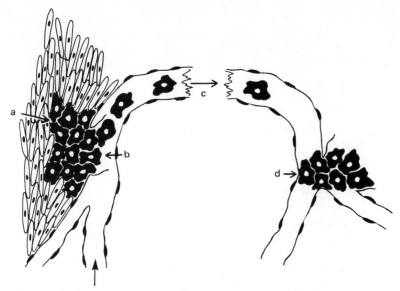

Figure 11.1 Invasion and Metastases. (a) Invasion of normal muscle by cancer cells. (b) Invasion of blood vessel by cancer cells. (c) Cancer cells carried in the bloodstream. (d) Lodgement and establishment of cancer cells in the lung - metastases.

HAS
THE TUMOR
SPREAD?

One of the most important questions for deciding what treatment is best is whether or not the tumor has already spread, or is likely to spread. (See Figure 11.1) Many tests and studies can help determine if the cancer has spread. This depends partly on the type of tumor. Some are far more aggressive about invading neighboring tissues while others appear to be quite capricious and unpredictable from one person to another. The location of the tumor is also a factor. Cancer of the pancreas is close to the liver and extension to the liver is hard to treat. Cancer of the bowel is usually further away from the liver. The size of the cancer is important since large tumors presumably have had more time to spread elsewhere than small cancers.

Cancers that rarely spread from where they begin and can usually be treated successfully with surgery or radiation include some of the most common skin cancers, cancer of the salivary gland, and cancer of the thyroid. Cancers which tend to spread gradually and predictably to the lymph nodes nearby, going to distant areas much later, include cancer of the cervix and many of the cancers of the face and mouth and neck. These, too, are usually treated by surgery or radiation. Cancers that often spread early to other parts of the body include some of the sarcomas, a rare cancer of the uterus (choriocarcinoma) and one type of cancer of the lung (small cell). For these chemotherapy is always used, sometimes in addition to surgery or radiation. Finally, there is a large group of common cancers which are relatively unpredictable, with a great deal of variation from one person to another. These include cancer of the breast, lung, bowel, stomach and melanoma of the skin. The treatment of these cancers is usually determined by stage of the disease at the time of treatment. Doctors rely heavily on some form of "staging" for most cancers to determine the best treatment, and to predict and evaluate results. Many systems are used to describe the extent or amount of disease in each individual.

In its simplest form Stage I is a tumor that is confined to the organ and tissue where it began. Stage II represents the same tumor which has spread to the lymph nodes nearby. This is common behavior for some cancers. Stage III, or Stage IV for some tumors with more complicated patterns of spread, describes spread to more distant parts of the body such as the lung, liver, brain, bones, etc. so that the cancer must be considered and treated as a more general disease.

The best chance for curing a cancer, usually by surgery or radiation therapy, is when it is still in Stage I. This is the value of early detection. Many cancers are curable at this early stage. For many cancers the chances of cure are reduced to about one-half if the tumor has already spread to nearby lymph nodes. Unfortunately, many of the most common cancers can only rarely be cured if they have spread to more distant parts of the body and involve other organs, such as the lung, liver, brain, or bones.

WHEN THERE IS A CHOICE OF TREATMENT

For some cancers there are two forms of treatment which are essentially equal. These are more often surgery or radiation, but occasionally radiation or drug therapy. Examples of this are some cancers of the face and mouth, cancer of the bladder, prostate, and several others. The choice of treatment depends not only on the location and type of tumor but also on its size. If there is any question about your own tumor, you should be sure to ask your doctor what other forms of treatment are available and have him explain them. If your doctor is a surgeon, you may ask him to arrange for you to talk to a radiation therapist or medical oncologist about the possibility of treating your tumor or vice versa. The doctor should advise, but you should decide.

COMBINED TREATMENTS FOR CANCER

A very important new trend in cancer treatment is to combine two or even three forms of treatment in an attempt to get better results than can be obtained by any one of them. The cure rate from surgery alone has not improved much for many cancers in recent years because they spread before the surgery is done. The logical step is to combine surgery with chemotherapy or radiation to try to change this. Various combinations include radiation before surgery to reduce the size of the cancer and to kill cells at the edge of the tumor that may escape at the time of surgery; or radiation following surgery to kill cancer cells that may have escaped to regional lymph nodes in the area; or drug therapy before or, more commonly, after surgery to kill tumor cells that have escaped elsewhere. This latter is the common type of adjuvant chemotherapy that is now being tested on a wide scale on cancer of the breast and several others. All three forms of therapy—surgery, chemotherapy, and radiation—have been used together to cure some children's tumors including Wilm's tumor of the kidney, and a sarcoma of muscle, and cancer of the testicle in the adult.

One of the most common questions asked is, "What are my chances?" The overall cure rate for all cancers taken together is about 40 percent. For some types of cancer it is much higher than this and for some it is lower. The published figures make it easy to see that cancer of the lung is a worse disease than cancer of the breast, which in turn is more serious than cancer of the lip. In describing the results of treatment, doctors often speak in terms of survival rates and the most commonly used term is the "five-year survival rate". A 50 percent five-year survival rate means that 50 percent of people with that particular tumor can be expected to be alive at the end of five years. Many cancers are unlikely to recur after five years, so that survival for that length of time is frequently considered to be equal to cure. This implies that a person who has such a cancer, is treated, and is well five years later can expect to have a normal life span and die of something other than his cancer. The "five-year survival rate" for *your* cancer, with its hope and implication of cure, is the figure that you, the patient, are most frequently interested in. It is an estimate that your doctor can provide for you, with respect to your own particular tumor. You have every right to this information.

THE RESULTS OF TREATMENT

For a few cancers the five-year survival rate is not an accurate description of the disease and is not the equivalent of cure because the cancers can come back ten or fifteen years later. These include cancer of the breast, thyroid, bladder, and melanoma of the skin. Most doctors avoid using the word "cure" in these cancers and prefer to speak of "control" since they know that they cannot predict accurately whether or not the cancer may come back years later. Even with these tumors, however, the likelihood of the tumor coming back decreases with time and late recurrences are uncommon.

When a cancer has spread or returned and cure is no longer likely, radiation or drug therapy may be used to reduce the size of the cancer and provide comfort and longer life. This is measured as a "response" rate. A complete response usually implies complete disappearance of all evidence of the tumor by physical examination or by x–ray for at least six months and possibly a year. A partial response rate is less easily defined and usually requires shrinkage of the cancer to one-half of its original size for a reasonable period of time, without pain or distressing signs of the tumor. On the premise that people reading this book want concrete information I have included facts and figures in the chapters on specific cancers. These figures should be understood for what they really are—*averages* of response to treatment or survival of large numbers of people with the same type of cancer. They give us an overall picture of how some cancers behave, how good our treatment is and if the results of treatment are improving over a period of years. Furthermore, five- and ten-year survival rates that are quoted today represent the results of treatment given more than five or ten years ago. For many tumors today's improved treatment will yield better results when they are tabulated five or ten years from now.

It is very important to realize that these figures represent statistics obtained from the treatment of large numbers of people and that they have little meaning for any individual. They are averages, and no one wants to be average. Each of us is unique and each cancer is unique. There is too much that we do not understand about this disease to expect uniform results, even when identical tumors are treated exactly the same way. A person whose cancer has a 90 percent five-year survival rate obviously has a better outlook than a person whose cancer has only a 10 percent five year survival rate. On the other hand, even with a discouraging tumor, it is impossible to predict who will respond well to treatment and will be in the 10 percent surviving and free of cancer in five years. Among the "good" and "bad" cancers there is none that is *never* fatal, nor is there any cancer that is always fatal. There is an element of hope, and even luck, in every aspect of life but nowhere is it stronger or more important than to the person with cancer.

UNPROVEN TREATMENTS

Desperate people do desperate things.

Unproven or unofficial forms of treatment of cancer are those which have not been adequately tested by qualified scientists or have been tested and found to be valueless. Considering the extent of our knowledge of this disease and the availability of many proven forms of treatment, you may wonder why so many people go far out of their way and spend thousands of dollars to obtain treatment that at best is useless and at worst may even be harmful. The answer is that they are afraid and desperate. Most unfortunate is the person who has early cancer that may be cured. In grasping blindly for hope instead of dealing with the reality of facts and figures, he may give up his only chance of survival. Fear alone is strong enough to drive some people to seek treatment when they do not have cancer at all.

Laetrile. Thought by most people to be new, this extract of apricot pits first appeared as amygdalin in 1920, then as Laetrile in 1952. Numerous animal studies of the kind used to test all anticancer drugs showed Laetrile to be of questionable or no value. In spite of this its use has caught on and it is estimated that 50,000 to 75,000 Americans spend millions of dollars each year to obtain it. The reason for this is the well-organized efforts of political groups, most notably the Committee for Freedom of Choice in Cancer Treatment. Organizations like this one use Laetrile in their efforts to protest government intervention into any aspect of life.

The political battle to legalize Laetrile has been long and surprisingly successful. To get around a ruling by the Food and Drug Administration (FDA) that drugs must not only be safe but effective, Laetrile producers called their product Vitamin B_{17}, considering it a food rather than a drug. Vitamins, however, are defined as chemicals that are essential to the diet to maintain normal health and growth. For example, lack of vitamin C causes scurvy, a disease common in sailors until it was found that it could be prevented by eating citrus fruits. Similarly, rickets, a bone disease of children, is prevented by vitamin D. Laetrile is not required in the diet and should not be considered a vitamin.

More recently, production and sale of Laetrile have been legalized in several states. The FDA has made it illegal to transport it across state lines, but cannot regulate its use within any state. The highest level of attack has been in Congress where a bill was introduced that would change the basic FDA ruling in such a way that it would no longer be necessary to prove that *any* drug is effective in doing what its manufacturer claims. Drugs for high blood pressure would not have to lower blood pressure and antibiotics would not have to be effective against infections. Most congressman are well informed, and such a bill is unlikely to pass.

Political pressure for Laetrile has been so intense that the National Cancer Institute has sponsored clinical trials of the drug at a recognized medical center, the Mayo Clinic, in spite of unconvincing tests in animals and the objections of the FDA. At the present time these trials have shown Laetrile to be relatively harmless at the doses suggested for treating cancer, but have failed to show any beneficial effects on the people treated, all of whom had advanced disease that had failed to respond to other forms of treatment.

Remedy or Treatment. No person who has cancer can escape

from the psychological effects of the disease and everyone—poor, wealthy, ignorant, or educated—is equally susceptible to promises of a sure cure. Many are aware of the side effects and limitations of conventional treatment as detailed in this book and prefer to take their chances with less drastic and relatively harmless forms of treatment. Others are skeptical of modern medical science and feel that it has little to offer them, often failing to realize how inconsistent this attitude is. The same people accept vaccinations against smallpox and polio, they take antibiotics for infections, insist on being put to sleep for operations, and even consent to having one or more artificial heart valves put in if needed. Some of these people, however, remain suspicious and skeptical when it comes to accepting the best treatment available for cancer, obviously reflecting the enormous fear caused by this disease.

Information about unproven forms of treatment may come from newspaper or magazine articles, advertising on television or radio, or in health magazines, notices in health organizations, health food stores, or even religious and political groups. The main sources, however, are well-meaning relatives and friends.

Table 11.1 lists just a few of the unofficial drugs that have been marketed in recent years. While drugs are the most common forms of unproven methods for treating cancer there are also many others. These include special diets, (often *confined* to vegetable and fruit juices), magic boxes, magnetic vibrating boards or similar devices, colonic irrigations (enemas) to "detoxify the body", and fever therapy induced by such agents as Coley's toxins. A popular approach now is creative visualization or imagery in which a person is asked to imagine his cancer cells as being insects or crabs and then concentrate his willpower on their destruction. When coupled with conventional therapy this may be helpful, but it is of no value alone.

Selling the Product. People who provide unproven forms of treatment usually look like doctors, often even more so. They are actors, and as such they may play their roles better than real doctors. They often have unusual titles and office walls plastered with unusual degrees, including just about everything except doctor of medicine (M.D.). The treatment offered may be available only from one person and may even be a "secret formula" bearing his name. Research leading to the treatment was usually carried out in an independent, privately funded laboratory, rather than with public funds, such as those provided by the National Cancer Institute or the American Cancer Society, which are competetive and harder to obtain. Moreover, the results of these studies are not published in reputable medical journals or presented at medical meetings.

Unfortunately, some quacks are harder to identify. They are

Table 11-1. A Few Unproven Methods of Treating Cancer

Name	Advocates	Date	What It Is	Route of Administration*
Coley's Toxins	W.B. Coley, M.D. H.C. Nauts	1893 1960	Strains of bacteria that cause fever	I
Gerson Method	M. Gerson, M.D.	1942	Diet of fruits, vegetables, oatmeal and vitamins	O
Hoxsey Chemotherapy	H.M. Hoxsey H.A. Galbraith H. Stegman	1920s	Herbs and harmless drugs	O
Kribiozen	S. Durovic, M.D. A.C. Ivy, Ph.D.	1950s	Extract of horse blood or meat	I
Laetrile	E.T. Kribs, M.D. E.T. Kribs, Jr. H.H. Beard E.L. McNaughton J. Beard	1920	Extract of apricot pits	I
Rand Antigen	H.J. Rand A.J. Lewis S.M. DeCarvalho, M.D.	1966	Extract of cancer tissues coupled to rabbit serum	I
Burton Treatment	L. Burton F. Friedman	1966	"Deblocking protein," an extract of normal blood	I

*I=Injection, O=Oral
From information provided by the American Cancer Society

bona fide M.D.'s who cannot be objective about their work or cannot accept eventual failure when early studies showed promise. It is to their credit and credibility that most doctors engaged in research acknowledge their failures publicly, retracting their original claims of success, and embark on new approaches that are more promising. Quacks obviously fail to do this and often resent any suggestion that their cures cannot be repeated by others using the same methods.

Unproven methods of treatment are usually much less expensive than conventional treatment. Also, the quack is usually willing to take your word that you have cancer. A biopsy that proves the presence of cancer is not necessary because it only confuses the issue. Besides, it is much easier to cure a person who does *not* have cancer in the first place. Second opinions from recognized medical doctors are discouraged or even forbidden on the grounds that you lack confidence in the treatment being proposed. Quacks are often in conflict with established medicine, feeling persecuted for their efforts, while they in turn ridicule established approaches to research and treatment.

The quack usually has a good salespitch. His language is apt to be extravagant in the use of psychological terms with a heavy emphasis on "trust", "natural defenses", "natural products", "relaxation", and "changing your attitude about your illness". The recommended treatment is often backed up with an elaborate explanation of what cancer is, how you got it, and why you have it. Your body may be unable to eliminate impurities or poisons adequately. It may be subject to unusual amounts of irritation or injuries. It may be deficient in some materials, such as a vitamin, or you may be reacting poorly to the unusual stresses in your life. Currently popular is the "immune surveillance" theory that your body normally develops resistance to small, early tumors and destroys them. If the body is somehow weakened so that this defense mechanism fails, cancer may develop. This theory was proposed by a very reputable scientist and has been extensively discussed and even studied experimentally. However, to date there is no clear evidence that surveillance or lack of surveillance play any role in human cancer.

Proof of the value of an unproven treatment is usually by anecdote or testimonial. Anecdotes, ("I knew a man who—"; "I heard of a woman who—"), are particularly convincing if they are told by well-known people: movie stars, politicians, atheletes, or musicians. We have become so used to this form of salesmanship that we often fail to realize that they are not speaking from personal experience or knowledge but only repeating something they have heard, or even been paid to say. A testimonial is more personal in that it represents an account by the person who received the treatment swearing to its effectiveness. However, rarely are the names available or can the people be interviewed directly.

A Doctor's Dilemma.   More difficult is the problem for the person who has received good treatment, only to be plagued by failure and recurrence. Here the desire to try *anything* new that *might* help is completely reasonable and understandable. The physician is in a difficult position when a patient insists on taking an unofficial remedy such as Laetrile, particularly if the disease is advanced. He realizes the importance of maintaining a good relationship in spite of the difference of opinion over unproven treatment. If the doctor is completely immovable the patient must "sneak off to Mexico" for treatment. When the treatment fails, the original relationship may be so damaged by guilt or anger that the patient is unable to bring himself to go back to his original doctor, who may *still* be able to help him. Many doctors find that the best compromise they can reach is to consent to having their patients get Laetrile if they want it, provided they continue on drugs that may be helping them.

The best that can be said for unproven methods of treating cancer is that they will not go away until conventional treatment becomes much better and our fear of this disease is greatly reduced. In the meantime, the best that you can do is obtain as much reliable information as possible about your illness and what *can* be done for it.

twelve
Removing Cancer by Surgery

Surgery is the oldest method of treatment for cancer and remains best for many cancers. There are three reasons for operating: to be sure that it *is* cancer and to learn exactly where it is; to remove the cancer completely if possible, in the hope of curing the disease; and to provide comfort. *The purpose of your operation should be discussed with your own doctor.*

If you have any doubts or questions about what is being proposed you should not hesitate to get a second opinion from another doctor. You may ask your own doctor to suggest one or more names of others who know a lot about your kind of cancer. Your questions should include your fears of any disfigurement or loss of normal function that may be caused by the surgery, as well as its chance of helping you.

There is rarely any emergency in surgery for cancer. An extra day or two to rest at home and get your affairs in order before surgery will free you of some unnecessary worries afterwards.

In the two week period between the diagnosis and surgery I felt as if I was outside of myself. It was like watching myself going through the motions of living. I was so glad when it was over.

BIOPSY The final proof that a disease is cancer comes from studying a small piece of suspicious tissue by microscope. A procedure called a biopsy is usually required to get this tissue. Since very little tissue is needed, the biopsy may be done under local anesthesia with a needle, or by making a small incision in the skin when the tumor is on or near the skin, or is easily felt. General anesthesia may be required to biopsy a tumor deep inside the body. In this case, the surgeon usually plans to remove the tumor at the same time so a second operation will not be

144

needed later. If the cancer cannot be removed, the necessary biopsy will show where the cancer is as a guide for other treatment.

For many cancers surgery offers the best chance for cure. The goal is to remove the entire cancer. Since many cancers spread to nearby lymph nodes, these are often removed at the same time. Surgery is the ideal approach for cancers that have not spread and where removal is possible without being too disfiguring or harmful to body function. These include cancer of the stomach, bowel, rectum, pancreas, kidney, prostate, breast, lung, brain, uterus, ovary, esophagus, thyroid gland, testicle, salivary glands, sarcomas of bones and fibrous tissues, and melanoma of the skin. In some cases, surgery is a high price to pay for possible cure. The possible benefits of completely removing the cancer must be weighed against the injury or loss from the operation. Surgery may also be used with radiation therapy and/or chemotherapy for treatment of some cancers. Radiation is clearly preferable in cases such as some tumors of the face, where there is a choice between surgery which may be disfiguring and radiation which usually is not.

SURGERY FOR CURE

Surgery may be required when the tumor is already known to have spread, in order to provide comfort (palliation) or avoid future complications. For example a cancer of the bowel known to have already spread to the liver would be removed because it is certain to cause obstruction or bleeding later.

SURGERY FOR COMFORT

The trend now is to try to replace destructive and disfiguring surgery with smaller operations combined with other forms of treatment in order to get better results. One example is cancer of the breast where the radical mastectomy developed around 1900 is being replaced by other procedures, with or without radiation therapy or chemotherapy. Major amputations for sarcomas of the arm or leg are being replaced by operations that preserve the limb but remove the tumor, followed by high doses of radiation to kill any tumor cells that may remain. These new approaches are the latest steps in the management of some cancers and represent serious attempts by the medical profession to combine various forms of treatment to get the best possible result while doing the least amount of harm.

Pain, the great horror of surgery, was brought under control over a century ago with the development of anesthesia. There are now three types of anesthesia: local, spinal and general. The choice is based on

ANESTHESIA

the type and extent of the operation and your general health. Except in the case of unusual allergies, which should be brought to the attention of your physician, local anesthesia carries little or no chance of complication. General anesthesia carries a low but significant level of complication, usually from problems with breathing. While a simple biopsy may require only a few minutes, a major operation may take several hours.

Local anesthesia, given by the dentist while working on the teeth is familiar to almost everyone. Injected into the area to be operated on, it is used primarily to biopsy tumors on or near the surface of the body or for biopsies of deep tumors that can be reached with a needle.

Spinal anesthesia involves the injection of a similar pain-killing drug near the main nerve center (spinal cord) in the middle of the back. This injection results in complete loss of feeling in the legs and body up to the lower ribs, for several hours. The advantage of spinal anesthesia is that you are awake, able to cough, and do other things that decrease the risk of complications after surgery. This is of particular importance for people with severe lung disease.

General anesthesia is used most widely. You are put to sleep by an injection in the arm and are kept asleep with a variety of drugs enabling you to rest peacefully throughout long and complicated operations. The anesthesiologist who administers these drugs sits at the head of the operating table where his or her sole function is to keep you comfortably but safely asleep.

BEFORE YOUR OPERATION

Like other major forms of cancer treatment, surgery requires careful evaluation to be sure you can tolerate the operation and to avoid complications. This includes a careful history and physical examination and special attention to the heart (by electrocardiogram, or EKG) and respiratory system (by chest x-ray), blood clotting, and general nutrition, all of which are important to the success of the operation. You should feel free to ask what these studies are and why they are being done.

Operations for cancer are rarely emergencies. There is usually plenty of time to make improvements in your condition so that the operation is safer. This may include giving intravenous fluids or blood before the operation, starting drugs that improve heart and respiratory function, and discontinuing drugs that may interfere with blood clotting. Occasionally days and even weeks are required to improve nutrition in a person who has been unable to eat.

A day or two before your operation your doctor should explain to you exactly what the operation will involve. This should be in terms that you can understand. If you have any questions, be sure that they are answered thoroughly. A great deal of the fear of surgery can be eliminated by knowing what the operation is all about. It is a good idea to have a member of your family or a friend present to meet your doctor and to help you think of questions you would like to ask. It is also a good time to find out when the operation is scheduled and when the surgeon would be available to your family following surgery.

Assuming your operation requires general anesthesia, several steps take place before your operation. In addition to evaluating your cancer and general health, other important things will be done. A sample of blood will be sent to the blood bank and if it is felt that you might need blood during the operation, several units (about a pint) will be set aside for you. You may be taught some special coughing and breathing exercises which will help you after your operation.

The afternoon or evening before surgery, a member of the anesthesia department will visit you to discuss the anesthesia that you will receive. She will be able to answer any questions that you have concerning that part of your care.

A nurse or a doctor will ask you to sign a consent form. It will include the name of the operation and will authorize your doctor to do whatever is necessary for your well-being should anything unexpected be found or occur during the operation. This does not replace getting a full explanation of the operation from your own surgeon. It is merely a legal form for the hospital.

Some operations require special preparation. For example, if your operation includes removing part of your bowel, you will be put on antibiotics for two to three days before surgery and given a laxative and enemas the night before surgery. This is to cleanse and empty the bowel to avoid infection. In the evening you will be asked to bathe carefully, with particular attention to the area to be operated upon. A nurse or orderly may shave the area before surgery or this may be done in the operating room after you are asleep. This is to avoid infection.

On the evening before your operation you may be given a sleeping pill. No one can go to bed very comfortably when faced with an operation the next day. You will be asked to take nothing by mouth after midnight so your stomach will be empty to avoid any possibility of vomiting when you are asleep during the surgery.

THE DAY OF THE OPERATION

If your surgery is scheduled for early in the morning, you will be awakened at about 6:00 a.m. for injections which will make you sleepy and your mouth dry. This dryness is to decrease the mucus that accumulates while you are asleep under anesthesia and unable to cough. The dryness is unpleasant but necessary. At about 7:00 a.m. you will be taken to the operating room. You should leave your valuables—including all jewelry, hairpins, glasses, false teeth, contact lenses, hairpieces, and hearing aid, etc.—in your room or with a family member. If your operation is to follow one or more earlier ones, the same sequence of events will take place later in the day.

You may be taken into a room where the anesthetic is given or directly into the operating room where you will be asked to move onto the operating table. It will be comfortable but narrow so a strap will be loosely placed over you to remind you not to roll over. If you look around you will notice that everyone is wearing a cap and mask to protect you from infection. A nurse will be setting up a table with linen and instruments needed for your operation.

You will be the center of attention for several people, mostly from the anesthesiology department. A needle will be placed in a vein in your arm in order to give you drugs, fluids, and blood throughout the operation. A blood pressure cuff will be placed on your arm so your blood pressure can be checked throughout the operation. You may receive a few instructions from the anesthesiologist, and when everything is ready to go, you will be given a drug, usually Pentothal, through the intravenous needle in your arm. By the time you count to five or ten you will drift off into a completely painless and dreamless sleep.

THE OPERATION ITSELF

It is not possible to outline how each surgical procedure is done and what it accomplishes. The exact details of your operation can only be explained to you by your own surgeon. However, we can take a look at what goes on behind the scenes while you are asleep.

Your surgeon will have one or two assistants who help with the operation and a specially trained nurse (scrub nurse) who handles the instruments. There is another nurse who can leave the room to get other things that are needed (the circulating nurse). The anesthesiologist is seated by your head where he or she can see that you are doing well by checking your blood pressure, pulse, breathing and urine output continuously throughout the operation, and giving you the drugs necessary to keep you safely and soundly asleep.

Because the exact limits of cancer are frequently not visible, the surgeon must often rely on the pathologist during the operation. When tissue is sent to the pathologist, he can freeze it and examine it by microscope quickly and tell the surgeon whether he has removed all the tumor with safe margins of normal tissue. In addition, your surgeon may encounter unexpected problems in other areas requiring different types of surgical experience. In most hospitals the operating rooms are clustered together making it easy to call on a colleague for consultation, advice, or help for some part of the operation.

When you begin to wake up you may still be in the operating room or in a special recovery room where you will remain until you are completely awake and able to take care of simple functions for yourself, particularly coughing and moving around in bed. This usually requres one to two hours. For several more hours you will feel very sleepy and find it hard to stay awake. The first thing you may notice is that your throat is sore from a tube that was placed in your windpipe to help you breathe during the operation. This may seem to be an extreme measure, but it is one of the greatest safety factors in modern surgery. Indeed, you may begin to wake up with the tube still in or while it is being removed. If you cannot breathe well enough alone, because of severe lung disease or after chest surgery, the tube may be left in for several hours or even days and your breathing will be assisted by a machine. Drugs are given to help you breathe with the machine rather than against it. This is not an uncomfortable experience but is frustrating because you are unable to talk while the tube is still in your throat. You will be encouraged to write notes so others can answer your questions and communicate with you.

While you are in the recovery room, and for a few more hours in your own room, your pulse and blood pressure will be taken frequently. You may also have wires from an electrocardiograph taped to your chest (EKG). All of these monitor your heart and breathing as you wake up from your surgery. You may also find that you are breathing oxygen through a plastic mask on your face or a small tube in your nose. This also helps your heart and lungs. It is not uncommon to feel quite cold for a few hours after surgery. If you are uncomfortable, be sure to ask for blankets.

Control of Pain after Surgery. Surgery always produces some pain. You will not have to be awake long before you realize you had an operation and know exactly where it was. The nerves that respond to pain are mostly on the surface of the body. During the first day or two following the operation, there will be pain in the area of the operation even when you lie perfectly still. You will soon find out that any motion at all makes the pain worse. This means that an operation on the arm, the leg or any other area that you can keep still is relatively free of pain. Surgery on the abdomen or the chest is more painful. Even breathing causes some discomfort and the coughing necessary to keep your lungs cleared out can really hurt. Fortunately, there are drugs which control this pain. They are usually given only at your request so you must ask for them when you need them.

One of the remarkable things about the pain following surgery is how quickly it goes away. You can expect discomfort on the day of the operation and the following day. By the second day after surgery the discomfort is usually reduced to about half of what it was and each day after that it decreases to about half of what it was the day before. This means by four or five days after a major operation there is little discomfort except upon real motion. Pain is usually gone in less than a week.

Soon after the operation, even in the recovery room, you will be asked to cough. The evening after your operation you will probably be asked to stand beside your bed and by the next day to take a few steps. You may wonder why such painful exercises are pushed so strongly. An operation is really an injury and not an illness. If you hit your finger with a hammer, you have injured your finger but the rest of you is alright. The same thing is true of an operation even though the area of injury may be much larger. The purpose of coughing, breathing deeply, getting out of bed and walking are to *keep* the rest of you alright. Deep breathing and coughing are to maintain good flow of air through your lungs and to clear your throat and windpipe of secretions which can lead to pneumonia if they are not constantly brought up and spit out. Getting out of bed and walking maintain general muscle tone and keep blood from pooling in certain areas of the body, particularly the legs, where it may form clots. Elastic stocking serve the same purpose.

Tubes. Many people remember the period after the operation because of the variety of tubes involved, many of which were put in while you were asleep. The most frequently used tube is a catheter in the bladder which allows your urine to be measured to see that you are getting enough fluid during and after the operation. This catheter may be removed shortly after the operation or may be kept in place for several days or even weeks if the bladder does not work properly. Another tube frequently used goes through the nostril and throat down into the stomach. This suction tube keeps your stomach and intestine empty of digestive juices and swallowed air. It is very important because abdominal operations are followed by several days of the intestine "taking a rest" and not working properly. Any materials taken by mouth, air swallowed, or backing up of juices produced by the stomach and bowel cause discomfort and eventually nausea and vomiting. All of these are avoided by the use of this tube (nasogastric or N.G. tube). Your doctor can tell when the tube should be removed by listening to your abdomen to hear when your intestine is "waking up". Three sure signs you can monitor yourself that indicate that your intestine is functioning are crampy gas pains that tend to move about in the abdomen, the passing of gas by rectum, and having a bowel movement. When these occur, and often even before, the tube can be removed.

While you are unable to eat, intravenous or I.V. fluid are given through a needle in the arm. Two quarts of fluid are required each day just to keep you comfortable and to provide good urine output. The fluids contain a mixture of salt and sugar. If the period when you need these is not expected to be long, and your nutrition before surgery was good, no attempt is made to give you a balanced diet by intravenous feeding. On the other hand, if intravenous feeding is needed for a long time, usually because the stomach or the intestine is not working properly, very good mixtures are available to maintain normal nutrition. The needle for giving fluids intravenously is kept in your arm until you can take what you need by mouth.

There are also a variety of special tubes associated with different operations. An operation on the chest requires the use of a chest suction tube which is attached to bottles which bubble continuously to regulate the amount of suction. This tube is removed a few days after the operation. In an area where blood or other fluids may collect following the operation, a special drain removes these so they do not become a source of infection. These may be soft rubber or plastic tubes covered with a dressing or they may be plastic tubes connected to small, spring-operated suction devices that pull the fluid out. The latter are used particularly in operations on the breast and neck where fluid tends to collect under the skin.

Dressings. Surgical wounds are usually covered with dressings while you are still in the operating room. The edges seal together quickly, however, and many surgeons remove the dressings one or two days after the operation. If it is necessary to continue to use dressings after you leave the hospital, your nurses will show you how to put them on and the necessary supplies will be sent home with you.

Any attempt to alter the function of the body, even by taking aspirin or penicillin, may occasionally cause an unexpected complication. Surgery is no exception. A great deal of attention that you receive focuses on preventing complications. In addition to the complications associated with particular operations for specific cancers, which your surgeon can explain to you, there are some which can occur after any operation.

Bleeding after an operation may be discovered by an unexplained fall in blood pressure or blood coming from one of the

COMPLICA-TIONS OF SURGERY

drainage tubes. Usually all that is needed is to replace the blood loss until the bleeding stops by itself. Very rarely is it necessary to go back to the operating room to find a blood vessel that will not give up.

The amount of water, salt, sugar, and blood that should be given intravenously can be calculated quite exactly. If not enough fluid is given, you notice dryness of the mouth and produce very little urine. Too much fluid results in difficulty breathing since the heart is unable to keep up with the extra load. Both of these can usually be corrected easily.

The accumulation of mucous in the throat and windpipe, eventually backing up into the lungs, is one of the most important and most serious complication that *you* can help prevent. Even though it hurts to cough, coughing is vital to prevent this from causing pneumonia.

Pooling of blood in the legs or other parts of the body can result in the formation of blood clots in the veins. This may cause soreness of the calf of the leg but frequently goes unnoticed until there is chest pain and a cough, and occasionally difficulty breathing. The sudden appearance of these signs following surgery is an indication to your doctor that a clot from the leg may have moved through the veins up to the lung. It can be checked by a chest x–ray and/or lung scan. If blood clots are found in the lung, drugs will be given for several days or weeks to prevent any more blood clots from forming.

Infection can occur any place where the skin is broken or cut and is no longer protecting the body. The most common places for infection are the wound itself and, less frequently, in tissues or organs deeper within the body. Sterile surgical techniques and antibiotics following some operations have greatly reduced the chances of infection, but they still occur occasionally. If the infection is in the wound, part or all of the skin over the wound may be reopened and covered with dressings to allow the infection to escape. If the infection is deep within the body, it may be necessary to re–operate and place a tube to drain the area of infection.

RECOVERY FROM SURGERY

Any operation takes a great deal of energy out of you. You realize this when you see how weak you are during the first few days after a major operation. Another measure of the stress that you have gone through is the amount of time required to regain *all* the energy you had before your operation. It is common to feel weak or tired for several days or even weeks. This requires you to limit your activities, increasing them gradually day after day. It is frequently not possible to go back to full–time work for several weeks. The rate of recovery is slower in an older person or someone who has been in bed for a long time. The major thing to look for is not immediate complete recovery, but rather a *continuous* gradual increase in strength and return of former energy. It does not really matter how long it takes. It also does not help to just sit and wait. Exercise and gradual resumption of activities speed up the process.

Family members or a close friend should meet your surgeon before the operation and be present when he explains to you what the operation will be and why it is to be done. They should also arrange to see him immediately following the surgery. Most hospitals have a waiting room for this purpose. At that time he should tell them exactly what he found and what he did. He should give you the same explanation when you wake up. He should also give you more details the next day when you are less sleepy and may have some questions you would like to discuss.

YOUR FAMILY AND YOUR SURGEON

thirteen
Treating Cancer with Drugs

Chemotherapy, the treatment of cancer with drugs, differs from surgery and radiation in that anti–cancer drugs spread throughout the entire body and are able to attack tumor cells wherever they may be. In this way chemotherapy reaches cancer cells that may have escaped surgery or radiation, the very cells that could later be responsible for recurrence of the tumor. Over fifty chemicals are used to treat cancer and some tumors can be cured.

Anti–cancer drugs have been developed from a variety of sources. In 1943, the sinking of a Liberty ship loaded with mustard gas resulted in illness and eventual death of several sailors under peculiar circumstances. The poisonous gas was found to have caused severe damage to their bone marrow, resulting in anemia, abnormal bleeding, and infections. These bad side-effects were the first clue that the compound may also have some potential as an anti–cancer agent. Mustard gas was never used for this purpose but its successors, nitrogen mustard and phenylalanene mustard are used today.

Shortly after World War II, two more discoveries opened the door still wider. Dr. Charles Huggins at the University of Chicago found that sex hormones could influence the growth of some tumors, a discovery for which he later won the Nobel Prize. At almost the same time at Harvard University, Dr. Sidney Farber showed that a drug called aminopterin could bring about dramatic but transient remissions in children with acute leukemia. This drug was later replaced by one closely related to it, amethopterin or methotrexate, which is currently used. New anti-cancer drugs are being investigated all the time and chemotherapy stands as one of the most important and promising areas of cancer research and treatment.

Treatment with chemotherapy is highly specialized. The drugs are powerful and, if not properly used, dangerous. Frequently, the margin between enough drug to injure the tumor and too much, doing serious harm, is a narrow one. Doctors with experience in the use of these drugs are invariably those who see many cancer patients. They may be medical oncologists, the new medical specialty dealing only with the use of drugs in the treatment of cancer, or hematologists, doctors specializing in diseases of the blood, or they may be surgeons or radiation therapists who have learned to use the available drugs well. The primary factor is the experience of the individual rather than his or her exact background and training, although they usually go together.

I was on Prednisone and lots of other stuff. It was a real roller coaster. Some days I felt great and other days I was super-depressed. I finally realized that there were days when I felt lousy, not because anything happened but just because I was in a bad mood and lonely. My body was in a bad mood. There was nothing to do but just accept the fact and get away from things that made it feel worse. In a few days it was gone. In fact I felt good, probably because it is so nice to feel up when you have been down. (A person treated for leukemia.)

Although anti–cancer drugs work in different ways, the net result of all of them is to kill cancer cells by preventing them from "growing up" and functioning properly or from dividing to form new cells. The ideal cancer drug would be one which damages only cancer cells and causes no harm to normal cells. Unfortunately such a drug does not exist. The drugs that are now used do significantly more harm to cancer cells but they may still produce unwanted side-effects by injuring normal cells. As with radiation therapy, the difference may be due to greater capacity of normal cells to repair themselves.

There are three main reasons for taking chemotherapy: to attempt to cure the tumor, to attempt to decrease the likelihood of recurrence (adjuvant chemotherapy) after surgery or radiation, or to control growth and relieve symptoms from recurrence (palliation).

WHY CHEMO-THERAPY?

You have every right to know why chemotherapy has been suggested for you. To understand your treatment fully you should ask your doctor to explain exactly which category you fall into, what his expectations for you are, and how he will judge whether the drugs are working. While you may benefit from these drugs, you may also have to endure their side effects. The ultimate decision of whether to start or continue or discontinue chemotherapy is yours.

Chemotherapy for Cure. The miracle of chemotherapy is that in the last few years a few types of cancer have responded so well that one can begin to speak of "cures". They include the following, some of which are treated by chemotherapy in combination with surgery or radiation.

- Acute leukemia (lymphocytic leukemia of childhood, 70 percent survive five years and may be cured.)
- Advanced Hodgkin's Disease (a tumor of the lymphatic system; 40 percent survive five years and may be cured. Many more are cured if the disease is treated early.)
- Testicular carcinoma (not including seminoma, 3 percent cured by chemotherapy with surgery and radiation. Seminoma has a higher rate of cure).
- Wilm's tumor (a kidney tumor of children; 30–40 percent cured by chemotherapy with surgery and radiation.)
- Burkitt's lymphoma (a disease of the lymphoid system seen most frequently in Africa, 50 percent cured by chemotherapy).
- Choriocarcinoma (an uncommon tumor of the uterus in which 90 percent of women can be cured by chemotherapy.)
- Retinoblastoma (a tumor of the eye, usually in infants or young children.)
- Osteogenic sarcoma in children (a bone tumor.)
- Ewing's sarcoma (a bone tumor.)

Just a few years ago, all of these tumors were fatal. At best, however, they account for only about 7 percent of all people treated with chemotherapy. Since many of them are rare tumors, their impact on the overall picture of cancer is not great. However the accomplishment that these results represent should not be underestimated. By proving that it can be done, chemotherapy has been raised to full partnership with surgery and radiation as approaches to the cure of cancer. These tumors are already serving as stimuli and models for treatment of many others.

Why Chemotherapy May Fail. There are several reasons why more cancers cannot be cured by chemotherapy. One of these is the number of cells to be confronted. In order to truly cure a cancer every single cell must be eliminated. A very good drug, which may kill 99.9 percent of the cancer cells could be expected to cure a person who only has 100 or even 1,000 cancer cells. The same drug could not cure a person who has a million cancer cells and may have very little effect on someone who has several billion cancer cells. For this reason it is often more desirable to use chemotherapy after most of a tumor has been removed surgically or destroyed by radiation.

Getting enough drug to the tumor can be difficult. A small

amount of drug undergoes enormous dilution when injected into the blood stream, and even more as it becomes distributed throughout the body tissues. Moreover, many tumors do not receive as much blood as most normal tissues. Some parts of the body, particularly the brain and central nervous system are relatively isolated and some drugs cannot get to tumors in these areas. Many drugs are rapidly broken down and detoxified in the body, and eventually eliminated in the urine. Timing is also a factor. Most anti–cancer drugs act on cells that are actively dividing rather than when they are resting, so that only a portion of the cells making up a tumor are sensitive to the drug during the few minutes that it is present. This has led to continuous administration of some drugs over several hours or days, or to repeated administration daily for several days or weeks. To counterbalance this, it is also necessary to include rest periods, when drugs are not given, to allow the normal tissues to recover. Since each drug has its own optimum timing and rest period, treatment with several drugs can require quite complicated schedules or "protocols".

Finally comes the problem of drug resistance. Some tumors are naturally resistant to all available drugs so that chemotherapy has little to offer. Tumors sensitive to one or a combination of drugs may eventually lose their sensitivity and become resistant. Each time the drug is given, the most sensitive cells are killed but less sensitive ones are not. These are cells that are able to bypass the drug. As this process is repeated the composition of the tumor changes until it is made up entirely of resistant cells. At this point it becomes time to use a different drug.

Chemotherapy Combined with Other Forms of Treatment (Adjuvant Chemotherapy). Because the chances of completely eliminating a tumor are greater when the tumor is small, drugs are often used after initial treatment by surgery or by radiation. It is hoped that at this early time, when no *detectable* tumor remains, any cancer cells still present can be eliminated before they have a chance to become established and grow. Encouraging results have come from studies of cancer of the breast and of osteogenic sarcoma, a bone tumor, and this approach is now being applied to other cancers. At the present state of our knowledge, adjuvant chemotherapy should be reserved for people who have a relatively high risk of recurrence and where drugs effective for the particular tumor are available. It should not be given to people whose cancer has probably been cured by the initial surgery or radiation. The reason for this is not only the toxicity of the drugs while they are being given but also the possibility that they may do harm years later.

Control of Recurrence. Unfortunately many cancers recur after initial treatment by surgery, radiation, or chemotherapy. If they recur in several places throughout the body and cannot be removed, the best method of continuing treatment is chemotherapy. The goal here is to control the growth of the tumor, slowing down its growth or stopping it temporarily, to provide a longer, more productive and comfortable life. Factors to be considered include the response rate of the particular type of cancer to the drugs available, the severity of the pain versus the expected drug toxicity, age, the expected duration of survival from the recurrent tumor, general physical condition, emotional factors, and even such things as the complexities of taking the drugs and the cost of the treatment (for example, hospitalization versus home care). Control of the disease implies slowing down or arresting the growth of the tumor, while palliation is aimed at providing comfort. Neither of these is an attempt to cure the tumor and there are times when continuing treatment may not be the best thing to do.

RECEIVING CHEMO-THERAPY

Chemotherapy should not be undertaken unless an absolute diagnosis has been made on the basis of microscopic studies of the tumor. X–ray studies help determine the location and size of the tumor, if it is known to be present, and for later evaluation of how the drugs are working. It is also necessary for your physician to evaluate your general condition since the drugs place some stress on your system. These include your general nutrition and digestion, blood counts, evidence of any infection, knowledge of any abnormal bleeding, and even psychological problems that could interfere with treatment. Drugs that you are taking for other conditions may be affected by your chemotherapy, so you should be sure to tell your doctor of any and all medications you are on. In addition, you should not have a vaccination with any live vaccine while you are receiving chemotherapy. These include smallpox, measles, polio, german measles, mumps and yellow fever.

What Drugs Will Be Used. By design and by testing and evaluation we have found that some drugs are more effective for certain tumors than others. This matching-up process continues as more drugs are being tried every year. Many cancers are now treated with what may seem like a cocktail of several drugs. These are selected to minimize the toxicity of each drug and to attack the cancer through different mechanisms such as direct killing, prevention of cell growth, or prevention of cell division. The combinations are frequently referred to by their initials, providing a language that would put some government agencies to shame (MOPP, COPP, CMB, and HEXACMF). For many tumors, these combinations are much more effective than any single drug alone.

Table 13.1 lists the drugs used to treat cancer. Listed below are the explanations of the abbreviations used in the table. There frequently are alternatives. While one drug or combination may be the first choice, often there are others that can be used, or held in reserve if the tumor fails to respond to the first treatment. These are important decisions and require the knowledge of a physician experienced in the use of these modern drugs.

How Chemotherapy is Taken. Each drug has its own best way to be taken. A few can be taken by mouth, but most of them are injected into a vein in the arm. Some drugs are taken intravenously for several hours or even days, and some are even administered directly into the blood vessels that go to the tumor. Some require hospitalization if they have to be taken over a long time, or if they may be quite toxic. Others may be taken in the office or clinic, while still others are started in the hospital but continued in the office. The exact schedule and duration of treatment depend on its purpose and how well it works. Treatment of recurrence is usually continued until one drug is no longer effective and then others may be tried. When chemotherapy is used as an adjuvant to surgery or radiation it is usually continued for a prescribed period of time, usually one or two years.

SIDE EFFECTS

Many people have little trouble from chemotherapy and some have none at all. Only rarely is it necessary to discontinue chemotherapy because of side effects. Individuals differ enormously in their reactions to anticancer drugs and it is impossible to predict who will have difficulty.

It will help you avoid unnecessary worry to know something about these possible side effects. A few drugs have very specific effects on the heart, lung, or the kidney. Doctors avoid these by regulating the amount carefully so the total cumulative dose does not exceed the maximum that can be tolerated. More general side effects are due to the fact that most drugs attack normal cells that are rapidly dividing with almost the same vigor that they attack cancer cells. These normal cells include the bone marrow and lymphoid cells responsible for control of infections, the lining of the bowel and bladder, hair and skin, and the reproductive glands—ovaries and testicles.

Digestive Tract. The stomach, the bowel, and even the mouth are lined with a sensitive membrane of cells which divide very frequently. Injury to these mucous membranes may cause nausea and vomiting one to two hours after the drug is taken and continue for several hours. Occasionally this injury causes diarrhea or bleeding

Table 13.1. Drugs Used to Treat Cancer

Drug	Other Names	Class	Taken	Tumors Treated	Acute Side Effects	Major Side Effects
Androgens	(Testosterone, Halotestine, many others)	H	I, O	Breast	—	Water retention, masculinization
Estrogens	(Diethylstilbestrol, many others)	H	O	Breast, Prostate	N, V (rare)	Water retention, feminization, vaginal bleeding
Anti-estrogen	(Tomoxifen)	H	O	Breast	N, V (rare)	—
Progestins	(Many)	H	I, O	Uterus, Kidney	—	Weight gain
Adrenal Steroids	(Many)	H	O, I	Leukemia, Breast, Lymphoma, Myeloma	—	Water retention, high blood pressure, diabetes, infections
Nitrogen Mustard	(Mustargen)	AK	I	Breast, Lymphoma, Lung, Ovary	N, V	Bone marrow, bleeding
Chlorambucil	(Leukeran)	AK	O	Breast, Leukemia, Lymphoma, Ovary	—	Bone marrow, bleeding
Phenylalanine Mustard	(Alkeran, L-PAM, Melphalan)	AK	O	Breast, Melanoma, Myeloma, Osteosarcoma, Ovary	—	Bone marrow, bleeding
Cyclophosphamide	(Cytoxan, Endoxan)	AK	I	Leukemia, Breast, Lymphoma, Lung, Myeloma, Neuroblastoma, Ovary	N, V	Bone marrow, bleeding, hair loss, bladder
Thio-TEPA	(TSPA)	AK	I	Bladder, Breast, Lymphoma, Ovary	—	Bone marrow, bleeding
Busulfan	(Myleran)	AK	O	Leukemia	—	Bone marrow, bleeding, lung
Methotrexate	(Amethopterin)	AM	O, I	Leukemia, Breast, Choriocarcinoma, Head & Neck, Osteosarcoma, Testicle	—	Mouth, digestive tract, bone marrow, bleeding
6-Mercaptopurine	(6-MP, Purinethal)	AM	O	Leukemia, Choriocarcinoma	—	Bone marrow

Table 13.1. Drugs Used to Treat Cancer (continued)

Drug	Other Name	Class	How Taken	Used For	Side Effects	Affects
6-Thioguanine	(6-TG) Thioguan	AM	O	Leukemia	—	Bone marrow
5-Fluorouracil	(5-FU)	AM	I	Bladder, Breast, Colon, Ovary, Stomach	—	Mouth, digestive tract, bone marrow
Cytosine Arabinoside	(Ara-C, Cytosar)	AM	I	Leukemia	N, V	Bone marrow
Adriamycin	—	AB	I	Leukemia, Bladder, Breast, Uterus, Lymphoma, Lung Myeloma, Neuroblastoma, Sarcomas, Wilm's Tumor	N, V	Mouth, digestive tract, hair loss, bone marrow, heart
Bleomycin	Blenoxane	AB	I	Head & Neck, Lymphoma, Testicle	N, V, chills, fever	Mouth, hair loss, lung
Dactinomycin	Actinomycin D Cosmegen	AB	I	Choriocarcinoma, Sarcoma, Testicle, Wilm's Tumor	N, V	Mouth, digestive tract, bone marrow, hair loss
*Daunomycin	Daunorubicin	AB	I	Leukemia	N, V, fever	Bone marrow, hair loss, mouth, heart

KEY TO ABBREVIATIONS

Class

- H = hormone
- AK = alkylating agent: (drug that blocks formation and replication of genes necessary for cell division).
- AM = anti-metabolic: (chemical counterfeits that are similar to normal cell constituents but do not function normally).
- AB = Antibiotic: (products of plants).
- M = miscellaneous drugs whose mode of action is not known.
- MI = mitotic inhibitor—drugs that prevent cell division.

How Taken

- O = by mouth
- I = by injection

Side Effects

- N, V = nausea and vomiting.

Table 13.1. Drugs Used to Treat Cancer (continued)

Mithramycin	Mithracin	AB	I	Testicle	N, V	Bone marrow, bleeding, liver
Mitomycin-C	Mutamycin	AB	I	Colon, Osteosarcoma, Stomach	N, V	Bone marrow
BCNU	—	M	I	Brain, Colon, Lymphoma, Lung, Melanoma, Myeloma	N, V	Bone marrow
CCNU	—	M	iv	Brain, Colon, Lymphoma, Lung, Myeloma		
*Methyl-CCNU	—	M	O	Brain, Colon, Lymphoma, Lung, Melanoma	N, V	
DTIC	Imidazol Carboxamide Dacarbozine	M	I	Lymphoma, (Hodgkins) Melanoma	N, V	Bone marrow
Hydroxyurea	Hydrea	M	O	Leukemia, Melanoma	—	Bone marrow
Cis-Platinum	Cisplatin Platinol	M	I	Testicle, ovary	N, V	Bone marrow, kidney, hearing
Procarbazine	Matulane	M	O	Lymphoma (Hodgkins)	N, V	Bone marrow, mental depression
Vinblastine	Velban	MI	I	Breast, Choriocarcinoma, Lymphoma	N, V	Hair loss, bone marrow, nerves (reflexes)
Vincristine	Oncovin	MI	I	Leukemia, Breast, Lymphoma, Neuroblastoma	—	Nerves (tingling, loss of reflexes) weakness, bone marrow
*Hexamethyl-melamine	—	M	O	Lung, ovary, breast, lymphoma	N, V	Bone marrow, mental depression
*L-Asparaginase	Elspar	AM	I	Leukemia, lymphoma	N, fever, abdominal pain	Liver, pancreas, blood clotting, mental depression

*Experimental drugs, available only at research centers

into the stool. A few drugs may cause sores in the mouth, usually near the corner of the lips. Treatment of these side effects is covered in the section on nutrition (see pp. 000).

Bone Marrow.   A less obvious complication of chemotherapy is damage to the bone marrow and lymphoid system. This may show up as weakness and tiredness from anemia when red cells are not made rapidly enough, abnormal bleeding if enough tiny platelet cells which help blood to clot are not present, or infections when the bone marrow or lymph nodes and spleen do not produce enough white cells. Your doctor will follow your blood counts very carefully. If your white count or your platelet count falls below a critical level, the dose of your drug will be decreased or stopped until your bone marrow has had a chance to recover. Infections may include local skin infections, deeper abscesses, or more serious infections such as pneumonia, kidney infections, and infections of the bladder. Any fever or sign of infection, including a cold, should be reported to your doctor. Antibiotics can prevent or treat infections. Occasionally, if the number of blood cells are too low, it is necessary to take special precautions including isolation from other people for a few days in the hospital, in order to avoid infections. In the treatment of leukemia it has become common to give transfusions of white blood cells, usually from close relatives, to help prevent infections. Anemia and bleeding from lack of platelets are also treated with transfusions of blood.

Hair and Skin.   Loss of hair on the body and head, referred to by one person as "instant aging", is a complication associated with a few drugs. It does not always happen, even with drugs such as Adriamycin, and the loss is often not complete. However, it should be considered in advance because buying a wig is a step that many women and some men will do as a simple precaution. The hair always grows back after the treatment has been discontinued, but it may be thinner and finer in texture than before.

"You're lucky! At least you didn't lose your hair." "Are you kidding? I've been wearing a wig for a year". (Two men talking in their doctor's office.)

Skin reactions are relatively rare. Skin cells are occasionally damaged by drugs. This may cause a rash, reddening, or slight discoloration of the skin. Occasionally these rashes cause itching and may peel like a sunburn does. They can be treated with medications and clear up when the chemotherapy is finished.

Bladder.   Occasionally the lining of the bladder, which is also made up of cells that divide rapidly, may be damaged, causing blood to appear in the urine. It helps to drink large quantities of water while receiving the drugs in order to decrease the concentration of the drug and the possibility of developing bleeding sores in the bladder.

Nerves and Muscles.   Weakness and fatigue are common side effects of many drugs. While this may be due to bone marrow damage, it can also be caused by direct effects of the drugs on nerves and muscles. Some drugs occasionally cause a feeling of tingling in the hands or feet similar to when your hand is asleep. Clumsiness and loss of balance are rare. A few drugs occasionally cause soreness and itching of the eyes, lasting a few days out of each course of treatment. We do not know if this is due to direct irritation or interference with tear formation.

Sexual Glands and Function.   When receiving chemotherapy, one may be too tired to have much interest in sex. The drugs also have a direct effect on the sexual glands. The vagina may become dry and sore. The testicles stop forming sperm and women may stop having their periods. These functions usually return to normal after the treatment has been completed, but there is a slight risk that fertility can be permanently impaired in young adults receiving chemotherapy. This should be discussed carefully with your doctor. Men may wish to attempt to have their sperm frozen to be available later for artificial insemination.

Long-Term Side Effects.   You may wonder why your doctor is reluctant to put you on adjuvant chemotherapy following surgery when the overall outlook is quite good but you realize that there is still some possibility that your cancer may recur. Why take a chance when the drug may help? The problem at the present time is that we do not know very much about the long-term side effects of these drugs years later. Drugs used for chemotherapy have been shown to actually cause cancers many years later, particularly leukemias. In young people who have long life expectancies ahead of them, the use of potentially dangerous drugs to treat a tumor that stands a good chance of being cured by surgery may be more of a risk than our present knowledge justifies. It is quite possible that in the future less dangerous drugs will allow adjuvant therapy to be applied to people with less serious tumors.

Another concern is the long term effect of chemotherapy given to a woman who is pregnant. Many of the drugs used can affect the unborn child, but the time when serious injury can take place is usually limited to the first three months of pregnancy. After that, treatment of the mother has little chance of injuring her child.

GETTING ALONG WITH CHEMO-THERAPY   Most people receiving chemotherapy find that they can continue their normal activities, including both work and play. This may require some cutback with extra days taken off to receive treatment, and perhaps a day of rest to let the effects wear off. Your doctor can tell you exactly what schedule you are going to be on so you can plan ahead. It is a good idea to keep a written record of any side effects to bring to your doctor's attention. He needs this information to regulate your treatment properly so do not feel you are bothering him or that your complaints are not important. More than one combination of drugs can be used and if the drugs you are on now are giving more trouble than they are worth, it may be possible to try others.

There are certain things that you can do to help yourself when receiving chemotherapy. There is no doubt that anxiety and anticipation can increase side reactions. Some people begin to have distressing symptoms, particularly nausea, vomiting, and weakness, *before* they received their monthly injection. A positive attitude can actually reduce toxicity and make treatment more tolerable. It helps to imagine what the drugs may be doing to the cancer cells, visualizing the cancer cells being dissolved like sugar in water, or killed off like bugs exposed to a spray. Anything that is more pleasant to think about than cancer and treatment can be a relief from the anxiety and stress of chemotherapy. Even if you feel weak and cannot keep it up every day, moderate exercise is very helpful to keep your body in good tone. Tell yourself that you can tolerate anything if it is doing some good and does not last too long. All of the side effects of chemotherapy clear up promptly after treatment is finished.

HORMONE TREATMENT

The hormone or endocrine system consists of a number of widely dispersed glands, each of which sends out its own chemical messenger through the bloodstream. Although these chemicals, known as hormones, are distributed throughout the entire body, each one affects only those cells or organs that have particular receptors for that hormone. Thus, one hormone, produced by the pituitary gland at the base of the brain, causes ovulation, while another causes milk to be produced in the breast. Taken together, the network is extensive, affecting many aspects of life, including digestion, energy levels, weight gain, water and salt balance, and sexual growth and activity. Of all the glands that produce hormones, only a few have been found to be significant in the treatment of cancer (See Figure 13.1).

In 1941, Charles Huggens showed that treatment of men with cancer of the prostate with large doses of the female hormone estrogen, caused marked regression of the original prostate tumor and also of metastases to bones. This opened the door to further studies of the effects of hormone manipulation on other tumors. Like chemotherapy, the effects of hormone changes extend throughout the body and can reach tumors that have spread far from their original location. The tumors most commonly treated with hormones include

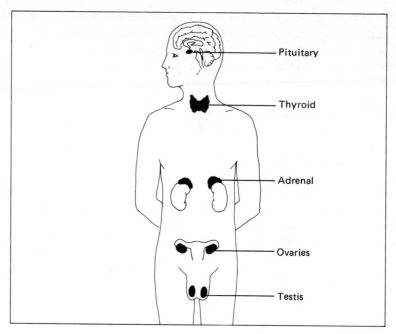

Figure 13.1 The endocrine or hormone system showing only the glands that are important in the hormonal treatment of cancer.

breast, prostate, brain, thyroid, uterus, and kidney, as well as leukemia. Hormone treatment can control or slow down the growth of these tumors but cannot cure them.

There are three main approaches to changing the hormone environment in the body. The first and most obvious is to remove the source of hormone. Removal of the testicles in advanced cancer of the prostate removes the source of male hormones that often stimulate growth of this tumor. Similarly, removal of the ovaries eliminates one of the major sources of estrogens that stimulate the growth of some breast cancers. A second source of estrogen that can be eliminated if necessary is the adrenal gland. This can be accomplished by removing the adrenal glands or by removing the pituitary gland which stimulates most of the functions of the adrenal glands. More recently, drugs have become available which interfere with the action of estrogen and may eventually make surgical removal of these sources of estrogen unnecessary.

The second common way of changing the hormone environment is to give abnormally large amounts of the hormone to which a particular tissue is sensitive. Paradoxically, a breast cancer which may be stimulated by low, physiological levels of estrogen may be slowed down significantly by much larger amounts taken artificially.

Finally, some tumors respond to the opposite hormone. Treatment of prostate cancer with female hormones or breast cancer with male hormones are examples of this.

The side effects of hormone treatment must also be reckoned with. The estrogens can cause nausea, weight gain due to retention of water and salt, uterine bleeding, and accentuation of secondary female characteristics. Men undergoing intensive estrogen treatment for prostate cancer often experience some growth of breast tissue. The male hormones or androgens cause virilization in women, with deepening of the voice and increased growth of facial hair. Both male and female sex hormones produce changes in libido and occasionally in personality. The adrenal corticosteroids, or cortisones, used widely in the treatment of leukemia, lymphoma, and some brain tumors, have a very wide range of side effects, particularly if taken for a long time. These include development of stomach ulcers; weight gain; salt and water retention that may lead to heart failure in people who already have heart trouble; diabetes; accumulation and redistribution of fat on the body and face; psychological changes; and increased susceptibility to infection. Growth may be retarded in children receiving adrenal steroids for leukemia.

The side effects of hormone treatment are usually less than those of many anti-cancer drugs and for this reason hormone treatment is often tried first for tumors where it may be of value. For at least one tumor, cancer of the breast, it is now possible to predict whether or not the tumor will respond to hormone changes. The presence of estrogen receptors in the tumor cells, as discussed in more detail in Chapter 16, indicates that the tumor may respond to hormone treatment. This approach is being extended to other hormones and other tumors.

IS TREATMENT HELPING YOU?

A fair amount is known about which drugs are most apt to be effective for different tumors. Statistics, however, cannot possibly predict how any individual will respond to a particular treatment. Even when the response rate is known to be low, it is often worth a try. Someone has to make up the lucky ten or twenty percent and it might as well be you. Follow-up in the course of your treatment will include x–rays and other examinations to evaluate the size of the tumor and to see whether it is shrinking, staying the same, or growing.

Doctors have their own words for measuring the response of tumors to different drugs. *Response rate* is the statistical chance, based on large numbers of people, that a particular tumor will respond to a given drug or combination. A good response or partial remission usually requires that the tumor decrease by at least 50 percent in size for more than six months, and that no new tumors appear. A complete remission is when no disease is detectable after completion of treatment.

It is obvious that a drug that can reduce a tumor to half of its original size may be very effective in relieving distress. You may be aware of a decrease in the symptoms, particularly pain, caused by your tumor giving you first-hand evidence that the drug is working. Most tumors eventually become resistant to one drug or combination after which a switch to different drugs may be of help. A point is reached in the treatment of many recurrent cancers where it is doubtful that chemotherapy is doing much good, and you and your doctor must decide whether to continue and accept the side effects, or discontinue chemotherapy. However, no area of cancer treatment is changing more rapidly than chemotherapy and who knows what new drugs will be available tomorrow?

THE VALUE OF CHEMO-THERAPY

Of all people treated with chemotherapy and hormone therapy, the picture is as follows:

- Improved to a normal lifespan and probably cured – 7%.
- Good response with relief of symptoms and increased survival – 26%.
- Some response with relief of symptoms but little or no change in survival – 15%.
- Little or no benefit – 52%.

These figures obviously leave a lot of room for improvement, but improvement may be close at hand. Only a few years ago chemotherapy was used as a last resort when all other forms of treatment had failed. This is no longer the case. There is now a gratifying list of cancers for which chemotherapy is the treatment of choice and where survival has been long enough to allow us to speak of cures from chemotherapy alone or in combination with surgery or radiation.

There are also a significant number of tumors for which chemotherapy can significantly prolong life and give relief of distress caused by the cancer. These include carcinoma of the prostate—70 percent respond; breast carcinoma—60–80 percent respond; chronic leukocytic leukemia of adults—50 percent respond; lymphosarcoma of adults–50 percent respond, acute myeloblastic leukemia of adults–65 percent respond; chronic granulocytic leukemia of adults—90 percent respond; multiple myeloma of adults—35–50 percent respond; carcinoma of the ovary—30–40 percent respond;

carcinoma of the lining of the uterus (endometrium)—25 percent respond; melanoma (an uncommon skin cancer)—30 percent respond.

Finally, there are several tumors for which chemotherapy appears to be worth trying, but where the response-rate is not great and the duration of response may be brief. They include the following: lung—30–40 percent respond; head and neck—20–30 percent respond; large bowel—10–30 percent respond; stomach—20–25 percent respond; pancreas—10 percent respond; liver—10 percent respond; cervix and uterus—30 percent respond; sarcomas of soft tissues and bone—40 percent respond; and brain—40 percent respond. Even for these tumors it would be hard to say that chemotherapy should not be tried. It takes only about six weeks to find out if the treatment is doing any good. If symptoms are relieved and the tumor grows smaller, the gamble was won. If there is no change, very little was lost.

Now that chemotherapy has shown its potential for actually curing some tumors, the door is open for continued progress in this area. Although the number of tumors that can be cured is small, for those patients, their families, and their doctors, these results are magnificent. The possibility clearly exists to cure any tumor if the right drug becomes available. Even as this is being written, newer drugs and methods are destined to improve the results.

fourteen
Destroying Cancer with Radiation

WHAT IS
RADIATION
THERAPY? The alternative to removing a cancer is to try to kill the cancer cells where they are. This is the goal of radiation therapy (also called radiotherapy, x-ray treatment, irradiation treatment or therapy, or cobalt therapy). Radiation therapy is the best form of treatment for some cancers. It is sometimes used *with* surgery or chemotherapy and often relieves discomfort from tumors that have recurred or cannot be removed completely.

Radiation bombards cancer cells with rays similar to light and heat, with an energy capable of penetrating deep into the body and damaging or destroying cancer cells. These rays, called x-rays and gamma rays, are not seen as light or felt as heat. An alternative method of bombardment may be by tiny invisible particles (alpha, beta, electrons, or neutrons).

Although there are several sources of these rays and particles, their effects on cancer cells are the same. They either kill them, or stop them from dividing and producing more cancer cells. In either case, the threat is eliminated; the cells eventually die and are removed by normal healing processes. Radiation damages normal cells along with cancer cells, but normal cells may be less sensitive or are able to repair the damage quickly. Radiation is targeted at a small area and does not spread throughout the body. More important, you are not made radioactive by receiving radiation therapy and no radiation remains after the treatment. These are what allow radiation to be used in the treatment of cancer.

The type of radiation used for cancer treatment is similar to the x-rays that take pictures of broken bones or tracer techniques that find cancers. The difference is that greater amounts of radiation are needed for treatment of a cancer than for these harmless studies. Examples of the relative amounts of radiation used for different purposes are given in Table 14.1.

Table 14.1. Relative Exposures to Radiation (in Rems)

Type or Purpose of Radiation	Dose of Radiation
Normal background, average in USA	0.1-0.13/year
Maximum allowed for general public	0.5/year
Maximum allowed for radiation workers	5.0/year
Average received by x-ray technicians	0.1-0.5/year
Diagnostic chest x-ray	0.05
Xeromammogram	2
Upper GI series or barium enema	25-50
Radiation treatment of cancer	3000-8000 (total treatment)

RADIATION FOR CURE

About half of all people who have cancer receive radiation treatment at some time. For some tumors radiation is the main treatment and offers the best chance of cure. These include many cancers of the head and neck, including the lip, tongue and cheek; skin cancers (with the exception of melanoma); cancers of the cervix and body of the womb (uterus); some bladder cancers; cancer of the vocal cords (voice box); some tumors of the testicle; some childhood tumors; and the lymphomas, particularly Hodgkin's disease. Skin cancers, although usually very slow growing and rarely fatal, are often on the face where they can be seen. Cancers of the mouth, lip, or tongue are also highly visible. Many of these can be treated by surgery or radiation. When there is a choice and radiation can cure the tumor, it has the advantage of causing little or no scarring. The same is true for early cancer of the vocal cords, where radiation can preserve the function of the voice. Radiation treatment of Hodgkins disease that has not spread has been so successful in the last twenty years that over 90 percent of patients are cured by radiation alone. Cancer of the cervix is treated by radiation or surgery, depending on its extent. The other tumors on this list are usually treated with radiation plus surgery with very good results.

Radiation offers an alternative for people who cannot have surgery. These include cancer of the breast, lung, brain, ovary, esophagus, thyroid, and some tumors of the testicle. For some of these, the cure rate is not as high with radiation as it is with surgery.

Many trials using combined forms of treatment are taking place throughout the world. Radiation therapy with surgery, or radiation therapy with chemotherapy, or all three are being used to improve on the results which can be obtained with any one form of treatment. The combination of radiation and surgery may not only give a higher cure rate, but preserve function and reduce scarring by allowing the surgeon to do a smaller operation. This combination has seen its best results in some of the sarcomas and brain tumors, and is now being looked at carefully as a better treatment for cancer of the breast.

Radiation and chemotherapy are being combined in treatment of cancer of the lung, ovary, more advanced Hodgkins disease, leukemia and many others.

RADIATION FOR COMFORT

When that heavy door closes I feel very alone. The machine is so big and I am so small. But then I begin to think about it killing my cancer and I feel better.

It is not always possible to completely remove a cancer by surgery or to cure it by radiation or chemotherapy. When the surgeon knows or suspects that some cancer has been left behind she will often ask for radiation treatment to eliminate the remaining cancer or slow its growth. When cancers do recur, either in their original location or other parts of the body, radiation is frequently used to relieve pain and restore normal function. Discomfort from cancers that spread to the bones, particularly from the breast or prostate, is usually relieved promptly by radiation of the involved bone. The amount of radiation needed is relatively small with little or no side effects.

PLANNING YOUR TREATMENT

The best treatment for you is planned by a radiation therapy specialist and may take several days after your first visit. She will want to look at slides from a biopsy of your tumor and at your hospital records. She will give you a physical exam based on the amount and type of treatment your cancer will require. Radiation therapy is strong medicine, and cancer cells do not give up easily. When the tumor is small and near the surface of the body the amount of radiation required may produce only a small amount of stress. On the other hand, if the tumor is big and a large amount of tissue must be radiated, the stress and side effects may also be great. For this reason, the very first step in treatment planning will be a careful evaluation of your general physical condition. This will include your level of nutrition, any evidence of infection or bleeding, and any abnormality in heart function, breathing, or digestion.

Exactly Where is the Cancer? The next step is to determine the exact location of the tumor and its margins, that is, where it begins and where it ends. Again, if the tumor is on the surface of the body and easily seen, this is no problem. If the tumor is deep within the body, such as the stomach, its exact location will be found by picture x–ray studies involving the swallowing of barium. Necessary studies, including x–rays, scans, and ultrasound, will determine the exact location and extent of the tumor in order to treat it completely while minimizing the amount of radiation to normal tissues.

What Kind of Radiation is Best for You? The type of cancer and its location will determine the type of radiation your doctor chooses. Cancers deep within the body require very high energy radiation. Different cancers have different sensitivities to radiation, just as normal tissues. Cancers of the blood, bone marrow (leukemias) and lymphomas are sensitive to radiation, while many tumors of harder tissues such as bone, fibrous tissues, and nerve tissues are not. This means that a less sensitive tumor will require more radiation to destroy most or all the cells. It is important to realize that complete destruction of a tumor is not always possible and that sometimes reducing the size of the tumor for relief of pain is all that can be hoped for.

Another decision concerns the best way to give the radiation. For most cancers, this involves external radiation from one of a variety of different machines that produce or release the appropriate rays or particles. For some other tumors, radiation is given by placing a potent source of radiation, usually radium or cesium, inside the body. A physician must be able to reach the organ involved for this type of application. It is most commonly used for cancer of the cervix or the body of the uterus.

Most people can receive external radiation treatment four or five times a week as outpatients. This is not true for internal radiation. In carcinoma of the cervix, the radiation source must be placed in the vagina in direct contact with the cervix. This is done in the operating room under local or general anesthesia. You may be asked to lie on your back continuously throughout the two or three days required for treatment. This becomes uncomfortable but helps keep the radium in the right place. Because strong radiation might constitute a danger to other people, visitors should be limited to family members. They sould not stay more than half an hour and should sit at least five feet from your bed. Removal of the internal radiation at the end of the treatment is done in your bed and is not painful. After that you can be up and around and have as many visitors as you like. You no longer have a radiation source inside you that is a hazard to anyone. Treatment of this type requires hospitalization for several days.

Important factors in planning radiation therapy include how often treatments should be given—usually daily for five days a week; how long each treatment should last—usually a very few minutes; and how much radiation should be given each time. A single large dose of radiation is much more destructive to both normal and tumor cells than the same total amount given in several doses over a longer period of time. Divided doses, however, have the advantage of allowing normal tissues to recover between treatments. Tumor cells are most sensitive to radiation at the time they are actually dividing. Since they are not all dividing at the same time, and there is no way of knowing when any particular cell is dividing, repeated treatments day after day is usually the best way to damage the largest number of cancer cells. This means that some treatment schedules can last for several weeks in order to give the total required dose to the cancer.

Some normal tissues such as the kidneys, lungs, heart, or ovaries—more easily injured by radiation than others—are avoided by directing the radiation past them or by protecting them with lead shields. The shields must be made for each person and are placed outside the body to block out part of the radiation beam during treatment.

The several types and sources of radiation available allow your doctor to select one that is best suited for your particular cancer. A tumor on or near the surface of the body does not need radiation that passes through and damages other tissues beyond the tumor. On the other hand, a tumor deep within the body should be radiated in such a way that the surface skin gets as little radiation as possible while the tumor itself gets a great deal. This is accomplished by giving the radiation from several directions or through several fields, decreasing the amount of radiation to any particular area of skin while concentrating the full effect on the tumor within the body (see Figure 14.1).

The area to be treated frequently includes not only the cancer but also the lymph node areas where the tumor may have spread. Since your treatment may involve radiation from different directions, and extend over a period of many days, it is important that the machines always be accurately aimed. This requires placing you in the same position each time for each individual exposure and marking on your skin the exact area where radiation will enter the body. It is usually done with a purple marking pen which leaves stains that do not wash off easily.

Choosing the Best Final Plan.   At this point, it is time for a test run in which a simulator is used instead of the treatment machine. It requires that you lie on an x–ray table and have pictures taken from several different directions. In this way, the best positions for treatment are determined.

Many different things are involved in determining the best treatment for any individual. These include the type of cancer; its location and size; body structure or build; general health; and nearby normal structures that should be avoided. This information and data from the simulator are computerized to suggest the best treatment for you. The computer determines the number of treatments, the

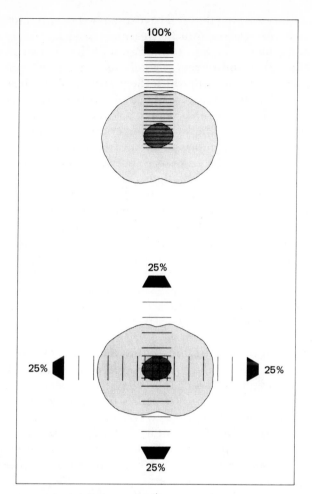

Figure 14.1 Use of multiple portals to treat tumors deep in the body. The same tumor dose divided between four portals reduces the radiation to any one area of skin or intervening tissue to 25% of that of a single portal.

amount of radiation at each treatment, and the exact direction from which each treatment should be given. In this way alternative plans can be arrived at quickly, work that could require several days without the computer. Sometimes there will be only one obvious treatment. Other times there may be a choice of treatments with the best selected by your doctor on the basis of his experience.

Now that the rehearsals are over and the planning is done, treatment can begin.

Sometime before your treatment begins you will be asked to sign

TREATING YOUR TUMOR

a consent form showing that you have discussed your illness with your doctor, that you understand the treatment, and have agreed to it.

Depending on the size and location of the area to be radiated you may be asked to undress partially or completely and put on a hospital gown. The room in which the treatment is given is different from that used in the simulation. It usually involves passing through a heavy door or curved tunnel behind a thick wall. This protects the staff from continuous exposure to high energy radiation. You will be positioned exactly as you were in the simulation. The treatment machine itself is apt to be very large and much of the moving around must be done by you rather than the machine. Once you are in position the area to be treated will be checked again by taking an x–ray picture. When it shows that everything is alright you will receive your first treatment. You should lie still for the two to five minutes the treatment lasts. There is no discomfort while the treatment is being given. For the safety of the people caring for you they are not able to stay in the treatment room at the time the machine is turned on. However, they can see you and talk with you by a television intercom system and keep track of exactly what is going on. For children it often helps to have a parent read to the child over the intercom.

Some cancers require only one treatment from one direction each day while others may require treatment from two or three different directions with a change of positions between each treatment each day. Treatments are usually given at the same time each day. The time can often fit your convenience so be sure to let your doctor, nurse, or technician know if you have a preference. Repeated treatments can be depressing at first as a constant reminder of your disease. This usually gets better as treatment ends and you begin to be aware that it has done some good.

Treatments are given by trained technicians under the supervision of your doctor. Generally you see the same technician each time and will get to know her quite well. The technician will ask how you feel each day and you should be sure to mention any changes so that the doctor can be called to see you. The doctor will see you frequently during your treatments and again one month later to be sure that you are recovering well. She may continue to see you or may refer you back to your own family doctor for follow-up.

What is Happening to the Cancer?   Usually you are not aware of any change taking place in the tumor, only of the side effects. Occasionally large tumors near the surface of the body, such as lymph nodes in Hodgkin's disease, may increase in size and cause some pain for a few days, before they shrink and the pain disappears. Occasionally bone tumors become more painful for a day or two after treatment is started before they begin to get better. With many tumors the good effects of radiation may continue for a week or two after the last treatment has been given. Damaged cells do not die right away and the healing process is not as rapid during treatment as it is after treatment is finished.

Side effects from radiation treatment differ. Since it is impossible to predict who will have side effects or what they will be, the following outline will help you understand what *may* happen, while hoping that it will not.

Side reactions to radiation therapy are due to normal tissue damage. Some tissues are particularly sensitive. These include the skin, the lining of the bowel, and the bone marrow cells and white cells in the blood. Other tissues, which are less sensitive but avoided in treatment if possible, include the liver, kidney, lung, and heart, and glands such as the thyroid, testicles, and ovaries.

Skin. Some skin is almost always exposed to radiation. Signs of injury similar to sunburn show up in about two weeks. At first there is reddening of the skin and hair loss in the treated area. Occasionally, there is even blistering. As radiated skin heals it shows a deep tan which may be more permanent than usual. There may be some itching and scaling of the skin during this healing phase. People differ greatly in their sensitivity to the sun just as they differ in sensitivity to radiation. In general, those with fair skin and hair react more easily. Healed areas of skin that received high doses often show permanent changes in which the color of the treated area is lighter or darker than normal, and the skin is thin and more easily injured. Occasionally the skin becomes thicker than normal and feels leathery. Minor injuries to areas that received high doses of radiation are apt to heal poorly.

A skin reaction in the radiated area is a normal response and is almost always temporary, showing little or no evidence of the treatment several months later. This is particularly true with the deeper penetrating forms of radiation which cause less skin damage. There are steps that can be taken to decrease discomfort of radiation damage to the skin while the treatment is being given. These include keeping the area dry; avoidance of washing the area, except under specific instructions from your doctor; *no* use of ointments or lotions unless they have been approved by your doctor; avoidance of the application of heat to the irritated area; and avoidance of direct sunshine or exposure to cold in the radiated area until it has become normal again. Any scabs or sores that form should be left alone but called to the attention of your doctor so that he can check for infection. Itching can be treated with corn starch or baby powder, but only on your doctor's advice. Other powders or ointments should be reserved until after the treatment has been completed since some of them interfere with radiation. Any irritation to the radiated area should be avoided. Although gentle washing is permissible, rough drying of the skin with a towel can be harmful. The marks painted on the skin should be carefully preserved and not washed away. Shaving with ordinary razors should be avoided but the careful use of an electric razor is permissible. Loose fitting clothing in the radiated area (open collars, no bra or tight girdle) helps avoid irritation.

After the treatments have been completed, the ink marks may be washed off and baby oil will help if your skin is dry or itchy. You may go back to wearing whatever is comfortable, but you will always have to be careful not to expose the radiated skin to sunlight because it will burn easily.

Internal Organs. Some organs and tissues beneath the skin are sensitive to radiation. If a tumor of the arm or leg is being treated, the deep tissues of bone and muscle are extremely resistant to radiation and little or no discomfort can be expected beyond the skin changes already mentioned. On the other hand, if radiation is being given to a tumor inside the body, organs sensitive to radiation may be injured. The injured tissues heal and the discomfort disappears promptly after the treatment is finished.

The lining of the digestive tract, including the mouth, esophagus, stomach, and bowel, is easily injured by radiation. Treatment of any part of the abdomen or bowel, while painless at the time of treatment, may be followed within hours by nausea and even vomiting. This may follow every treatment. A more severe side effect may be diarrhea or dark bloody material in the stool. These problems should be reported to your doctor. Fresh fruits and vegetables, spicy or greasy foods, and milk should be avoided because they tend to give diarrhea. Nausea and vomiting are helped by avoiding fatty foods and drinking skim milk or carbonated drinks such as ginger ale. Frequent small meals, snacks of toast or crackers, and sucking on hard candy all help to combat nausea. Several drugs are also available to reduce the discomforts of nausea, vomiting, and diarrhea and can be used without danger.

When the lower abdomen or pelvis is treated, the lining of the bladder may be damaged, resulting in pain on urination and occasionally blood in the urine. Drinking lots of water (eight or more glasses per day) helps prevent irritation of the bladder. There are drugs for these problems too, so be sure to ask. Women should not have intercourse during the several weeks they are having abdominal radiation. Vaginal discharge may increase with pelvic radiation and douching should be done at least twice a week or as often as necessary (one tablespoon of vingear in one quart of warm, not hot, water). Menstrual periods usually stop at this time, either temporarily or permanently, depending on how much radiation is given. You should report any vaginal bleeding.

The Mouth.   The linings of the mouth, throat, and esophagus are easily injured by radiation. Treatment of tumors of the mouth and neck is usually associated with dryness of the mouth, loss of taste, sore throat, and pain on swallowing. Radiation of the chest may also cause pain in the area of the esophagus and difficulty swallowing. Before treating tumors in or near the mouth, it is necessary to remove any teeth that are not in good condition. The reason for this is that the blood supply and health of these teeth is damaged by the radiation, making dental treatment painful and difficult.

To reduce irritation in the mouth, it helps to brush your teeth gently after every meal with a soft brush and toothpaste or baking soda. The use of a water pick, frequent gargles, mouth washes, and sprays also help. Dentures should fit well and be left out as much as possible. Your doctor can prescribe other ointments, lozenges, or sprays that work well. These should be used before meals and at bedtime. A bland diet of frequent small meals which do not require much chewing are more comfortable to eat. Depending on how sore your mouth is or how difficult it is to swallow, you may prefer ground or pureed foods or even liquids. Spicy or sour foods may be hard to swallow. Your food should contain plenty of calories and should be eaten warm but not hot.

Blood.   The other important cells which are very sensitive to radiation are the blood cells and bone marrow, where the cells are produced. If the area being radiated is small, the amount of bone marrow exposed to the treatment is too small to give any trouble. However, if the area is large, the bone marrow is temporarily damaged and the blood count must be watched carefully. This is particularly true of the white cells which help to fight infections, and the platelets that are responsible for blood clotting. Because these tissues recover very rapidly when treatment is stopped your doctor will check these levels frequently during treatment to be sure that they are staying at a high enough level. This only requires a drop of blood from your finger. If the count falls too low, treatment will be stopped temporarily.

Other organs which are relatively sensitive to radiation are protected by lead shields, unless they are involved with the cancer. These include the eye, the kidneys, the lungs, and the heart. Reproductive organs—the ovaries in women and the testicles in the men—can be damaged by radiation and must be protected unless they are being treated.

Radiation Sickness. Radiation sickness, a general reaction to radiation therapy, can occur in anyone if a large area is being radiated. Similar in effect to seasickness, it includes nausea, vomiting, weakness, headache, and general tiredness. If a person is already quite debilitated, this may be severe enough to require hospitalization or interruption of treatment. While several drugs are available to combat these various problems, it is most important to maintain your general health. Keeping up your nutrition, even when your appetite is gone and you feel nauseated, increases your tolerance for treatment and speeds up recovery after the treatment is over. Try new foods or old favorites prepared in any way that makes them acceptable. A nutritionally balanced diet is so important that you should be sure to discuss any eating problems with your doctor.

Most people tolerate radiation very well, with few side effects. Treatment can always be discontinued for a few days or stopped if necessary.

fifteen

Caring for a Person with Cancer

"The secret of care is caring".
We never thought we could do it but we did, and it made us feel very good.
Looking back, even his death was less frightening than it would have been in
the hospital.

HOME CARE

Many families wish to take care of a member who is ill at home as long as possible, even to the time of death. The requirements for this include having adequate day-to-day help, medical and nursing help, instruction in medical and nursing techniques, and availability of appropriate equipment and supplies. There is no type of cancer that categorically cannot be cared for at home.

Help.   Good home care requires constant supervision and support by a trained nurse with backup from a physician whenever necessary. Most communities can provide this. Many hospitals have developed their own home nursing services for patients who have left the hospital, while other communities rely on visiting nurses or public health nurses.

Most people are surprised at how little technical knowledge is needed to provide good home care, and how easily it is acquired. Learning should begin in the hospital where staff nurses can teach you whatever daily techniques may be required. These may include care of the skin, care of wounds and sores, care of the mouth, suctioning of respiratory secretions, administration of pain medication, the safe use of oxygen, irrigation of urinary catheters and other drainage devices, even the changing of bottles for intravenous feedings, and many more.

Many families feel that they do not have enough help within the family to care for someone who is seriously ill. The fact is that spouses often provide excellent care almost alone. Most families can go outside for help. Close friends or neighbors, practical nurses, or home aids are sources of day-to-day help.

Supplies and Equipment.   Much of the equipment commonly used in the hospital is also available for use at home. Supplies for bed care that save on work and laundry include large absorbent cotton pads backed with plastic, which are waterproof (Chux), and large cotton bandages (ABD pads). A hospital bed that can be raised and lowered, a table that fits over the bed, and a wheelchair are often important items for home care. A special alternating pressure mattress or a thick piece of lamb's wool may be necessary to prevent pressure sores from developing on a person who is confined to bed. With proper instruction, oxygen equipment can be used at home. Other things include special bandages, catheters, feeding tubes, irrigating and suction equipment, and cleansing solutions. Many items of equipment or supplies can be obtained free from your local American Cancer Society. Others can be obtained through your hospital or through a medical supply company on a rental basis.

Careful records should be kept because the cost of all of these can be deducted for tax purposes and many of them are included in good health insurance plans. As more people want to try home care, there is pressure on insurance companies to provide adequate coverage, particularly since it is much less expensive than hospitalization. You should check with your own insurance agent to see what aspects of home care are covered and with your doctor or nurse to see what hospital and community resources may be available to you.

NUTRITION

Many illnesses cause loss of appetite. This presents no problem when the illness is of short duration since the body can go for several days with little or no food, as long as there is adequate intake of fluid. In a longterm illness, such as cancer, a cycle is easily established in which the tumor or its treatment causes a loss of appetite. This results in weight loss and weakness, leading to further loss of appetite. Since poor intake can actually decrease tolerance for treatment, maintaining good nutrition is an important responsibility that must be shared by patients and families together.

Causes of Loss of Appetite

The causes of loss of appetite and poor nutrition in cancer include obstruction by the tumor, depression, pain, side reactions of treatment, and poorly understood but often severe loss of appetite and loss of weight associated with advanced disease.

Obstruction by the Tumor.   Tumors that involve any part of the digestive tract can interfere with eating or the digestion of food.

Cancer of the mouth, throat, or esophagus can make swallowing difficult or painful, particularly during treatment. Any tumor of the stomach, small bowel, or large bowel can cause obstruction, usually making itself known as crampy pain, nausea, vomiting. Even tumors of other organs in the abdomen, such as ovary or pancreas, can obstruct the digestive tract.

Depression. Purely emotional causes of loss of appetite are usually easily identified and, fortunately, of short duration. Anxiety and depression are common when a tumor is first discovered, when it has been found to recur, when surgery is necessary, or when treatment must be changed. Usually the course of events, including starting or changing treatment, provides an emotional lift in a few days and appetite returns.

Pain. Chronic pain presents a serious obstacle to good nutrition. It is almost impossible to eat when you are uncomfortable, and one of the major blessings of pain relief is return of your desire to face food.

Treatment. Unfortunately the treatment of cancer can also interfere with good nutrition. It is in this area that the need to maintain a good dietary intake is most obviously important. Surgery with general anesthesia always prevents eating for a day or two. Abdominal operations, even when they do not directly involve the digestive tract, may require as long as a week before the digestive tract functions properly again. This relatively short time is well tolerated by anyone who is well nourished to begin with.

Radiation therapy poses a greater problem because it is usually given over a period of several weeks. Many tumors of the head, neck, and mouth, are treated with radiation. The mucous membranes that line the mouth and the throat are very sensitive and may become sore enough to make swallowing painful. Radiation of the abdomen is often associated with loss of appetite, nausea, vomiting, and diarrhea.

Many drugs used to treat cancer cause loss of appetite, nausea, or vomiting in *some* people. These side effects of chemotherapy may be experienced off and on for months or even as long as treatment continues. For reasons that are not known, many people have no trouble at all. Usually these symptoms come on soon after the drug is received and wear off within twenty-four hours. Drugs that are taken daily can obviously give more prolonged distress. Although every effort should be made to do so, most people find it hard to maintain good nutrition at the height of the side effects of either chemotherapy or radiation, so that it becomes all the more important to make it up between treatments when you are feeling well.

Weight Loss in Advanced Cancer. Severe loss of appetite and weight are common in advanced disease. The reasons for this are not known, but the observation that some people lose weight even when their food intake appears to be adequate suggests that the tumor may use more than its share. This late effect is distressing to see, and it is very hard to combat. Moreover, there is no evidence that forced feeding or any other artificial methods of providing nutrition can lengthen life. Since this loss of weight is not associated with any discomfort from hunger, it is probably better to accept it as being unavoidable.

Getting Enough to Eat
The treatment of cancer has many ways of interfering with good nutrition. For each of them there are a variety of simple steps that can help you stay ahead.

Loss of Appetite. Loss of appetite implies lack of interest in food or a feeling of fullness when you have eaten very little. Many drugs, as well as radiation, can cause this.

In addition to supplying bodies with necessary energy, most people consider eating an aesthetic experience. When the desire for food is decreased, it can often be revived by emphasizing this aspect. Food that is cooked nicely, attractively arranged, and served with flowers, a bright napkin, or simple table decorations can make every meal slightly festive. A small serving on a dessert plate, which can be finished, may be more appetizing than a large serving on a large plate.

Eating is also a social function and most people do not like to eat alone. A leisurely meal with members of your family, occasionally inviting in a friend, emphasizes this. The surroundings should be quiet and mealtimes should not be used to air grievances or for confrontations.

Light exercise between meals, as well as a cocktail or wine before eating may stimulate an appetite. Washing before you eat makes you feel clean and prepared. Comfort is also important and pain medication should be timed to give maximum relief at mealtime. It is easier to eat sitting up than lying down, and it is more distracting to eat in the dining room or in the living room in front of the television set with others, than to sit alone in a bedroom.

People respond differently to the odors of cooking food. Strong food odors may depress the appetite or cause nausea in which case it is better to stay away from the kitchen before mealtime. On the other hand, many people find the smell of baking bread, brownies, or cookies irresistible. The child who is ill may take more interest in his food if he can help prepare it.

Some foods are more tiring to eat than others. If chewing and swallowing are difficult, most foods can be cut into smaller pieces that are easier to eat without losing their flavor.

Finally, we should recognize how greatly our eating habits are influenced by our culture. The established patterns of what and when we eat are convenient but hardly necessary. Illness requires experimentation and flexibility. The person who is too sleepy to eat anything at 7:00 a.m. may be ready for a good breakfast by nine. Similarly, a large meal or dinner can just as well be eaten in the middle of the day as in the evening. Indeed, five or six small meals, with the last one just before bedtime, may be better than attempting to make any one meal particularly large.

Nausea and Vomiting.   Many drugs as well as radiation therapy cause nausea and vomiting. At the height of these distressing side effects, eat whatever you can whenever you can. Concern about nutritional standards should be put off until you feel better. If nausea and vomiting come on soon after receiving a certain drug, you may plan your mealtimes around that, knowing that you are going to feel ill for a few hours.

Clear soups, water, and cold soft drinks are usually tolerated. Toast and salty foods, such as crackers, can add a little nourishment. Some people tolerate rice, potatoes, or soft boiled eggs. You should avoid any foods that seem to cause nausea. These often include greasy or very sweet foods and those with strong odors. Bottled water which has no chlorine in it is often better-tasting than tap water. An alternative is to let the tap water stand in a pitcher at room temperature overnight and serve it chilled with ice. Most of the chlorine escapes in a few hours.

It helps to eat slowly, taking small frequent meals, and some people get relief by lying down for a few minutes after eating. Your doctor can prescribe anti-nausea drugs for severe distress. Marijuana has been tried for this purpose and found useful by some people.

Change of Taste.   Radiation therapy often causes a loss of taste for food which may last two or three months. Chemotherapy can go a step further and actually change the taste of food. People differ enormously in this respect, but in general there is a tendency for sweet foods not to taste sweet enough while bitter foods taste too bitter. The use of additional sugar and of nonbitter spices can make foods taste less bland. Meats pose a particular problem for many people because they tend to taste unusually strong and bitter. To cover this up, strong seasonings such as tomato or oriental sauces can be used. Even the odors of meat cooking can be distressing. Fish, eggs, poultry, and mild cheeses are good substitutes for beef and pork. Foods that taste too sweet can be toned down with small amounts of vinegar or lemon juice. Salt also helps to tone down sweet or acid foods. Other ways to boost flavor include orange slices, lemon on chicken or fish, fresh vegetables instead of canned or frozen ones, combining soups or making your own from almost anything on hand, the addition of cinnamon, raisins, or other fruits, as well as brown sugar or honey on hot cereals. Bacon bits, sliced almonds, small pieces of ham, onion, or mushrooms add flavor to vegetables.

Dry Mouth, Sore Mouth, Sore Throat. Radiation of tumors of the head and neck area injures the glands that produce saliva, resulting in dryness of the mouth which is usually permanent. This can be overcome by using soups, gravies, and sauces to moisten the food. Dry foods such as toast, bread, or cakes can be dunked in tea or coffee or swallowed with sips of liquid. Chewing gum and hard candies stimulate production of saliva.

Both radiation and chemotherapy can cause soreness of the mouth while treatment is in progress. A soft diet, including finely chopped meats, vegetables, and fruits served cold are easier to handle. Ice cream, popsicles, melons, and grapes are soothing. Using a straw may help to get liquids far back in the mouth where they go down quickly without bothering the sore areas. Sweet drinks may be soothing, while spices and acid foods such as tomatoes and fruit juices may be painful. If pain on eating and swallowing are severe, your doctor can give you medication that will numb the mouth and throat at mealtime.

Cramps and Diarrhea. Radiation to the abdomen and some chemotherapy drugs can cause cramps and diarrhea. If this is a problem you should avoid rough foods such as bran, whole grain cereals, seeds, beans, vegetables, dry or raw fruits, or nuts. The exception to this is bananas which are soothing and provide the mineral potassium which is lost in diarrhea. Large quantities of fluids should be taken and extra salt should be added to make up for losses. Clear liquids, crackers, and rice are good to start with. Potatoes, meat, and milk may also be tried. Your doctor can give you a medicine to control severe diarrhea.

Constipation. Constipation may be a problem for people who are on morphine-like pain drugs or who are already taking soft or liquid diets. The changes in diet are just the opposite of those listed for diarrhea in that your food should include more fiber. If possible you should eat whole grain cereals, bran, raw and dried fruits or vegetables and nuts. If these are painful to chew or swallow they may be replaced by prune juice, adding bran to cooked cereals, and adding grated raw fruits or vegetables to the soft diet.

Weight Loss, Protein, and Calories

The net result of anything that interferes with good nutrition is weight loss due to lack of protein and calories. Calories are necessary to provide energy for the demands of everyday life, and to spare the body from having to break down its own tissues to meet these demands. Extra protein is needed in the diet to help the body replace normal cells that are damaged or destroyed by treatment. The cells must be given every chance to recover between treatments. The following are suggestions to help you boost your intake of protein and calories.

Meat is our usual source of protein but other very good ones include: cheese, eggs, nuts, peanut butter, avocado, lentils, beans, yogurt, powdered milk, cereals, all kinds of fish, milkshakes, eggnog, and sandwich meats. Homemade milkshakes can include almost anything besides milk: fresh fruits (particularly banana), ice cream, peanutbutter, eggs, nuts, honey, maple syrup, fruit juices and many more.

Skim milk powder added to regular milk increases the protein and caloric content. Powdered milk can also be added to sauces and gravies with the same effect. Raw egg or chopped hardboiled egg can be added to gravy without changing the taste. Extra calories can be obtained by using milk or even half milk and half cream in making up cocoa and canned soups, or puddings. Meat, fish, or poultry breaded and fried in fat contain more calories than the same foods broiled or roasted.

Margarine or butter can be added whenever possible, including hot cereals, mashed potatoes, cooked vegetables, or rice. Sour cream adds a lot of calories to soups or baked potatoes, and can be served as dips for raw vegetables. Peanut butter can be spread on raw fruits and vegetables.

Some additional hints: Candy and many desserts are rich sources of calories. Sauces and gravies boost the calorie content of meats. Hot bread or rolls soak up more butter than cold ones. Marshmallows or whipped cream should be added to cocoa. Mayonnaise has more calories than most salad dressings.

A variety of food supplements are available, including Carnation Instant Breakfast preparation, Ensure in fruit flavors, Susta-Cal in chocolate, Lital, Precision High Nitrogen, Isotonic and Meritene. Extra vitamins should be taken only on your doctor's recommendation since large amounts of vitamins may interfere with chemotherapy.

The dietician in your hospital can help you pick out foods that you need for good nutrition and suggest many ways of preparing them. Nutrition can be of great concern to people who have cancer and their families, even leading to anger and frustration, neither of which help one to want to eat. The best advice is to do what you can and then relax.

Other methods of eating include the use of elemental diets, intravenous feeding, and tube feedings. Elemental diets are foods that have been broken down to their simplest and most elementary components to provide nourishment for people who are not able to digest normal food. Vivonex, Flexical, and other similar products used for this

Other Ways of Getting Nutrition

purpose are relatively expensive and have a chemical taste that many people find difficult to accept. Elemental diets have a very limited place in the treatment of cancer.

Intravenous feeding can provide very good nutrition for long periods of time by means of a small tube or catheter inserted directly into a vein. Complete maintenance feeding by this route can be carried out for weeks or even months at a time and is used when the digestive tract is unable to process and digest food. When the digestive tract must be at rest for only a few days, as following surgery, intravenous feedings consist only of sugar, salt, and water. However, when the digestive tract must rest for longer, very nutritious mixtures are available. Intravenous feeding is also occasionally used to supplement the oral intake of people receiving radiation or chemotherapy, when nutrition and weight loss are severe problems.

Tube feedings are used when there is severe difficulty swallowing, or obstruction in the throat, esophagus, or stomach, but when the remainder of the digestive tract functions normally. The tube usually goes into the stomach by way of the nose and the foodpipe (nasogastric tube) or through a small hole in the wall of the abdomen directly into the stomach (gastrostomy). In both cases, the food mixture is blenderized with milk and injected or allowed to drip into the stomach through the tube.

The most important thing for me is to be in control, to be able to take my own pain medication when I need it, without having to ask anybody for help.

RELIEF OF PAIN

Although half of the people who have cancer have little or no pain, everyone fears it, often more than any other aspect of the disease. When present, pain can disrupt the lives of individuals and families. Relief of pain is an important part of the treatment of cancer and certainly one of the most sacred responsibilities of the physician. This chapter will help you understand how pain may be caused by cancer and the steps that are taken to contol it.

Ordinarily we think of pain as an important form of protection. It tells us that we are injured, that we should let go of something that is too hot, that we should go to the dentist or the doctor. This kind of acute pain, rapid to appear and of short duration, is a warning that something is wrong, and a demand that we do something about it. More important, we have learned to ascribe meaning to pain and to look behind it for a cause that can be treated. Over the years experience provides each pain with its own message and gives us confidence in those who can relieve it with proper treatment.

The chronic pain of cancer, like that of arthritis and many other diseases, is entirely different. It is meaningless as well as endless, and treatment must often be directed at the pain itself rather than the disease causing it. The cause remains and, without constant attention, the pain returns. This kind of pain is demoralizing because it carries no important message and has no obvious value. It is just there.

Pain is a very complex sensation with physical and psychological components. From the source of the pain, whether it is a cut finger or a tumor in a bone, the distress signals are carried as electrical impulses by tiny nerve fibers to the spinal cord, where nerves from all over the body are bundled together to form a sort of cable. These travel up to the part of the brain that records the electrical impulse as pain. Side by side with nerves that carry pain, and also distributed throughout the entire body, are other nerves that carry the pleasant sensations of warmth, coolness, and touch. It is in the brain that the various messages, good and bad, pleasant and unpleasant, are sorted out, and that pain is recognized and felt.

How We Feel Pain

The sorting-out process is critical, because it is in the mind that pain may be subjected to filters that reduce or eliminate it, or increase it out of proportion to the cause. The brain can even be tricked into overlooking some bad messages in favor of more pleasant ones. One may consider the sorting-out process as a very small opening or gate through which only a few messages can pass at one time. If all of the messages arriving at the gate at the same time are painful, they will be perceived as pain. On the other hand, if many pleasant messages are coming along with the painful messages, the pain will be diluted by pleasant signals and the perception of pain may be greatly reduced. There are even situations where pleasant signals can crowd out the pain altogether. Another way to control the traffic is to make the gate larger or smaller. Anxiety appears to make the gate larger, allowing more painful sensations to come through, while general comfort and emotional well-being make the gate smaller, keeping the pain out. Finally, it must be realized that the gate is not a one way street and that pleasant signals can force their way through the gate against the current of painful sensations. If people are coming out of a narrow doorway, it is hard to get in. The distraction provided by music, conversation, or games, may work in this way. The brain has even been found to produce its own morphine-like chemicals, called endorphins, which suppress the sensation of pain, perhaps very much the same way the drug morphine does.

Studies of the psychological aspects of pain have provided clues to the mechanisms of pain perception and have contributed to its treatment. In medicine we see people who have no pain when we know they should, and we see people who have intense pain with no obvious cause. It is a common experience to feel more pain at one time than

The Psychology of Pain

another, even though the cause remains constant, and everyone is aware that many types of pain are worse at night when other incoming stimuli are greatly reduced. The reverse of this is that pain can often be relieved by a variety of forms of distraction such as heat, cold, music, conversation, or having something important or helpful to do.

Punishment for wrongdoings in childhood can create an unfortunate partnership between pain and guilt. Some people see their disease as punishment for which they should feel guilty, creating a cycle in which guilt feeds on pain and pain feeds on guilt, each making the other worse.

In some cultures, people are taught as children to express their feelings of joy and distress openly, and they appear to be sensitive to pain. Other cultures reward suppression of these same feelings, and such people appear to be stoical and insensitive to pain.

Pain is made worse by fear and anxiety. The child begins to cry in the doctor's office long before he is hurt. Many adults would like to do the same thing as they too begin to feel the pain before they need to. If severe enough, anxiety and fear of the unknown can cause distressing symptoms that are not related to cancer at all. We are less fearful if the intensity and duration of the pain are predictable and we know that it will end. The discomfort associated with cancer can have the opposite effect since we may not know when it will end. Even this anxiety, however, can be relieved by understanding the physical basis of the pain, and what steps are being done to relieve it.

How Cancer Causes Pain

People are surprised when they are told that cancer is a *painless* lump in the breast or a *painless* sore in the mouth. Indeed, any discomfort associated with cancer does not come from the tumor itself but is caused by pressure of the tumor against other normal structures. The most obvious of these are nerves that may be pushed, stretched, or actually invaded by the tumor. Although bone is a hard and relatively insensitive tissue, the thin tissue that covers the bone (periosteum) is very sensitive. Pressure on blood vessels can obstruct the flow of blood to an area, depriving the tissues of oxygen, causing pain. Growth of a tumor in the wall of any hollow or tubular organ may cause obstruction, with backing up, overfilling, and stretching of the tissues. Examples of this are obstruction of the bladder by cancer of the prostate, or obstruction of the bowel. Finally, inflammation or infection can cause swelling of the tissues and irritation of nearby nerves. In each case, the pain has a specific and local physical cause. When possible the pain is treated at its source, the tumor itself. When this is not possible, the pain must be treated at a higher level where it is perceived.

Many factors, both psychological and physical, contribute to the complex sensation of pain, and control of pain must take all of them into consideration. These include general comfort, relief of fear and anxiety, attacking the source of the pain directly, blocking the flow of painful sensations to the brain, crowding out the pain with pleasant sensations, and the use of drugs to obtain relief. Everyone is aware that if you sit in an awkward position long enough it becomes painful. The opposite is also true. Reaching an optimum level of general comfort by positioning, the use of pillows, appropriate clothing, the correct temperature, and many other seemingly minor things can all contribute to the relief of real pain.

Anxiety and fear, including fear of pain itself, greatly increase pain. Familiar surroundings, friendly and helpful people, and mutual trust are vital factors. Understanding your disease and its treatment eliminates much fear of the unknown. Finally, your doctors and nurses have many ways to relieve pain and should assure you that they will do whatever is necessary to provide comfort.

Treating Pain at the Source.   The best approach is usually to prevent or relieve pain by attacking the tumor itself. This may be through surgery to relieve obstruction of the bowel, radiation to tumor that has spread to the bones, particularly if it is localized in one or two places, or chemotherapy if the tumor is in several places and is known to respond to the drugs. Since this kind of treatment is given to relieve pain caused by the tumor (palliation) and not for cure, the side effects of the treatment must be weighed against the benefits it may provide. These should be discussed carefully with your doctor because sometimes it is clearly better to relieve the pain by some other method without trying to attack the tumor.

Interrupting Nerve Pathways for Pain.   The very precise organization of the nervous system makes it possible to relieve pain by interrupting the tiny nerve fibers that carry the sensations. The neurosurgical procedures required to do this have largely been abandoned now because of the development of better methods of controlling pain by the use of drugs. Neurosurgical operations to relieve pain, however, have a place when drugs fail to give adequate relief, or when the side-effects of the drugs (usually drowsiness) are not acceptable, and when life expectancy is greater than three or four months. Most of the operations have side effects and risks of their own that require careful consideration. These may include muscle weakness and loss of control of the bladder or bowels. The latter is particularly apt to be a problem when the tumor causing the pain is near the midline of the body, requiring interruption of nerve pathways on both sides. The procedures most frequently used include:

1. Nerve blocks, in which the nerve is injected with alcohol to deaden it permanently.
2. Chordotomy, in which the nerve pathways are interrupted high in the neck.
3. Myelotomy, in which the nerve fibers are interrupted in the midback.
4. Singulotomy, in which a small area of brain is destroyed, relieving anxiety and fear of pain more than the pain itself.

It is beyond the scope of this book to go into these procedures in detail since they are new and still being tested.

Drugs that Relieve Pain. The most common approach to relieving pain is through drugs. These range from common analgesics familiar to everyone, such as aspirin, to a variety of narcotics that can be obtained only by prescription. Factors that are considered in choosing the best drug include particularly the potency of the drug, or how powerful it is as a pain reliever, and what side effects or risks the drug carries. The narcotics, which include the most potent pain killers, all cause drug dependence or addiction if taken long enough. When these potent drugs are used to relieve the acute pain following surgery, they are usually discontinued four or five days after surgery to avoid this possibility. By this time the pain is gone and no drugs are needed.

Pain from cancer is obviously different, and comfort is far more important than concern about drug dependency. The dependency that occurs in this situation is unavoidable and hardly qualifies one as a drug addict. Along with this dependence goes a gradual increased tolerance for the drug so that over a matter of weeks, more drug may be needed to obtain the same amount of relief. This, too; is a natural phenomenon that cannot be avoided.

A still different situation is encountered by the person who has pain for several weeks, often during treatment, although the tumor responds to treatment and the long-term outlook is good. Here the development of drug dependence could continue to be a problem after the pain is gone. To avoid this, drugs are given in low doses, just enough to give relief, and are rotated, using no one drug for more than a few days or a week at a time. In this way, dependency on any one drug and unnecessary addiction are avoided.

Another important factor in the choice of drugs is the route of administration. Those that can be taken by mouth are easier to handle at home, less expensive, require no equipment, are less time-consuming and less uncomfortable to take. They also have fewer complications because there is no possibility of injecting the drug directly into the bloodstream or causing an infection in the area of the injection.

The frequency with which a drug must be taken reflects the amount of time that a single dose remains active as a pain reliever. For many drugs this is four to six hours, but for some it may be as little as two hours, particularly when there is some tolerance for the drug. Pain medication is more effective if it is taken *before* the pain becomes severe, and doctors often adjust the schedule so that medication is given *regularly* every four hours.

One of the most important aspects of pain control is being in control yourself. Having to call on others for relief places you in a very dependent relationship. At home this requires that you or your family be responsible for the drugs. This is easy when the drug is taken by mouth, but most people can also be taught to administer drugs by injection if necessary. Many hospitals now teach people to handle their own pain medication even while in the hospital.

Most narcotics cause some drowsiness and a few people find that they prefer to be uncomfortable to feeling "knocked out" by pain medication. Other side effects may include difficulty coughing, nausea, vomiting, or constipation. These side effects are not as common or as severe as those caused by drugs used for chemotherapy, and they can usually be relieved by simple measures.

Good pain control also requires relief of anxiety and fear. Part of this is accomplished by learning that the drugs can indeed produce comfort quickly. In addition, however, anxiety can be treated with tranquilizers such as Librium, Valium, Equanil, Sparine, Phenergan, Thorazine, or Vistaril. Severe depression also aggravates the perception of pain and can be relieved with drugs such as Elavil, Sinequin, or Tofranil.

Table 15.1 lists the drugs most commonly used for pain relief in order of their relative potency. Those drugs listed as narcotics can be habit-forming and require a prescription. Codeine, Demerol, and morphine, are the potent drugs most frequently used for short-term relief of pain after surgery where relief is usually needed for only a few days. Brompton's Mixture, an oral preparation of morphine and a tranquilizer, is widely used for chronic pain in cancer because it can be taken by mouth in a liquid form. Its disadvantage is that it must be taken frequently, and since morphine is much less effective by mouth than by injection, more of the drug is needed to get the same relief.

Dilaudid, Levo-Dromoran, and Methodone are the drugs most frequently used for relief of chronic pain. They can all be taken by mouth. Levo-Dromoran and Methodone have the added advantage

Table 15.1. Drugs Commonly Used to Relieve Pain

Name of Drug	Type of Pain	Danger of Dependence (Narcotic)	How Taken	Onset of Relief	Duration of Relief
Aspirin	Mild	None	Oral	30 Min.	2-4 Hours
Tylenol	Mild	None	Oral	30 Min.	2-4 Hours
Talwin	Mild-Moderate	Yes	Oral	30 Min.	2-4 Hours
Codeine	Mild-Moderate	Yes	Oral, Inject	30 Min.	4-6 Hours
Demerol	Moderate	Yes	Inject, Oral	15-30 Min.	2-4 Hours
Morphine	Severe	Yes	Inject, Oral	15-30 Min.	2-4 Hours
Brompton's Mixture	Severe, Chronic	Yes	Oral	15-30 Min.	2-4 Hours
Dilaudid	Severe, Chronic	Yes	Oral, Inject	15-30 Min.	4-6 Hours
Levo-Dromoran	Severe, Chronic	Yes	Oral, Inject	30 Min.	6-8 Hours
Methadone	Severe, Chronic	Yes	Oral, Inject	1 Hour	6-8 Hours

of being very long acting so that they need only be taken three times a day. They both give steady, continuous pain relief compared to drugs such as morphine, where the effect wears off relatively quickly.

Common Cancers

sixteen
Cancer of the Breast

Cancer of the breast is the most common cancer of women, and virtually everybody knows someone who has had it. Each year in the United States there are approximately 100,000 new cases and almost 40,000 women die of breast cancer. From a more personal perspective, one out of thirteen, or about 7 percent of all women in this country will eventually develop this disease. Breast cancer can occur in men, where it has many features in common with the same disease in women. Since it is a rare disease in men, it will not be included here.

Frequency and Causes

Although the cause of cancer of the breast is not known, several factors have been identified which increase the risk for some women. One is a *family history* of breast cancer in a sister, mother, aunt, or grandmother. The occurrence in the family of *other* cancers, with the possible exception of cancer of the uterus, does not increase the risk of a woman developing breast cancer. The increased incidence of breast cancer within families has been considered evidence (but far from conclusive) that this cancer could be caused by a virus that may be transmitted from mother to daughter, perhaps even before birth. Of more direct importance is that female relatives of breast cancer patients, particularly sisters and daughters, realize that they do have a higher than average risk of this disease. They should be sure to tell their physicians about this family history and learn and practice breast self-examination regularly.

A personal history of previous breast disease is associated with increased risk of developing cancer of the breast. This is highest in women whose earlier disease actually was *cancer of the breast*. Approximately 10 percent of these women will some day develop a second cancer in the other breast.

A history of *fibrocystic disease* of the breast is associated with slightly increased risk of eventually developing cancer. In fibrocystic disease usually both breasts have several or even many small sacs (cysts) that are filled with clear fluid and feel like lumps. This disease is common in women in their twenties and thirties and tends to disappear after the menopause. If you have been told that you have this problem, you should be followed closely by your physician and examined at least once a year. Removal of the breast tissue underneath the skin (subcutaneous mastectomy), replacing it with artificial breast implants, is occasionally recommended, to avoid the possibility of developing cancer. However, most doctors feel this is excessive treatment for fibrocystic disease.

Sexual and *hormonal* factors are of great importance. Cancer of the breast is more common in women who begin to menstruate at an early age but who have no children, or who defer sexual activity or childbearing until after age 35. Late menopause also appears to be a factor, as is the long-term use of some hormones, particularly female hormones, estrogens. These are used in large quantities for birth control, avoidance of menopausal symptoms, or in the hope of slowing down the process of aging. Whether prolonged use of female hormones constitutes a risk by itself for the woman who has no *other* risk factors is not known. It is certain, however, that hormones increase the risk for the woman who has other significant factors such as family history or benign breast disease. If you have such risk factors, you should avoid prolonged use of estrogens for any reason whatsoever.

Excessive radiation to the breast can cause tumors many years later. This was more commonly seen when x–ray was used to treat acne, and when some women with tuberculosis received a great many chest x–rays. Today the use of mammography for early detection of breast tumors is being looked at carefully because of the conflict over its risk-benefit value. This controversy is discussed in more detail below.

There are other less important factors which may contribute to breast cancer. It is more common in women who are overweight and eat large amounts of animal fat, butter, milk, cheese, and ice cream. Another factor is ethnic background. Cancer of the breast is more common in Jews of European ancestry and in whites living in the Western Hemisphere or in colder climates. For reasons that are not known the incidence is also higher in women in the upper socio-economic brackets. There is no evidence that nursing one's children offers any protection against this disease.

Signs   Although cancer of the breast may make itself known in a variety of ways, the most common sign is a *painless lump,* usually discovered by the woman, her husband, or her physician during a routine examination.

I was taking a bath and I noticed this hard lump in one of my breasts. I just couldn't believe it, I was shocked!

I was putting my glasses on right after I'd showered, and I noticed something in the movement, noticed a deviation in the right breast.

I felt a lump in my breast on my regular self-examination.

My husband found it. We were lying in bed talking and he had his hand on my breast and all of a sudden he said, "What's that?" I had never felt anything before but after he found it I could certainly feel a lump.

Many diseases of the breast present themselves as a "lump". Cancer is only one of them. Statistically cancer is rare in women in their twenties; it begins to make its appearance when a woman is between thirty and forty years old. The risk increases after age forty and is highest between the ages of fifty and seventy. As more women routinely examine their own breasts, suspicious lumps are being brought to the attention of doctors earlier when they are smaller and when the chance of curing the disease may be significantly greater.

It should be noted that cancer of the breast can present itself in other ways, much less common but harder to overlook than the innocuous little lump. These include discharge from the nipple, pulling in of the nipple, scaling of the skin around the nipple, dimpling or redness of the skin anywhere over the breast, change in the size or shape of the breast, ulceration of the skin over the breast, or occasionally a persistent aching in the breast.

Cancer of the breast may spread to other areas before the original tumor is even discovered. The abnormality to be noted first may be large hard lumps in the armpit from involvement of the lymph nodes, swelling of the arm, or even signs of more distant disease frequently associated with recurrence (see below).

Self-Examination of the Breast. Techniques for examining the breast are illustrated in Figure 16.1 but a few points are worth mentioning. The most important part of examining your breasts is to know how *you* look and feel. The first simple step is to make a habit of looking at yourself in the mirror and to raise your arms over your head. Your breasts should be symmetrical and move symmetrically when you do this.

Examining your breast when your skin is slippery with soap in the shower or bathtub can make small abnormalities easier to feel. It is important to remember that breast tissue is normally a little lumpy. This means that you are trying to find a somewhat larger lump against a background of small glands that make up the normal tissue. If you pinch the tissue with your finger tips you will easily feel lumps almost everywhere. Instead the breast should be examined with the flat of the fingers, by holding the fingers together to make a flat surface. The pressure should be against the chest wall rather than

Step 1

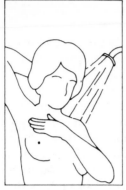

Step 2

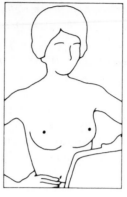

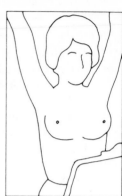

Step 3

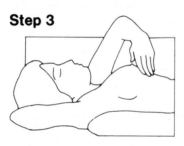

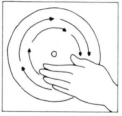

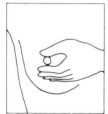

Figure 16.1 Monthly Breast Self-Examination.

Step 1: Examine your breasts during bath or shower; hands glide easier over wet skin. With fingers flat, move gently over every part of each breast. Check for any lump, hard knot or thickening.

Step 2: Inspect your breasts with arms at your sides. Then raise your arms overhead. Look for any changes in contour of each breast, a swelling, dimpling of skin or changes in the nipple. Then rest palms on hips and press down firmly to flex your chest muscles. (In most women, left and right breasts don't exactly match.)

Step 3: To examine your right breast, put a pillow or folded towel under your right shoulder. Place right hand behind your head to distribute breast tissue more evenly on the chest. Using your left hand, fingers flat, press gently in small circular motions around an imaginary clock face. A ridge of firm tissue in the lower curve of each breast is normal. Then move in an inch, toward nipple, and keep circling to examine every part of your breast; this will require at least three more circles. Repeat procedure on your left breast. Finally, gently squeeze the nipple of each breast and look for any discharge, clear or bloody.

Reproduced by permission of the American Cancer Society, which recommends this procedure.

trying to pinch the breast tissue. Coating the hands with soap or oil makes the examination much more sensitive when you are lying down, just as it does in the shower. You should also be sure to check the armpits since the "tail" of the breast extends far out in this direction. The lymph nodes that drain the breast (see Fig. 16.1) are also in the armpit.

Examining yourself on a routine basis, at the same time of the month, gives you information against which to compare even the slightest change or abnormality. For women who are still menstruating, about ten days after the start of the period is the best time, since changes in size and consistency of the breast are minimal at that time.

It is difficult to describe the way abnormal breast lumps feel. Some are very discrete and even quite movable within the breast tissue. Others are more like thickenings of the tissue. *Any* and all abnormalities of this kind should be brought to the attention of a physician.

When *anything* causes you to suspect an abnormality of the breast, the first thing to do is to see a physician. The real tragedy is the unfortunate woman who cannot bring herself to do this even though she suspects something is wrong. While a lapse of a few days is of little consequence, putting it off for months and months is asking for serious trouble. Furthermore, most lumps are *not* cancer. **Is It Breast Cancer?**

If a doctor is seeing you for the first time for a suspicious breast lump, his questions should include the risk factors for cancer of the breast given above, as well as other aspects of your general health. His examination should include a careful examination of both breasts, including the armpits and the areas above the collar bone. While the examination in the office may be brief and not a complete physical, you should mention any other area in which you have had pain or unusual signs that developed recently.

Mammograms. In addition to the physical examination, your doctor may wish to have an x–ray study of your breasts. This is called a mammogram or, if a xerox technique is used, a xeromammogram. The major value of the procedure is its ability to distinguish between solid lumps which may be cancer and fluid-filled lumps or cysts which are not cancer. The procedure is of much greater value in older women. After menopause, the gland tissue is largely replaced by fat which is lighter and against which a solid tumor can be much more easily and accurately recognized. In young women, where a major portion of the breast tissue is dense, active gland tissue with a relatively small amount of background fat, a solid breast tumor is hard to distinguish from solid normal breast tissue.

Mammography is painless. The breast is placed on a shelf-like apparatus containing the film while the x–ray tube takes a picture of the breast from above, and then again across the breast from the side. In this way the breasts can be compared from two points of view to pinpoint anything suspicious. The amount of radiation used to obtain a single study is not significant and should not be of concern to the women for whom reasons for doing the procedure are clear, such as the presence of a lump. Mammography is an important diagnostic aid for evaluation of a suspicious lump, regardless of your age.

Because of the risk of radiation causing cancer, there has been public concern about the use of xeromammograms as a screening technique for breast cancer in normal women when *no* obvious lumps can be found on examination. The current recommendation is that yearly xeromammograms be used as a routine screening technique only for women over fifty and in high risk women between thirty five and fifty, namely those who have already had cancer in one breast and those whose mothers or sisters had breast cancer. Yearly mammograms for detecting cancer at an early stage are not very reliable in younger women, and may give a potentially dangerous amount of radiation over a period of years. Meanwhile attempts are being made to develop better equipment that produces good pictures of the breast with much lower doses of radiation so that this technique can be used safely to screen all women.

When a suspicious area is found by mammography but no lump can be felt, the area should be biopsied and the tissue examined carefully by one or more pathologists. Under no circumstances should more extensive surgery (that is, mastectomy) be carried out until the diagnosis from the biopsy is absolutely certain.

Biopsy. Unfortunately, very little can be told about a breast lump by how it feels. The single most important step is a biopsy. The lump can often be biopsied by inserting a special needle into the breast tissue after first freezing the skin with a local anesthetic. The alternative method is to remove the entire lump in a so-called open biopsy. This is done by freezing the skin and removing the lump if it is relatively small and close to the surface of the breast, or it may be done under general anesthesia if the lump is large or deep in the breast. The first is an office procedure while the second may require being in the hospital for at least one day because of the anesthesia.

For many years, it was customary to do the biopsy in the hospital under general anesthesia, informing the woman in advance that if the biopsy proved to be cancer, a mastectomy would be done while she was still asleep. The pathologist examined frozen slices of the tissue (frozen sections) and could identify cancer within minutes. This sequence of events had the disadvantage of subjecting all women to the psychological stress of the *possibility* of waking up with a breast removed while in fact eight out of ten need only to have a biopsy. Since most of the lumps biopsied are not cancer, it seems more reasonable to separate the two procedures of biopsy and mastectomy. In this way every woman who has a biopsy knows that she is only going to have a biopsy at this time and will not wake up with her breast gone. More important, the woman whose biopsy proves to be malignant will have time to find out more about her disease, discuss her treatment with her doctor and family, prepare herself for a mastectomy, if that is what is to be done, and consider the possibility of reconstruction. There is no rush!

I only signed for a biopsy. I felt I wanted to know what I was getting in for. I knew that way would be better for me. The next day my doctor came in and I could tell without him saying anything. I could see it on his face, so he never really told me. I said, "It's bad news", and he said, "yes", and then he sat down and talked to me quite a bit.

I talked my doctor into an extra day because I know me, and I wanted to be emotionally prepared before I went into the hospital. When I went in I knew and I was ready to face it. I didn't have any problems after that.

Another compelling reason for separating the biopsy from the mastectomy is to search carefully for spread of the disease beyond the breast (see Fig. 16.2). Examination of the several areas where breast cancer may spread is unnecessary, expensive, and rarely done in every woman biopsied for a breast lump. On the other hand, such a search is very important for the woman found to have cancer, since spread to other parts of the body could make removal of the breast unnecessary. The most common studies to evaluate spread of the disease beyond the breast are careful examination of the armpit, a bone scan to detect possible spread of disease to bones, a bone survey by conventional x–ray studies of the bones, *if* the scan shows any suspicious areas, a liver scan to detect possible spread to the liver and a chest x–ray to detect spread to the lungs. Innumerable other studies could be done but because of the predictable nature of breast cancer and its patterns of spread, these are the studies that are most frequently helpful.

What Treatment?

For the one or two woman in ten whose biopsy shows cancer the best treatment by far is some operation that removes all or part of the breast. However, there is controversy over what is the best operation. Going from the *least extensive* to the *most extensive*, the operations used are as follows:

Partial mastectomy (also known as lumpectomy or tylectomy)—In this operation up to a third of the breast is removed, including a margin of normal tissue around the lump. This leaves enough breast

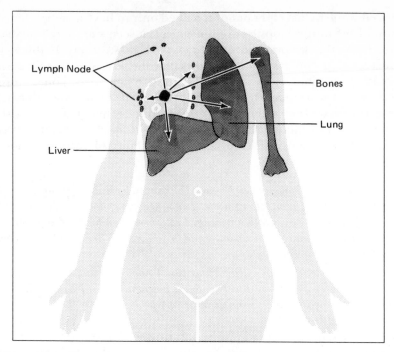

Figure 16.2 Cancer of the breast tends to spread to nearby lymph nodes and to bones, lungs, and liver.

Lymph Node

Bones

Lung

Liver

tissue to be cosmetically acceptable but is applicable only for small tumors which are near the surface and near the edges of the breast, away from the central area behind the nipple. Because of the apparent value of adjuvant chemotherapy (see below), it is advisable to remove the lymph nodes from the armpit as part of this procedure, even though it frequently means a separate incision in the armpit. Examination of these lymph nodes is important in determining the overall likelihood of cure and in selecting appropriate follow-up treatment. Lumpectomy is often followed by radiation therapy.

Simple mastectomy—This operation is rarely done. It involves removing all of the breast tissue but preserving the underlying muscles and the lymph nodes in the armpit.

Modified mastectomy—In this operation the breast is removed as well as the lymph nodes from the armpit. The underlying muscles at the front of the shoulder and the chest wall are preserved and the deformity is somewhat less than that associated with the following procedures. It is also better suited for reconstruction of the breast after mastectomy.

Standard (Radical) mastectomy—This is similar to the modified mastectomy except that the large muscle on the front of the chest wall is also removed along with the breast tissue and lymph nodes. This was standard procedure for over fifty years in the United States and Europe, but is rapidly being replaced by the modified mastectomy since it is more deforming and does not offer any increase in survival for most women.

Extended–radical mastectomy—This is an extension of the standard mastectomy which includes removal of the inner segments of four ribs to gain access to a chain of lymph nodes just *inside* the chest. This procedure has not gained great popularity because it has a high rate of complications and its advantage over the standard mastectomy is not proven.

The real controversy centers around standard mastectomy versus the lesser procedures. The standard mastectomy is the operation about which we have the most information and by which all others are measured. It is unlikely that any lesser operation is going to give *better* results than the standard mastectomy. The question is whether lesser procedures will give results that are *just as good,* in which case a less extensive operation would clearly be preferable. Evidence is accumulating to indicate that the modified mastectomy is just as good and it is rapidly replacing the standard mastectomy. Partial mastectomy has begun to be looked at more seriously. The question is whether this procedure can usually get all of the tumor. There is evidence that some women have two or three separate tumors in the same breast, in which case removal of only part of the breast with one tumor would obviously not include the others and recurrence would be likely. The use of radiation before or after partial mastectomy is being looked at as a possible solution to this with encouraging results.

In discussing the choice between partial, modified, and standard mastectomy with your surgeon, the two main factors are the results of each operation, in terms of survival, and deformity. The standard or modified mastectomies are of proven value when the tumor is confined to the breast but they are deforming operations. Lumpectomy is much less deforming but has not *yet* been shown to be the equal to the other procedures in ability to cure the disease.

It is not surprising that many other factors may play a role in determining what type of operation a woman chooses. Indeed, a small but significant number of women elect to have no surgery or more rarely no treatment at all. Concern about quality of life is very important and influences different women in different ways. Every woman, regardless of whether she is married, single, divorced, widowed, young or old has *some* concern about her self-image and feels threatened by mastectomy. This is where some of the other factors may come in.

The unmarried or recently divorced woman, or one who has relied upon her physical appearance for her feelings of self-esteem may have such a strong desire for an intact body image and sexual appearance that she may be willing to accept some risk to her life and choose a less disfiguring operation.

The young mother who faces a mastectomy obviously also has concern for her body integrity, but such feelings about physical beauty may be outweighed by her desire to live to see her children grow up; therefore she chooses a larger operation which seems to offer the best chance for her survival, in spite of the greater deformity.

By that time I was running real scared thinking that it might be more than just in my breast. Everything got so relative to me. My main thought was that I was going to "pop off" because I had it everywhere. Losing my breast was the least of my worries. I was afraid I was going to die. Everything in my life was going very well and I didn't want to die. So there was no debate for me.

Complications of Mastectomy.   During surgery one or two small plastic tubes are placed under the skin flaps to drain any fluid that may accumulate into a simple mechanical suction apparatus. This is emptied at least once a day and is removed after a few days when fluid stops appearing. Occasionally, this may take a week or more. Until it has been removed, motion of the arm is usually limited to movements required for eating, brushing the teeth, etc. This is the normal sequence of events. Like any operation, mastectomy can be followed by rare complications that require longer hospitalization or may result in permanent disability. These include local infection, which can complicate any major operation, or loss of part of the skin if the blood supply to the edge of the scar is not adequate.

A later complication which is noticeable and may even cause some disability is swelling of the arm (lymphedema). This is due to the the long-term collection of fluid in the arm because tiny lymphatic channels that normally drain this fluid were interrupted by the surgery. This complication occurs in about 10 percent of women undergoing mastectomy when the lymph nodes are removed. Infection and radiation following surgery tend to increase the incidence of swelling of the arm.

While swelling of the arm cannot be predicted or completely corrected, some simple steps should be taken to avoid unnecessary injury to the arm that may produce swelling. These include: a) avoiding injections on that side, b) not wearing constricting jewelry, c) having blood pressures taken in the uninvolved arm, d) not holding cigarettes in that hand, e) avoiding injury to the affected arm, f) treating burns, cuts, and scratches immediately and carefully, g) wearing gloves when injury is possible, (i.e., while gardening), h) avoiding sunburn, i) wearing a thimble when sewing, j) using an electric shaver, k) avoiding burns from cooking, l) not picking at cuticles or hangnails on the hand, m) wearing loose rubber gloves while washing dishes, and n) in general, avoiding any unnecessary injuries to that hand. If you have no evidence of any swelling in the arm one year after the operation, the likelihood of having future difficulty is smaller, but it is still wise to take these precautions.

The Psychological Hurt of Mastectomy

When I began to relax more about the possibility of dying I began to think more about the breast loss. I felt it as a loss of part of me, a part that I really liked. I think I went through a period almost like grieving for it. It was a sadness that was very deep. I used to cry for my breast and I wanted it back. Eventually I came to realize that I had lost my breast but this didn't change me or my life. It took me a while to realize that in order to live I had to lose it.

In our society the breast is the most identifiable and important female symbol. The adolescent responds to the development of her breasts with a mixture of pride and shyness, but they are obvious and sought-after signs of developing womanhood which she sees and by which she is seen. To many women, breasts symbolize womanhood, motherhood, beauty, and sexual desirability. One can easily understand the impact that the loss of a breast represents. In addition to the common reaction of depression, anger, and fear of recurrence or possible death, a woman who has had a mastectomy may experience a real feeling of grief over the loss of a very significant portion of her body. However, the very special fear associated with mastectomy is the fear of sexual rejection. Fortunately there are several things that can be done to lessen this fear.

For Women: The *real* you has not been changed through your operation and you certainly are not "damaged goods". There is nothing you could do before that you could not do again. You are still able to see, hear, think, work, and play, to give and to receive, and above all, to love and be loved. Do not underestimate the man in your life. He will react very much the way you do. He has to adjust, too, so give him some help and understanding yourself. Help him to help you by sharing the experience and your recovery together. The barrier that you feel will become real if you do not give him the opportunity that he needs.

For Men: You can help a lot! In the simplest of terms, your wife is afraid that you will no longer be able to love her, and that she will lose you. She has lost something that is very important to her and with it some of her self-confidence. It will take time for her to get over this. Understanding, love, and sympathy from you can do more than anything else.

I can honestly say that my cancer never affected my relationship with my husband at all. I can credit my surgeon for that. He took my husband aside and said, "Look, she may be missing a breast but she's no different inside". He has been wonderful and my feelings about sex have not changed at all.

For Both: Do not shut each other out and do not let yourself be shut out. It will take each of you time to accept and adjust to the situation but you can do it better and more quickly together. Behave as you always have together and avoid the trap of hiding from each other, physically or psychologically. The scar is not pretty but only by looking at it and touching it can you learn to live with it instead of around it. Dress and undress together and resume sex as soon as it is comfortable. Above all share your fears and feelings openly with each other. If you are afraid, say so.

We made love right away, as soon as I got home. I felt that I wanted to and I felt that I should do it now. The longer I waited the more uptight I would get about it, so I didn't wait at all.

For the Woman Who Has No Partner at the Time: Having no sexual partner at the time deprives you of a very helpful support since you cannot gain immediate confirmation of your sexuality. It is hard not to be afraid that the loss of your breast will jeopardize your chances of establishing a meaningful relationship in the future. If you are a little lonely now, it is impossible not to be afraid that you will always be lonely.

I still get a little uptight with somebody who didn't know me before. I think that anybody who didn't know me well might not take the chance to know me now just because of this. Maybe I won't have a chance for a real friendship if they find out. Maybe they won't try to see me for who I am.

You must in turn rely more on yourself to re-establish your self-confidence, getting support from your family and from other friends. You may not want to risk sexual encounters until you are quite sure of yourself in other areas, and then you will always be faced with the problem of how to bring up your mastectomy with someone you like. You will probably feel the need to have a deeper relationship with more preparation before getting into sex. Whenever the time comes explain your situation gently and help him to get used to the idea. Do not expect a miracle of instant acceptance. You were not capable of that yourself. He will need some time and understanding on your part.

It is tricky to say that there is an arbitrary time to bring it up. I came to feel that the deciding point for me would be my comfort level. I think that you can tell somebody too soon. You don't want to say, "how do you do, oh, by the way, I have breast cancer". By the same token, you can't wait until you are really starting to get involved. I think I would try to ease into it slowly.

If rejection occurs the first time, give him a chance to change his mind. If he really likes you as a person he may feel badly and guilty about not being able to accept your mastectomy right away. On the other hand if he cannot cope with it at all, he is obviously not the right person for you and there is nothing to do but pick up your hurt and angry feelings and try again.

A major step in psychological recovery from this operation begins with physical recovery and the realization that you really are okay, that the soreness is temporary, and that recovery of complete use of your arm is prompt. Understanding the importance of physical and emotional recovery prompted the organization of Reach to Recovery, the Encore program of the YWCA and others. Reach to Recovery is a volunteer group of the American Cancer Society which is active in most major cities. It is made up of women who had mastectomies and who have had instruction and training in physical rehabilitation. In order to have a Reach to Recovery volunteer visit you, she must be invited by your doctor. If your surgeon does not mention Reach to Recovery, it is up to you to ask her to make the arrangements when she feels you are ready. This is usually a few days after the operation. A volunteer will make two or more visits to teach exercises that will help you regain full use of your arm. She will also provide a great deal of first-hand information about temporary, and later, more permanent prostheses and clothing. More important, the volunteer provides you with a living example that a woman can survive mastectomy and resume a normal life, both in appearance and in fact.

Rehabilitation

     The exercises that help regain normal use of your arm include: combing your hair, swinging your arm, grasping objects in your hand, climbing the wall with your fingertips, reaching behind the neck, and several others. These exercises are begun gradually while still in the hospital. Complete range of motion of the arm is usually regained within two to four weeks after surgery. However, if exercises are not started within at least two weeks of surgery, complete range of motion may be difficult to regain. Diligent attention to the exercises as soon as you are comfortable enough to do them is important.

Results of Treatment.   In addition to early recognition and adequate removal of the tumor, several other factors affect the chances of cure. Foremost among these is involvement of the lymph nodes in the armpit with tumor. The lymph nodes are removed by the surgeon and turned over to the pathologist who requires two to four days to examine them. If the lymph nodes are free of cancer cells, the chances are relatively small that the tumor has escaped beyond the area of the operation. Seventy percent of women with this "Stage I" disease survive free of cancer for five years. On the other hand, if several lymph nodes in the armpit are found to be involved with tumor at the time of the original operation, the likelihood that the tumor has escaped beyond the limits of the surgical procedure is greater and only 30 percent of women with "positive lymph nodes" are alive and free of disease five years later. When only one or two nodes are involved, the figures are almost as good as if no nodes are involved.

Adjuvant Therapy.   Attempts are now being made to improve the results of surgery by combining it with chemotherapy and/or radiation. Adjuvant chemotherapy is used extensively in women with positive lymph nodes to try to "mop up" any tumor cells that may have escaped beyond the limits of the operation before they have a chance to become established and grow. The drugs used include the combination of cytoxan, methotrexate and fluorouracil, known as CMF; phenylalanine mustard, known as melphalan or L-PAM; and adriamycin and vincristine. New drugs and combinations are being tried all the time. At present, adjuvant chemotherapy appears to be particularly beneficial for premenopausal women with positive lymph nodes, and now similar regimens are also being tried with women who do *not* have positive nodes. Here the goal is to increase their five-year survival rate to 80–90 percent, or higher.

Radiation therapy is often used for women who have several positive lymph nodes, tumors that involve the skin or chest wall, or large tumors on the inner side of the breast. Although radiation has not been shown to decrease distant spread or prolong life, it definitely reduces recurrence in the area of the original operation. Radiation may be expected to assume an even greater role if it gives good results when combined with partial mastectomy.

Reconstruction.   The plastic surgeon now offers a new option to the woman who has lost her breast to cancer. It is possible to place a permanent artificial breast under the skin to simulate a real breast. The materials that are used are heavy plastic envelopes (silastic) filled with a gelatinous fluid or water, giving it very much the same weight and consistency of normal breast tissue. The artificial breast is usually not inserted at the time of the original operation or when on chemotherapy because of the risk of infection. It can be put in three or four months later, when the scar is well healed and the skin has softened and stretched. On the other hand some women have had reconstruction as late as twenty years after the original operation.

While reconstruction is the ideal solution for some, this new procedure also has some disadvantages. The implant operation requires a separate surgery and hospitalization with all the associated discomfort and expenses. Indeed by the time a few months have elapsed since the original operation many women who plan to have reconstructions find that they have adjusted well and do not want to go through any more surgery.

It is important to understand what can and what cannot be done so as not to expect too much. Breast reconstruction after a mastectomy is not perfect; the artificial breast cannot be made to look exactly like the remaining normal breast. It is occasionally even desirable to change the normal breast, usually at the same operation, making it smaller to get a more even appearance. All of these possibilities should be discussed with a plastic surgeon and you should ask her to show you photographs of women with reconstructed breasts so that you will know what to expect.

It is not always possible to do a satisfactory reconstructive operation. If the mastectomy left too little skin and a tight scar, or required a skin graft, or was followed by radiation to the area, reconstruction can be very difficult. While something may be possible, it often requires several complicated operations and yields a result that is far from ideal. Finally, reconstruction can be followed by complications. Most are minor and easily treated but some may require removal of the implanted material, sometimes with the possibility of trying again later and sometimes not. In spite of these restrictions many women who feel strongly about regaining their normal sexual image find implantation of an artificial breast an excellent compromise.

I'm so delighted with my new breast I wish I could show it to everybody. I didn't know anything about reconstruction when I had my first operation. Women could be spared a lot of grief if they knew about the possibility of reconstruction before they have a mastectomy.

After breast surgery, a follow-up routine is established which usually consists of examinations every three months for one year, every six months for two or three years, and then every year. The places where cancers of the breast are most likely to recur are the scar, lymph nodes in the axilla (if they were not removed) or low in the neck, bones, liver, and lung. About 10 percent of women with breast cancer eventually develop a similar tumor in the other breast. It is difficult to say if this is recurrence or a brand new cancer. Most of these areas can be

Follow-Up
and
Recurrence

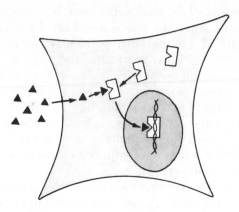

Figure 16.3 Estrogen receptors. The female hormone, estrogen, enters the cell where it is bound to estrogen receptors, if they are present. The estrogen receptor complex then go into the nucleus of the cell where they stimulate some genes to function, often causing the cell to grow and divide. To test a tissue such as a breast cancer biopsy for estrogen receptors, a small piece of tissue is exposed to estrogen that has been "tagged" with a radioactive isotope. The tissue is then tested to see if it binds the tagged estrogen. Tumors that have estrogen receptors (receptor positive) are often sensitive to treatment that change the hormone levels, while those that do not have receptors (receptor negative) usually do not respond.

examined by physical examination or x–ray. Recurrence in the scar or lymph node are painless lumps, while those in the liver or lungs are usually detected by x–ray long before they give any symptoms. Spread to bones causes an ache or pain in the involved area. These are harder to detect before they cause symptoms because the number of x–rays required to examine all bones routinely would be excessive. Bone scans are better for detecting early spread to bones.

The woman who has recurrence of her breast cancer, perhaps more than most others, has several good forms of treatment available. First of all, if the tumor is found to have already spread when it is first detected in the breast, a mastectomy is usually not necessary. If the recurrence is localized to one or a few areas, such as the scar or bones, radiation can give relief from discomfort in a matter of days. For other recurrences, the choice of treatment is the use of hormones or chemotherapy, and often eventually both.

Hormone treatment of cancer of the breast is based on the knowledge that normal breast tissue is strongly influenced by female and male hormones and that some cancers of the breast retain the characteristics of normal breast tissue. Recently it has become possible to evaluate this on an individual basis by measuring in the laboratory the appetite that the tumor cells have for the female hormone estrogen.

Tumors that have estrogen receptors (ER) are said to be ER positive and, like normal breast tissue, are more apt to be sensitive to alterations in the hormonal environment than those that do not. Estrogen receptors can be measured from samples of the original tumor or, less frequently because they are harder to get at, from metastases. About half of all breast cancers are ER positive. The most significant hormonal alteration that can be done is to reduce the amount of estrogen by the drug Tamoxifen, or by removing the ovaries. If this gives good relief of symptoms it may be followed by removal of the adrenal glands, or now more frequently the pituitary gland (hypophysectomy), to further decrease estrogen production. These procedures are of greatest value in premenopausal women whose tumors are estrogen receptor positive, of whom 70 percent have a good response.

The other side of hormone treatment is to *increase* the amount of hormone in the body. Estrogens, and sometimes the male hormones, androgens, can be taken by mouth or injection. They are of greatest value in postmenopausal women whose tumors are estrogen receptor positive, of whom more than half get relief of discomfort from this treatment. Although many breast cancers that are ER positive respond well to hormonal alterations, very few of those that are ER negative respond. Chemotherapy is usually a better choice for these women than hormonal treatment. Chemotherapy can also be of great help for women whose tumors are first treated with hormone alterations but later become resistant to this.

The drugs most frequently used are various combinations of cytoxan, fluorouracil (5FU), methotrexate, vincristine, prednisone and adriamycin. Relief of discomfort and shrinkage of the tumor are experienced by up to 70 percent of women receiving chemotherapy.

I know I'm not absolutely free of cancer but I'm certainly better than I was a few months ago. I'm much more comfortable. Chemotherapy helped a lot.

Women today know more about breast cancer than any other cancer. Most are aware that the best treatment is far from perfect and that there are now alternatives to the standard mastectomy of yesterday. The results of these alternatives are not yet known but they may turn out to be as good or better. Early detection, separate biopsy, the possibility of reconstruction, and the effectiveness of additional treatment all help to make this a less fearful disease. Moreover, the medical profession is gradually developing better understanding of the psychological problems associated with breast cancer. With this will come greater flexibility and more sensitivity to help each woman obtain the highest quality of life that good treatment can provide.

seventeen
Cancer of the Colon and Rectum

Frequency and Causes

The large bowel or colon is the last five or six feet of the intestinal tract, with the rectum making up the last six inches and opening to the outside (Figure 17.1). Most digestion takes place higher up in the stomach and small bowel. The main functions of the colon and rectum are to remove water and store the solid waste products so they can be eliminated daily. Cancer begins in the lining or mucosa and eventually spreads outward through the muscular walls of the bowel.

Cancer of the bowel is the second most common cancer in men and women. There are over 100,000 new cases and 40,000–50,000 deaths from this disease in the United States each year. It is rare in children and young adults, but begins to make its appearance in the forties and is most frequent in people between age sixty and eighty. Cancer is exceedingly rare in the small bowel and the anus. This chapter will be confined to cancer of the larger bowel and the rectum because they are common.

Clues to the causes of cancer of the bowel point towards *diet*, particularly the amount of animal fat eaten. Cancer of the bowel is common in the United States and Western Europe where large amounts of animal fat are eaten, but uncommon in other parts of the world where diets are significantly different.

Another dietary factor is the amount of roughage. Large amounts tend to speed waste materials through the bowel so that potentially dangerous products from bile and bacteria are not in contact with the lining of the bowel for long periods of time. In societies where large quantities of roughage are eaten, solid wastes remain in the colon only a few hours. In our more constipated society, with a diet that contains little roughage, waste products may rest in contact with the lining of the bowel for two or three days.

Polyps are also related to cancer of the bowel. These are small

214

mushroom-like growths of the bowel lining which frequently give no signs at all. They occasionally call attention to themselves by bleeding or causing diarrhea or a mucous discharge from the rectum. Polyps are much more common than cancer of the bowel and while most are not considered early cancers, there is increasing evidence that some eventually turn into cancer. It is currently thought that most polyps should be removed and this is easily done if they are in the rectum or in the lower portion of the bowel. When they are higher up they can often be reached with a colonoscope. The problem becomes more complicated if the polyp cannot be removed without an operation. The decision is then frequently based on the size and shape of the polyp and results of a biopsy, if it can be obtained. Small round polyps, under one-half inch in diameter, are rarely malignant.

Familial polyposis is a very rare hereditary disease in which the bowel is literally studded with small polyps. These begin to appear in adolescence in about half of the members of affected families, and almost invariably turn to cancer in the twenties and thirties if not treated. The treatment for the affected members of these families is removal of the entire colon and rectum.

Inflammatory disease of the bowel or ulcerative colitis, a relatively uncommon disease of young adults, is associated with subsequent development of cancer. This disease can frequently be treated medically, without requiring surgery. However, people who have ulcerative colitis should be followed carefully with yearly examinations of the bowel to look for any changes that suggest cancer.

Hemorrhoids are essentialy "varicose veins" of the rectum and have no relationship to cancer. They are a very common rectal problem that can cause pain and bleeding and my be mistaken for cancer. To eliminate any confusion they should be called to the attention of your physician any time that you have a physical examination to make sure that any minor bleeding is indeed from the hemorrhoids and not from something more serious.

Since everyone has occasional bowel problems, the earliest signs of cancer are frequently overlooked. They are often vague, with a tendency to come and go, prompting one to say "If I'm not better tomorrow, I will call the doctor". For this reason, the *recurrence* of *any* change in bowel habits should be looked upon with suspicion. The importance of attention to early signs of cancer of the bowel cannot be overstated.

The signs of cancers of the bowel often depend on where the cancer is (see Figure 17.1). Cancer of the rectum usually shows up as red blood on the surface of the stool and occasionally as pain, change

Signs

in the size of the stool (caliber), and a feeling of having to move the bowels without being able to do so. Cancers on the left side of the colon tend to narrow the bowel just at the place where the stool is solid. This frequently causes bouts of crampy pain, constipation, or diarrhea, or even diarrhea alternating with constipation, as the normal bowel above the tumor works harder to try to force material past the obstruction. Bleeding from these tumors may not be noticeable. Cancers on the right side of the bowel tend to bleed, often slowly but continuously so that the first sign of anything wrong may be weakness and fatigue due to anemia from blood loss. Usually this blood cannot be recognized and the bleeding is unsuspected. These cancers can grow to a large size before they give any other signs, but eventually cause dull pain on the right side of the abdomen, or weight loss and loss of appetite.

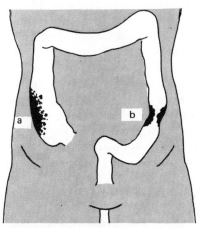

Figure 17.1 Cancer of the large bowel or colon. Tumors on the right side (a) often cause anemia by bleeding slowly. Those on the left side (b) often cause changes in bowel habits from obstruction.

Early Detection.   The key to early detection of cancer of the bowel is careful routine physical examination and detection of bleeding. Bleeding from anywhere in the digestive tract above the rectum is frequently not recognized because the blood is partly digested and turns black. Any black discoloration of the stools (not associated with taking iron by mouth, which also turns the stools black) should be investigated. More frequently, however, bleeding from cancer is so slow and small in amount that it cannot be recognized at all by looking at the stool. It can, however, be detected by a simple biochemical test. The test most frequently used, the Hemoccult test, requires applying a small amount of stool to paper slides on three successive days and mailing the slides to a laboratory where the stool sample is tested for blood. This test is inexpensive and slides can be obtained from your hospital or doctor's office. To make the test more accurate, it is recommended that meat not be eaten for the two or three days while the test is being carried out and that the food that is eaten include a large amount of coarse foods such as salads, vegetables, and fruits to add bulk to stool and to increase the likelihood of irritating a small tumor to make it bleed when one is looking for it. Fish and chicken can be eaten on the meatless days.

The second method of early detection is part of the physical exam done by your doctor. About two-thirds of these cancers are near the far end of the bowel where they can be felt or seen by direct examination with a lighted instrument or proctosigmoidoscope. These examinations are not painful and their value in early detection of cancer of the bowel cannot be overestimated. They should be part of the physical examination for anyone who has signs suggestive of cancer of the colon or rectum.

The studies that indicate if suspicious signs are indeed cancer of the bowel include:

Is it Cancer of the Colon?

Rectal Examination. The rectum can be examined easily by a gloved finger. If you push down at the time that the examination is being done, it is completely painless. Since about 12 percent of cancers of the bowel are low enough to be *felt,* this examination is a very important one.

Unsuspected Blood in the Stool. At the same time that the rectum is being examined your doctor usually has a chance to obtain a small amount of stool to test for unsuspected blood. This should always be included as part of this examination.

X–ray Study of the Bowel. The bowel can be examined by filling it with an x–ray dye (barium enema). The bowel must first be cleaned out completely so that it will contain only the barium. This requires taking a laxative and/or regular enemas before the examination. The x–ray study itself is carried out in a fluoroscopy room where the radiologist can watch dye entering the bowel and can look for any abnormalities throughout the course of the filling and emptying of the bowel.

Direct Examination. The rectum, lower bowel (sigmoid), and even the upper portion of the large bowel (colon) can be examined directly by three lighted instruments: the protoscope, sigmoidoscope, and colonoscope. These examinations also require that the bowel first be cleaned out. They are usually carried out in a head-down kneeling position, frequently on a special table that tilts forward. The instrument to be used is inserted slowly so that the examiner can look for any abnormalities along the way. Although this procedure is not a pleasant one, it is rarely painful. The advantage is that a suspicious area can be biopsied through the instrument without requiring surgery. Moreover, polyps can often be removed with these instruments to be sure that they are not cancer and to eliminate any possibility that they may become cancer. When a tumor is suspected but cannot be identified clearly for a biopsy, cells can be brushed off or washed off in the suspicious area and examined for cancerous changes.

Searching for Spread of the Tumor. When a cancer is found several tests are usually done to see if it has spread. A liver scan is frequently done. If the cancer is low in the bowel or in the rectum, the bladder, the ureters, the uterus, and the vagina can be examined if the location and size of the tumor suggests they may be involved. There is a biochemical test for a material produced by several cancers, including colon cancer, which is found in the blood. The test for CEA (carcinoembryonic antigen) is done on a small sample of blood. It is of no value for early detection of cancer of the bowel but can be useful for prompt recognition of recurrence. This requires, however, that it be followed at regular intervals starting before and continuing after surgery. In general, the level of CEA in the blood falls after surgery if the tumor has been completely removed, and does not go back up again unless there is a recurrence. Occasionally it rises early in the course of recurrence, before there are any other signs, when the tumor can still be completely removed.

Treatment   Surgery is the best treatment for cancer of the bowel. Usually a piece of bowel can be removed and the remaining bowel hooked up again (anastomosis). The portion of the bowel removed depends, of course, on the location of the cancer. When the cancer is low in the rectum the problem is more complicated because there is no more bowel below it to hook up to. When the entire rectum must be removed, the end of the bowel is brought out through a hole on the abdominal wall, forming a colostomy (see below). Occasionally a cancer of the bowel may be overlooked until it causes complete blockage of the bowel. In this case, the bowel is usually full of material and must first be cleaned out before the cancer can be removed. When the blockage is complete this again requires a colostomy above the blockage. In this case, however, the colostomy is a temporary one and can be closed after the obstructing cancer has been removed. This sequence may require two or even three operations several days or weeks apart. It is usually advisable to remove a cancer of the bowel, even when it is known to have spread to other areas such as the liver, to avoid bleeding or complete blockage of the bowel.

Two other forms of treatment for cancer of the rectum are

reserved for the person who is a poor risk for major surgery or who cannot accept living with a colostomy. Cancer of the rectum has been treated with radiation or by destroying most of the tumor with an electric instrument. Neither of these procedures is as good as completely removing the tumor surgically when it is possible to do so.

Before having an operation, there are important questions to discuss with your surgeon. Ask to see a drawing showing exactly where the tumor is and what part of the bowel must be removed. If the cancer is in the rectum, he should tell you if he plans to do a colostomy, or even if he may have to do one. In either case learn what the colostomy involves. Your doctor should provide you with information about it, including whether it will be temporary or permanent. It is also very important to have *time* to get used to the idea. Except when there is complete blockage of the bowel, there is no emergency and an extra day or two to learn about a colostomy from your doctor, an "ostomy" nurse or someone who has a colostomy is time well spent.

For two or three days before surgery on the bowel or rectum, you will be placed on a special diet consisting mostly of liquids, and you will be given enemas and drugs to kill the bacteria that normally live in the bowel. All of these steps are to empty the bowel and to cleanse it to avoid infection after the operation. When the rectum is removed, a defect remains which has to heal in gradually. Some surgeons close this completely and put in a small suction tube to help collapse the space. Others prefer to place gauze inside the wound, removing it a few days after surgery and then having you keep the area clean by sitting in a tub half full of water (sitz bath) several times a day until it is completely healed.

A very common side-effect of removal of part of the lower colon or rectum is impotence in men. This is due to unavoidable damage to nerves in the pelvis, resulting in inability to have an erection, to ejaculate, or both. Men should discuss this with their doctors before surgery. Sexual prostheses are being developed with can partially correct impotence. Nerves that go to the bladder are also injured in operations for rectal cancer and require a catheter to empty the bladder for several days or weeks until they heal.

The most frequent complication is infection from a leak where the bowel was sewn together. This usually clears up with the use of antibiotics but may require a subsequent operation to drain the infection to the outside. While this complication may prolong one's stay in the hospital, it is usually not life threatening.

Getting to Know your Colostomy

There are perhaps thousands every year who undergo surgery and a colostomy without fear or trepidation; there are others who are concerned about the

*physical, social, and emotional impact of the procedure; and, most unfortu-
nately, there are other countless thousands who choose to pay little or no
attention to warning signs and their ultimate consequences. I found myself in
the middle group. While not trying to make it sound ludicrously simple, life is
beautiful and well worth living thanks to the science of surgery. (From a letter
in 1977 from a patient with cancer of the rectum, operated on in 1955.)*

A colostomy is neither a disease nor a disaster but a life-saving procedure for thousands of people every year. It does represent a major
change. It takes time, patience, and a little bit of "grit" to undertake
toilet training as an adult, particularly when the bowel movement
comes out on the front of the abdomen and is not always completely
under control. However, a colostomy should not prevent anyone
from living a perfectly normal life and thousands of people with
colostomies go about their normal activities without even their closest
associates suspecting that they have been treated for cancer. A colostomy need not interfere with normal eating, work, social life, sexual
activities, exercise and sports, travel or the clothing that you wear. In
short, a colostomy allows you to function normally, but differently.
Friendships or love relationships are rarely altered by the addition of
a colostomy. Moreover, there is plenty of help available. People with
colostomies are so numerous, so resourceful, and so interested in
their own well-being and that of others that they have done much to
make the experience more tolerable. This includes the development
of ostomy clubs in many cities and the training of personnel with
experience in managing all of the problems that colostomies can
present.

Regardless of how well you prepared for it, a colostomy can
hardly be considered welcome and it takes several weeks to get to
know it. A few days after surgery the colostomy begins to "work". At
this time, it usually is covered with a plastic bag backed with adhesive
so when a stool does come out it does not soil you or the bed. Such
disposable bags are worn by most colostomy patients all the time.
They allow you to be free of worry about accidents, or the escape of
gas, or odors. A few people find that they can regulate their colostomies so well that they can wear just a small patch of cloth over the
colostomy to protect their clothing and do away with the bag altogether. This is completely optional and depends entirely on how
well the colostomy behaves.

The time to learn techniques of colostomy management is while
you are still in the hospital and can get help from your doctor or
nurse. About one week after surgery, usually after you are up and
around, it will be time to begin to "irrigate" your colostomy. This is
usually carried out sitting on the toilet. A small rubber tube or cathe-

ter is inserted into the opening (stoma) of the colostomy and about a quart of warm water is allowed to run in slowly. This stretches the bowel and stimulates it to squeeze down and push out the water and the waste material inside. The annoying part about colostomy irrigation as opposed to a normal bowel movement is that it can take up to thirty minutes for the bowel to empty itself completely. An appliance is used to catch the material that comes out so you can move about the bathroom a little but you cannot stray very far. A little light reading for this daily occasion is helpful. Your first irrigations will be done for you to show you how, but soon you must take over the responsibility yourself. Be sure you feel confident about it *before* you leave the hospital. Most people prefer to make a regular habit of irrigating their colostomies every day or two. This places you in control of the colostomy, leaving you free of worry between irrigations. A few people find that their colostomies work perfectly, every morning after coffee, without requiring irrigation. This should not be tried until you are at home and well and have established a normal colostomy schedule. Each individual develops his own pattern in the first few months after surgery. This does not come overnight and requires patience and some trial and error.

Colostomy Problems. In addition to being the wrong thing in the wrong place, a colostomy can cause a few problems of its own, *all* of which can be prevented with experience. These include irritation of the skin, odor, passage of gas, the production of unwanted noise, accidents between irrigations, and bleeding from the colostomy. Each of these are encountered at least once by everyone and a little experience will soon teach you how to avoid them. Skin care is rarely a problem with a permanent colostomy on the left side because the stool is solid there and free of digestive juices which irritate the skin. The temporary colostomy, particularly on the right side, continuously passes liquid material rich in digestive juices which are irritating. Special ointments and a bag that fits close to the colostomy are essential for protecting the surrounding skin. Odor, gas, and noise are all related to diet. While everyone should try to return to a customary diet, trial and error will show that some foods produce more gas and odor than others. These include beans, nuts, onions, melons, vegetables of the cabbage family, and sugar-containing drinks. There is no colostomy diet and you should take plenty of time to experiment with the foods you like and eliminate only those which cause trouble. Odor can also be prevented by some oral medicines, by using a deodorant such as chlorophyll in the colostomy bag, and by careful attention to cleanliness. Accidents between irrigations are usually due to incomplete or infrequent irrigations. People who go without irrigations at all are obviously taking a greater chance. The lining of the bowel that makes up a colostomy is a delicate tissue which occasionally bleeds when it is wiped or the appliance is removed. This is a common occurrence and not cause for alarm.

While you and your colostomy may never become real friends, you should soon be reasonable companions. Once you have established your own pattern you will be better able to recognize if the colostomy is not functioning properly. It is a simple organ and can only malfunction in one or two ways: either it goes too much or it does not go at all. If either of these two situations occurs and causes distress or pain, you should notify your doctor.

Results of Treatment. Treatment of cancer of the bowel is much more successful when a tumor is found early and is still small. If the tumor is confined to the lining of the bowel, the five year survival rate is 70 percent for bowel and 64 percent for rectum. If the cancer has penetrated into the wall of the bowel, these figures are 65 percent and 40 percent respectively. If the tumor has penetrated all the way through the wall of the bowel or involves the lymph nodes nearby, these figures drop to 40 percent and 30 percent respectively. Finally, if the tumor has spread further, usually to the liver, the outlook is not as good.

Follow-Up and Recurrence

Follow-up for cancer of the colon should be for life, with visits as often as every three months during the first year, decreasing to once a year after three years. In addition to history and physical examination, routine follow-up studies should include examination of the stool for blood, chest x–ray, an x–ray study of the bowel (barium enema), and direct examination of the remaining bowel by sigmoidoscopy or colonoscopy. If CEA studies were done following surgery, they can be continued and may help to predict recurrence. The most common places for cancer of the bowel to spread to are the liver and the lungs. Spread to the liver may make itself known by pain under the ribs on the right side or by yellowing of the skin (jaundice). When spread to the liver is suspected, a liver scan is usually done. Spread to the lungs is usually seen on a chest x–ray long before it gives any signs. Cancer of the rectum also spreads to the liver and the lungs but has a tendency to recur in the area where the rectum was. This usually shows up by discomfort or pain in the area of the rectum, and occasionally pain in the legs from nearby nerves.

Treatment for Spread or Recurrence. Spread of cancer of the bowel to the liver or the lung is treated with chemotherapy with quite good results. The combination of drugs currently being used are 5FU and methyl-CCNU, but other combinations are being tried. Recurrence of rectal cancer is best treated by radiation if it is localized in the rectal area, or by the same drugs if it has spread to the liver or lungs.

Occasionally, recurrence of bowel cancer can cause blockage when some other portion of the bowel is caught in the growth of the tumor. This type of obstruction gives cramps in the abdomen, nausea, and vomiting. A relatively simple operation can frequently bypass the obstruction and give prompt relief.

Surgery for cancer of the bowel is not adequate treatment if the tumor has spread. To try to improve the results of surgery, adjuvant chemotherapy is being evaluated following surgery, in national trials. At the present time the results suggest that a combination of drugs, particularly 5FU and methyl-CCNU, may improve the overall results. Additional treatment being tried now is radiation before or after surgery. It is clear that early detection of this cancer, when it is limited to the lining of the bowel, would be the best way to improve the results of treatment.

eighteen
Cancer of the Lung

The lungs take in oxygen to feed body tissues, and remove a waste product, carbon dioxide. This requires moving a large amount of air in and out (see Figure 18.1). The total respiratory system is like a tree, with a main trunk, the windpipe or trachea, two main branches and numerous small branches or bronchi going to each side. At the end of each branch are clusters of small air sacks, the alveoli, which are like bunches of grapes. They are surrounded by blood vessels with thin walls where the exchange of these two important gases takes place as the blood is pumped through the lungs by the heart. Because dust and smoke and other small particles frequently get into the lungs, the respiratory system has an efficient way of clearing itself. Some cells that line the respiratory passages produce a sticky mucus which traps the particles of dust. Other cells have tiny brushes on their surface which act like a carpetsweeper and move the mucus and dust up from the smaller to the larger branches and out the main windpipe to the throat where it is swallowed or coughed out. Cancer can begin in the cells that line the respiratory passages, the cells that produce the mucus for trapping the dust particles, or the cells that line the air sacks themselves.

Frequency and Causes

Each year over 100,000 people develop cancer of the lung in the United States. Eighty thousand of them are men. Unfortunately, less than 10 percent can be cured. These figures tell the sad story of a modern disease. Today, cancer of the lung is twenty times more common in men and six times more common in women that it was 40 years ago (see Figure 18.2). Moreover, the frequency in women is catching up fast. It has doubled in the last twenty years, and is now the Number Two cancer killer of American women, behind breast cancer. While there are many possible causes of cancer of the lung,

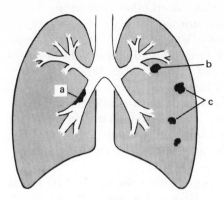

Figure 18.1 Cancer of the lung. Most lung cancers begin in the lining of the main bronchi (a) or its branches (b). Tumors arising further out in the lung (c) are more apt to be small cell (Oat cell) cancer or tumors that originate elsewhere and spread to the lung by the bloodstream.

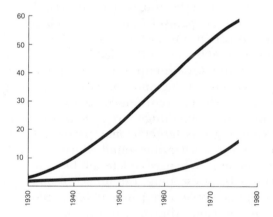

Figure 18.2 The Incidence of Lung Cancer (number of new cases per year per 100,000 population). The frequency of this disease continues to rise in men and is now increasing rapidly in women. Both of these correspond to increases in cigarette smoking (data from US National Center for Health Statistics and US Bureau of the Census).

the most common is the cigarette. Heavy smokers have about *twenty-three times* greater chance of developing lung cancer than nonsmokers. It has been said that one pack a day for twenty years will cause cancer. By the same calculation, half a pack per day would require forty years and two packs a day might require as little as ten years. Heavy smoking changes cells that line the respiratory passages. This sequence of changes includes decreased action and eventual disappearance of the small hairs that sweep mucus out of the lungs. The long column shaped cells that normally line these passages are gradually replaced by cells which are flattened out and tend to pile on top of each other, forming thick layers. Finally these cells begin to grow in an uncontrolled fashion and form a cancer. When the heavy smoker stops smoking, these changes may improve.

Other causes of lung cancer include industrial exposure to asbestos, some radioactive ores, and other poisonous materials. When two or three high risk factors are combined, such as a heavy smoker, who works in an industry involving asbestos, the risk becomes extremely high.

Cancer of the lung begins to appear after the age of forty and is most frequent between the ages of fifty and seventy.

Signs   Signs of lung cancer are late and variable. Very few are discovered by routine chest x–ray examination before they begin to give noticeable trouble. Cancers that begin in the alveoli or small bronchi near the edge of the lung may go unnoticed until they become large enough to reach the outer surface of the lung or to invade the chest wall. At that point the tumor becomes painful. Cancer in the cells lining the middle size and larger bronchi produces earlier signs. An open ulceration in the air passages caused by cancer can bleed. This shows up as streaks of blood in the sputum brought up on coughing. Irritation of the air passage and backing up of the mucus also cause coughing. A change of cough in a person who has a chronic cough from heavy smoking is a common warning that something more serious may be taking place.

As the cancer grows larger it may partially block off an air passage and produce a wheezing sound which can be heard when taking a deep breath. When complete air blockage prevents any mucus secretions from escaping, the lung will quickly become infected, causing pneumonia, with pain and fever. Blockage of a large air passage may also cause shortness of breath.

Other structures in the chest near the lung may be involved with cancer of the lung. Invasion of the esophagus causes difficulty in swallowing. Involvement of a small nerve that passes close to the lung can cause paralysis of one vocal chord and hoarseness. One of the big problems with cancer of the lung is its tendency to spread early to other parts of the body. For this reason the first signs may be dizziness, fainting, or headaches if it has spread to the brain; enlarged and hard lymph nodes in the neck above the collar bone if they have become involved; or pain caused by the cancer's spread to bones anywhere in the body. Abnormal signs in any of these places in a heavy smoker will make your doctor suspect lung cancer as the real problem.

When a doctor sees a person with any of these signs and learns the person is a heavy smoker or has been exposed to certain industrial poisons he cannot fail to think of lung cancer. In addition to a physical examination, a series of special studies are required. A chest x–ray will usually show a lung cancer by the time it causes any symptoms. Special x–ray techniques, or tomograms, can examine small portions of the lung and show the tumor clearly. If the tumor is close to large blood vessels, an x–ray dye study, or angiogram, may help to show if these vessels are involved with the tumor.

Malignant cells from lung cancer, particularly if it is in one of the larger air passages, frequently can be identified in the sputum. The sputum is collected over a period of hours and then examined by microscope for cancer cells.

The larger air passages can be looked at directly by bronchoscopy, through a tube with a light on the end of it. This is the single most important study since it often allows the doctor to see the tumor and obtain cells for a biopsy at the same time. The procedure is carried out under general anesthesia or after the throat and windpipe have been sprayed with a local anesthetic.

A cancer near the surface of the lung may cause fluid to collect between the lung and the chest wall. If fluid is found by chest x–ray, a small amount can be removed under local anesthesia to be examined for cancer cells.

Occasionally, if the tumor does not involve a major air passage, a full-scale operation is required just to get a small piece or biopsy of tumor for diagnosis. Once a biopsy has been obtained, it is sent to the pathologist to determine if it is cancer and if so, what type. This is important information because lung cancers are not all treated in the same way.

The next step is to determine if the tumor has already spread into the center part of the chest, the opposite lung, or to other parts of the body. The center of the chest is examined by mediastinoscopy, where a lighted instrument is inserted through a small incision low in the neck under general anesthesia to look for lymph nodes beside the trachea. A bone scan will usually show if the tumor has spread to bones, and a liver scan may be done if blood studies indicate the tumor may have spread to the liver.

The preferred treatment for most lung cancers is surgical removal. However, this should be done only when the tumor is still inside the lung and has not spread. About half the people with cancer of the lung are *not* operated on because the cancer is known to have already spread beyond the point where an operation would do any good. Of the people operated on, half have only a biopsy because the surgeon finds that the tumor has spread too far to be removed. This means that only 25 percent of all people with cancer of the lung can be operated on to attempt to remove all of the cancer and possibly cure the disease.

Operations for cancer of the lung include removal of part of the lung (lobectomy) or removal of all of one lung (pneumonectomy), depending on the location of the tumor. Removal of an entire lung requires better reserve function in the remaining lung. Removal of part or all of a lung is a stress not only at the time of surgery, but for the remainder of life. Preliminary studies are done to make sure you can withstand the operation and then get along comfortably on the remaining lung.

Chest surgery causes discomfort which makes coughing difficult. Instruction and practice before the operation on how to cough, along with medication to control the discomfort, will help. Occasionally, it is necessary to stimulate coughing by introducing a small tube into the nose and tickling the windpipe. This tube is attached to a suction device through which secretions brought up part way can be removed. If breathing is difficult immediately after the operation, the tube that was placed inside the windpipe to control breathing during the operation may be left in. The tube is attached to a machine which can help you breathe for several hours or even days, until you are comfortable enough to breathe without it. To check your progress, the doctors will take you off the machine from time to time and ask you to breathe on your own. They will then check the level of oxygen in your blood to determine when your remaining lung is functioning well. The discomfort following a chest operation is usually almost gone by the end of two weeks.

When only part of the lung has been removed, it is important to keep the remaining portion filled completely with air. This is done with a large plastic "chest tube", which enters the chest below the incision and is hooked up to a suction apparatus which bubbles continuously. This tube removes blood, fluid, and air and can be removed a few days after the operation.

Results after surgery, even when it was thought the tumor had been completely removed have been discouraging; about 25 percent survive five years. The main reason for this is the strong tendency for this tumor to spread to other places very early, before it causes any symptoms. Several trials of adjuvant therapy are being conducted to try to improve the results. These include the use of radiation or chemotherapy after surgery. At the present time no form of adjuvant treatment is of proven value.

Results of Treatment. One type of cancer of the lung, small cell or oat cell cancer (because of the shape of the cells as seen under the microscope), is not operated on at all. The treatment is chemotherapy. Several combinations of drugs greatly extend the survival of people with small cell carcinoma of the lung, even to the point where we now hope that some of them are being cured.

Many people with lung cancer eventually need treatment for spread or recurrence of their disease. Symptoms again depend on the location of the tumor. Recurrence inside the chest is most apt to give pain when it involves the nerves of the chest wall, or bleeding if it recurs in one of the air passages. Spread to bones causes pain in those affected. Spread to the brain causes headaches, nausea, vomiting, double vision, and occasionally weakness of an arm or a leg. Spread to the liver can cause pain in the right upper corner of the abdomen, near the ribs, and yellowing of the skin (jaundice). Spread to the esophagus can interfere with swallowing, giving the sensation that food is sticking in one's throat. Pressure on the windpipe can cause a feeling of shortness of breath. The treatment of all of these is radiation therapy or chemotherapy or a combination of both. While treatment at this stage usually does not prolong life, it can give very real relief.

Follow-Up and Recurrence

nineteen
Cancer of the Upper Digestive Tract

The upper digestive tract is responsible for digestion and absorption of food (See Figure 19.1). The esophagus conveys food from the throat to the stomach, passing through the chest behind the heart and lungs. The stomach is a reservoir where the food collects, allowing us to eat a few regular meals a day rather than continuously. Digestion begins in the stomach and continues as the food moves on through the duodenum and small bowel. Digestive juices formed in the liver and stored in the gallbladder (bile), and others formed in the pancreas meet the food in the duodenum. As the food is broken down it is absorbed through the wall of the small and large bowel to provide energy and building materials for the body.

Tumors to be considered in this chapter include those of the esophagus, stomach, liver, and pancreas. These four organs have one thing in common: they are situated deep within the body where they are relatively inaccessible to physical examination. Subsequently, their tumors are often very silent, giving little or no distress until they have grown to a large size. Although they occur, cancers of the gall bladder, common duct, duodenum, and small bowel are very rare and will not be considered here.

CANCER OF THE ESOPHAGUS

About 8,000 people develop cancer of the esophagus in the United States each year. The tumor begins in the lining of the esophagus and extends around and up and down the tube-like organ. Later it invades the muscular walls and eventually goes to neighboring structures, lymph nodes, and liver. The cause is not known but this tumor is frequently associated with heavy use of tobacco, strong alcoholic drinks, and untreated infections of the mouth. It is much more common in men.

230

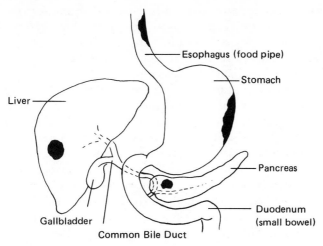

Figure 19.1 The upper digestive tract showing locations of the more common tumors.

The usual sign of this disease is difficulty swallowing. At first this is felt as sticking of large pieces of food in the throat or chest. Gradually this progresses until well-chewed food and even liquids fail to get through. As the degree of blockage increases, nutrition becomes a problem and weight loss is often severe. Except for mild discomfort which is often overlooked, pain is usually not a problem early in this disease. The diagnosis of cancer of the esophagus is made by an x-ray study (barium swallow) which outlines the entire esophagus and shows the area of narrowing. Once its presence is suspected, the tumor can be examined directly by means of an esophagoscope, a flexible tube through which a biopsy can be taken.

If general condition permits and there is no evidence that the tumor has spread, the best treatment for cancer of the esophagus is to remove the portion of the esophagus containing the tumor, bringing the stomach up into the chest and connecting it to the normal esophagus above the tumor. Occasionally a piece of large bowel is used to bridge the distance between the upper esophagus and the stomach if the tumor is high in the esophagus. These are large operations requiring two incisions. The first is in the abdomen to free up the stomach or large bowel, and the second is in the right chest to remove the tumor and re-establish continuity. Under the best of circumstances the cure rate from surgery is not very high, with less than 10 percent survival for five years. This is probably due to the central location of the esophagus near many other important organs, with easy and early spread of the tumor.

Radiation therapy can greatly improve the ability to swallow and is occasionally curative, particularly for tumors high in the esophagus where surgery is most difficult. Attempts to combine surgery with radiation therapy have failed to improve results. Chemotherapy has very little to offer for this disease.

Two small operations are occasionally done to relieve symptoms. The first of these is to put a funnel-shaped tube into the esophagus, passing the stem through the area of the tumor and anchoring it to the inside of the stomach so that it is held in place. This allows food to pass through the area narrowed by the tumor but obviously does nothing to alter the growth of the tumor itself. The second procedure is to insert a tube directly into the stomach through the abdominal wall so that pureed food and milk can be fed directly into the stomach (gastrostomy). There is little to recommend this procedure for cancer of the esophagus since it does not prolong life and certainly does not allow one to eat normally.

CANCER OF THE STOMACH

About 23,000 people develop cancer of the stomach in the United States each year and two thirds are men. This disease is rare before the age of forty and reaches its peak incidence in the sixties to eighties. The tumor originates in the cells that line the stomach from where it penetrates into the muscular wall of the stomach, often to involve the adjacent organs such as the spleen, pancreas, liver, or large bowel. It can also spread within the wall to involve most of the stomach, often before it is recognized.

Cancer of the stomach has *decreased* dramatically over the past several decades. In 1930, this was the most frequently fatal cancer in the United States. It is now a relatively uncommon tumor. Many efforts to identify changes in lifestyle or eating habits have failed to provide convincing answers and the reason for this remains completely unknown. This decrease has not been seen everywhere in the world. More than half of the cancer deaths in Japanese men are due to stomach cancer and the disease is almost as common in several other countries.

In spite of the fact that we do not know the direct cause, several factors are known to be associated with cancer of the stomach. Normally the lining of the stomach presents a relatively corrugated appearance. Smoothness of the lining of the stomach, seen in some older people (atrophic gastritis), is associated with a higher incidence of cancer. Similarly, failure of the lining of the stomach to produce normal quantities of acid digestive juice is associated with greater than four times increased risk of cancer of the stomach. Finally, people who have pernicious anemia *and* who fail to produce acid have an eighteen times greater risk of developing cancer of the stomach. Cancer of the stomach is more common in some families, so that people who have relatives who had this disease are at a higher risk. Blood types are also genetically controlled and individuals of blood group A appear to be at slightly greater risk. While none of these help us understand the cause of this disease they do make it possible to identify people at risk who should be followed closely after the age of sixty.

Ulcer disease is not related to cancer of the stomach. The most common type of ulcer, duodenal ulcer, is a different entity altogether. Ulcers that appear in the stomach are usually not cancer but should be studied carefully because stomach cancer can appear as an ulcer. The problem is to determine which ulcer is benign and which is cancer. In addition to the steps used to make a diagnosis of stomach cancer, prompt and permanent healing on good medical care usually indicates that an ulcer is benign.

Cancer of the stomach often presents with vague symptoms of indigestion, familiar to everyone and therefore not taken seriously until very severe or present for a long time. These include the sensation of fullness in the upper abdomen, discomfort or mild pain, nausea, heartburn, loss of appetite, belching, or regurgitation of food. Vomiting, weight loss, and anemia from unsuspected bleeding may be the first signs of this disease. Difficulty swallowing, as seen in cancer of the esophagus, can be the first sign if the tumor is located high in the stomach where it obstructs the opening of the esophagus.

The diagnosis of cancer of the stomach is made by an x-ray study using barium to outline the stomach, (Upper G.I. Series) showing when the wall of the stomach has some abnormal shape or appears to be rigid rather than soft and pliable. The flexible gastroscope makes it possible to see inside the stomach and biopsy any suspicious areas.

Signs

The best treatment for cancer of the stomach is to remove that portion of the stomach involved with the tumor. If necessary, the entire stomach can be removed. Loss of most or all of the stomach makes it necessary to take small frequent feedings in order to maintain adequate nutrition. The success of surgery for cancer of the stomach depends very much in the size of the tumor. If the tumor is small and has not spread to the regional lymph nodes the five year survival is greater than 50 percent. Large tumors or those that have spread to other organs have a poorer outlook. While radiation therapy has little to offer in this disease, chemotherapy including

Treatment

5FU, adriamycin, methyl-CCNU, and mitomycin-C, or some combination of these can give considerable relief of symptoms, particularly when there has been spread to the liver.

CANCER OF THE LIVER

The great majority of cancers that appear in the liver are actually tumors that originate elsewhere and spread to the liver by means of the bloodstream. These are not really liver cancers but must be distinguished from them by biopsy and by looking elsewhere for the original tumor. True liver cancer is relatively rare, affecting about 13,000 people in the United States per year, including men and women about equally. It is uncommon before the age of forty and reaches a peak in the sixties. Cirrhosis of the liver, either from excessive alcohol intake or a recent bout with hepatitis, is often associated with the eventual development of liver cancer. However, it is one of the most common tumors in Africa and the Far East, suggesting that nutritional deficiencies or contamination of food may be contributing factors.

Signs

Cancer of the liver usually shows up as pain in the right upper portion of the abdomen, often made worse by coughing or breathing deeply. Yellowing of the skin (jaundice) may be an early sign if the tumor is located where it can obstruct the bile duct as it leaves the liver. The diagnosis of cancer of the liver is made by a radioactive dye injected into an arm vein to outline the tumor in the liver (liver scan). An x-ray study in which dye is injected into the artery that goes to the liver can show whether the blood vessels that supply the liver have been pushed aside by the tumor. Finally, a biopsy can be done by means of a needle, after freezing the skin, or at the time of surgery.

Treatment

Surgical removal of the portion of the liver that contains the tumor is the only way this tumor can be cured. Unfortunately, these tumors often involve much of the liver before they are discovered or may even be present as two or three separate tumors, making curative surgery impossible. When the tumor can be removed, the five year survival rate is about 15 percent. Chemotherapy, usually with adriamycin, can give some relief of symptoms and occasionally prolong life but in general is not very effective against liver cancer.

CANCER OF THE PANCREAS

In contrast to cancer of the stomach which has been decreasing over the past years, the incidence of cancer of the pancreas has been increasing, also for reasons that are not known. About 23,000 people develop this disease each year in the United States, an increase of almost three times in the past forty years. This disease is rare in young people and most commonly seen between the ages of forty and seventy. Although little is known about the cause, it is more frequent in heavy smokers, people with chronic pancreatitis, diabetes (sugar diabetes), or alcoholism. It is definitely increased by exposure to some industrial carcinogens. Spread of this tumor is to nearby lymph nodes and liver, and less commonly to the lungs and bones.

If the tumor is located in the head of the pancreas (see Fig. 19.1) it may begin to compress the common bile duct before getting very large. In this case obstruction to the flow of bile results in yellowing of the skin (jaundice). This is associated with two other characteristic changes. The urine usually becomes a dark amber color and the stools become a light clay color because bile is no longer getting into the digestive tract. These signs may lead to detection of a tumor that is still relatively small. Tumors that are further out in the body or tail of the pancreas are much more silent until they become painful, producing an aching pain in the upper abdomen, sometimes more on the right and often with a component of pain in the middle of the back. Other symptoms include weight loss, loss of appetite, and the development of diabetes which was not previously present. **Signs**

The diagnosis of cancer of the pancreas is difficult and requires several different studies. X-ray of the upper digestive tract using barium taken by mouth may show pressure on the stomach or duodenum from the pancreas. The opening of the pancreatic and common bile duct into the duodenum (see Fig. 19.1) can usually be seen by a flexible optical instrument (duodenoscope) passed by mouth into the stomach. X-ray dye injected into these two ducts may show the point of obstruction to be in the head of the pancreas. X-ray studies of the blood vessels to the pancreas occasionally help to localize this tumor. The exact diagnosis usually can be made only by biopsy at surgery.

Treatment of cancer of the pancreas is to remove most or all of the pancreas along with the adjacent portion of the stomach and the duodenum. This is an extensive operation and is undertaken only in people whose tumors have not spread elsewhere, even to the neighboring lymph nodes, and whose general condition is good. Unfortunately, almost 90 percent of people who are operated on for cancer of the pancreas are found to have tumors that cannot be removed. Even when the tumor can be removed, the cure rate is distressingly low, about 5–10 percent. When the tumor cannot be removed, blockage to the common bile duct and the duodenum from the pressure from the tumor can often be bypassed by lesser operations that carry the bile or **Treatment** the food around the area of obstruction. While these operations do not prolong life they can provide a great deal of relief. Chemotherapy and radiation have been used to relieve symptoms of this tumor but with limited success.

twenty

Cancer of the Urinary System

The function of the urinary system is to cleanse the blood of waste and regulate the amount of water and salt in the body. This system is made up of 1) the kidney, which is the actual filter: 2) the ureters, which carry the urine from the kidney to the bladder: 3) the bladder, which stores urine and 4) the urethra, through which the urine passes to the outside. In the male, two other organs, the prostate and the testicles, are usually included because of their anatomical relationship to the bladder. The organs most frequently involved with cancer are the kidney, bladder, prostate, and testicle (See Figure 20.1).

CANCER OF THE KIDNEY

The kidney includes the filtration system and the upper end of the collection system. Cancer of the kidney, or renal cell carcinoma, occurs in the filtration system. This is not a common tumor, and comprises only about one or two percent of all cancers, but still adds up to 15,000 new cases each year. For unknown reasons, cancers of the urinary system are more frequent in men than women and cancer of the kidney is seen about twice as often in men. Its peak incidence is between the ages of thirty-five and sixty-five. The cause is not known but because of its greater frequency in men, sex hormones, and industrial chemicals have been suggested.

Cancer of the collecting system of the kidney involves a different type of cell known as transitional epithelium. Although cancer of the collecting system of the kidney accounts for a small percent of kidney cancers, its behavior is more like cancer of the bladder.

Signs

Cancer of the kidney is one of several tumors that may produce no signs until it is quite large. Fifty percent of these tumors are felt either by the individual or by a physician on routine physical examination.

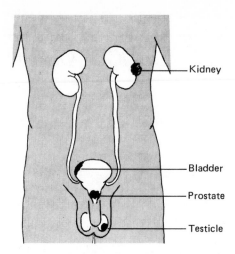

Figure 20.1 Cancers of the kidney and male genital system.

Symptoms may include pain in the flank or near the lower ribs in the back, or blood in the urine. More rarely fever, a general feeling of not being well, increased blood pressure or unexplained weight loss may be the first clues to cancer of the kidney.

Is it Cancer of the Kidney? Your physician may be the first person to discover this tumor when he feels a mass in the side of the abdomen. The initial x-ray study used to examine the urinary system is an intravenous pyelogram or IVP. This is a painless procedure, requiring only injection of a small amount of dye into a vein in the arm. A series of x-ray pictures is taken to watch the dye outline the kidneys and then follow it down into the bladder. A second x-ray study, a renal angiogram or arteriogram, involves the injection of a dye into the blood supply going to the kidney. A small catheter is inserted through a needle into an artery in the groin so that the dye can be injected directly into the branch that goes to the kidney. The x-ray pictures show the blood distribution in the kidney and indicate if vessels are involved or have been pushed aside by a tumor. A chest x-ray, bone scan, and liver scan are usually done to see if the suspected tumor has spread to these organs. Once an abnormal mass has been found in the kidney, it is necessary to get a biopsy. Because of the location of the kidney this requires an operation.

Treatment The best treatment is to remove the kidney and surrounding tissues. This may be followed by radiation to the area, particularly if the cancer extends beyond the kidney. Five and ten year survival rates are greatly influenced by whether the cancer is confined to the kidney, extends outside of the kidney, or includes the blood vessels leading to and from the kidney. These survival rates range from 35–50 percent for five years and 20–30 percent for ten years. Occasionally the kidney is removed when cure is not possible. This is to provide comfort or avoid loss of blood into the urine.

Cancer of the kidney is unusual in that it can grow very slowly, giving little or no trouble for many years. The most common places for it to spread are the lungs or bones and, much less frequently, to the brain or the skin. Because of its slow rate of growth, the spread may not be evident for a long time. There have been some unusual situations where cancer of the kidney was known to have spread to the lung, but disappeared completely after the involved kidney was removed. The peculiar behavior of this cancer, particularly when it has spread to the lung, has justified more aggressive treatment than is often used for other tumors. This behavior also raises the question of whether cancer of the kidney may be influenced by hormones or the immune system.

People with cancer of the kidney should be followed for many years because recurrence can be treated to greatly prolong life. It has been known to recur as late as fifteen to twenty years after the original tumor was removed. Follow-up should be every three to four months during the first year or two and then every year. Each followup should include a chest x-ray.

CANCER OF THE BLADDER

Cancer of the bladder is about three times more common in males than females and is more frequent in older people. The frequency of cancer of the bladder in the population is increasing steadily and now amounts to 30,000 new cases per year in the United States. At the same time, the death rate from this cancer is decreasing slightly, probably due to earlier detection and better treatment.

As long ago as 1895 it was first realized that workers in the aniline dye industry had an unusually high incidence of bladder cancer. Today a great deal is known about the causes of this tumor and of cancer of the collecting system of the kidney. Several industries, including chemicals, rubber, and cable manufacturing are all associated with increased risk of cancer of the bladder among their workers. There are also some foods (tryptophane from meats and other proteins) whose products may not be broken down and disposed of properly by some people. Cigarette smoking is definitely associated with an increased incidence of cancer of the bladder.

Signs

The most frequent and unmistakable sign of cancer of the bladder or any other part of the urinary collecting system is blood in the urine.

The bleeding is usually painless and is frequently a sign of a very early stage of cancer. Other less common signs of cancer of the bladder are frequent urination, pain on urination, inability to urinate, or pain in the flank or side.

Is it Cancer of the Bladder?

The bladder and the collecting system of the kidney are in direct contact with the urine so it is occasionally possible to detect these cancers by finding abnormal cells in the urine. The next step is to look into the bladder by means of a lighted instrument or cystoscope. This is done under general anesthesia and a biopsy may be taken at the same time. Two x-ray studies determine if any other parts of the collecting system are involved. In one, dye injected into a vein (intravenous pyelogram), is excreted by the kidney, and outlines the kidney and the entire collecting system. In the other (retrograde pyelogram), a dye is injected through a tiny catheter into the lower end of each ureter under general anesthesia to show the ureters and the collecting system of the kidneys.

A biopsy from the bladder is important because the choice of treatment and results are greatly influenced by the type of tumor, the degree of malignancy (that is, activity or grade of tumor), and particularly the depth that the cancer extends into the wall of the bladder. If the cancer is confined to the layers of cells that line the bladder or the collecting system, the long-term outlook is considerably better than when the tumor invades the muscular wall of the bladder. Two other factors are the location and extent of tumor involvement within the bladder. There is often more than one tumor of the bladder and there may be more cancers higher in the collecting system at the same time.

Treatment

The best treatment for cancer of the bladder is usually surgery. One of three procedures may be done depending on location and extent of the tumor. All require general anesthesia. The tumor may be removed from inside the bladder by means of a cystoscope-like instrument which is passed up through the urethra (transurethral resection or TUR). This can be done if the tumor is limited to the superficial layers of cells lining the bladder and is a low-grade malignancy. The tumor must be located in the portion of the bladder where it can be reached easily with this instrument. The bladder is not removed and recovery is quick. However, many tumors tend to be present in several places in the bladder and to recur after they have been removed. For this reason, very close followup is absolutely necessary. Follow-up consists of direct examination of the bladder by cystoscopy, frequently during the first few years and then less frequently.

In the second operation, partial cystectomy, part of the bladder is removed. This is done if the tumor invades the wall deeply or cannot be removed from inside. It is also preferred when the tumor is more malignant or appears to have spread to nearby lymph nodes. This operation retains nearly normal bladder function.

Occasionally it is necessary to remove the bladder completely (total cystectomy). This is the case when the tumor is near the point where the two ureters enter or the urethra leaves the bladder, or when a tumor penetrates deeply into or through the muscle of the bladder wall and neighboring lymph nodes are involved. Removal of the entire bladder requires re-routing the urine. Usually the ureters are inserted into a loop of bowel which has been separated from the rest of the bowel to make a blind pouch or "loop ileostomy" inside the abdomen. The opening to this pouch is on the skin of the abdominal wall where it can easily be fitted with an appliance to collect the urine. Any procedure of this type, which alters one's normal body habits so drastically, requires a period of adjustment. People undergoing these operations should have the same trained help before and after the surgery that is given to patients requiring a colostomy (see Cancer of the Bowel).

Radiation therapy is occasionally used when cancer of the bladder has not spread. It appears to be of particular value for cancer cells that are rapidly dividing. Close followup is required because cancers of the bladder and other parts of the urinary collecting system often recur. Chemotherapy, by injection or by mouth, is used when the cancer has spread. The overall five-year survival rate for all types and extent of bladder cancer is 60 percent and improving with earlier diagnosis and better treatment.

The prostate gland is located at the bottom of the bladder in men and makes the fluid in which sperm live. It is located just in front of the rectum where part of it can be examined by finger. The urethra, through which urine leaves the bladder, passes through the center of the prostate gland so enlargement of the gland causes obstruction to the passage of urine.

CANCER OF THE PROSTATE

Cancer of the prostate is common in elderly men, increasing in incidence through the age of eighty. It is more common in black people. Nine out of ten cases are found in men who are over the age of sixty. It has been estimated that 14 percent of all men over the age of fifty have some degree of cancer of the prostate but most are slowly growing tumors of very low grade malignancy and never give any trouble. On the other hand, of the 60,000 new cases reported each year of prostatic cancers that grow more vigorously and become a serious disease, most are not detected early enough to be completely cured. The cause of cancer of the prostate is not known.

Signs   In many men cancer of the prostate appears to be a slowly progressive disease which may be present for a long time without any symptoms. Because it is more common in older men, many probably die of other causes without realizing that they have cancer of the prostate. Indeed, quite a few of these tumors are found by accident when part of the prostate is removed for different reasons. Enlargement of the entire prostate (benign prostatic hyperplasia) is very common in elderly men and causes obstruction to the passage of urine. It is treated by removing the central portion of the prostate surrounding the urethra. About five percent of cancers of the prostate are found in this way. These incidental cancers are often slow growing, and are unlikely to spread or give further trouble. The doctor may even elect to do no more than follow the disease by regular repeated rectal examinations, reserving additional surgery for the few men whose tumors show signs of further growth. Helpful information can be obtained from the size of the tumor, the amount of cancer in the tissue removed, the number of separate areas of cancer, and the level of malignancy of the cells seen.

Another five percent of all cancers of the prostate are found as hard lumps in the prostate on rectal examination. These cancers are considered to be a stage beyond those found by accident, because they have grown into a separate lump within the prostate gland. The percent of cancers detected in this way would probably be increased by making rectal examinations routine for all men over forty-five. When these tumors are found early, they can usually be cured.

The remaining 90 percent of cancers of the prostate are found when they cause distressing signs. These include difficulty urinating or emptying the bladder completely or frequent urination. Pain in the area of the rectum or blood in the urine are usually symptoms of more advanced cancer. Cancer of the prostate has a strong tendency to spread to bones, almost anywhere in the body, causing pain in the bones or from pressure on nearby nerves.

Is it Cancer of the Prostate?   Cancer of the prostate is determined by rectal examination and needle biopsy. This is done under local anesthesia, usually through the rectum and is not a painful procedure. Cancer of the prostate also produces chemicals (alkaline and acid phosphatase) which may be present in the blood, particularly if the cancer has spread. About 50 percent of these tumors have already spread to bones by the time they are first discovered. For this reason a bone scan and x-rays of suspicious areas of bones are done routinely. An x-ray study of the urinary tract by IVP can show if a ureter is blocked or lymph nodes are involved.

Treatment for cancer of the prostate includes surgical removal of part or all of the prostate gland, radiation, or hormone alterations. Chemotherapy, other than the use of hormones, is of little value. The choice of treatment depends on age, general condition, and the extent of the disease. There is often a *choice* of treatment for cancer of the prostate and these alternatives should be discussed with your doctor before a decision is made.

Treatment

The usual treatment for early cancer, found as a lump within the gland, is removal of the prostate under general anesthesia. This is reserved for men who are not too old, who are in good general health, and where there is no evidence that the cancer may have spread beyond the prostate gland. A good alternative to surgery for early cancer of the prostate is radiation therapy. This has the advantage of maintaining sexual potency in about 70 percent of men treated. The five year survival for this stage of the disease is 50–75% after either treatment.

If the cancer appears to have spread beyond the wall of the prostate gland but not to the bones, the treatment of choice is radiation. This is often accompanied by limited surgery in which the central portion of the enlarged prostate is removed through the urethra to relieve obstruction. Radiation may be given by injecting radioactive material directly into the prostate under general anesthesia, or by external radiation.

Changing the hormone balance in those with widespread prostate cancer can greatly influence the course of the disease. These alterations consist of removing the source of the male hormone, which stimulates growth of cancer of the prostate, and replacing it with female hormones which have the opposite effect, slowing down the growth of prostate cancer. This is accomplished by removing the testicles (castration), or at least the part of the testicles that produces male hormones, and giving the female hormone, estrogen, by mouth or injection. These alterations in hormone balance can give prompt relief of bone pain or urinary obstruction, usually lasting two or three years and sometimes much longer. However, they cannot cure the cancer.

Side Effects of Treatment.   Removal of the prostate results in complete impotence. This should be discussed by husband, wife, and doctor before any surgery is done. The operation rarely results in loss of bladder control so that an appliance must be worn to collect the urine. Radiation may also cause problems. The rectum, which is behind the prostate, receives a heavy dose of radiation. This can result in diarrhea, crampy pain, a feeling of having to move the bowels, and occasionally bleeding. Similarly, the bladder is just above the prostrate and also receives some radiation which can cause increased frequency or pain on urination. These symptoms usually clear up soon after the radiation treatment has been completed. Female hormones used to treat prostate cancer cause breast development. This is usually more noticeable to the man being treated than anyone else and can be prevented by treating the breast tissue with a small dose of radiation before starting the hormone treatment. Hormones can also cause fluid to be retained in the body, resulting in some weight gain, swelling of the ankles, and occasionally shortness of breath.

Cancer of the prostate can recur long after removal of the original tumor. Close follow-up is important because if there is recurrence it often responds well to treatment with hormones or radiation.

CANCER OF THE TESTICLE

Cancer of the testicle is one of the more common tumors of young men between the ages of twenty and forty. The testicle is actually made up of at least four different types of cells which in turn produce four different types of cancer, each with its own name, its own form of treatment, and its own outlook.

Signs

The most frequent sign of cancer of the testicle is enlargement, causing a dragging or heavy sensation in the scrotum. The signs of advanced disease are related to where it has spread. These may include back pain, a mass in the groin, a mass in the neck above the collar bone, blood in the sputum, or shortness of breath.

Is it Cancer of the Testicle?

A solid mass in the testicle of a young man has a high chance of being a malignant tumor. For this reason and in order to avoid spread of the tumor, the usual biopsy is bypassed and the entire testicle is removed through a small incision in the groin. Examination of the tissue will determine the type of cancer and then the physician will search for further spread. This includes careful examination of lymph nodes, sometimes by lymphangiography, and of the lungs by chest x-ray.

Treatment

Treatment for cancer of the testicle always includes removal of the testicle. Further treatment depends on the type of tumor. The most common is seminoma which is usually treated with radiation to the lymph node area where this tumor most frequently spreads. The five year survival from this tumor is over 90 percent if it has not already spread. When it has spread beyond the area of the surgery and radiation, chemotherapy is added to the treatment.

Two more tumors of the testicle, embryonal carcinoma and teratocarcinoma, tend to spread to the lymph nodes along the spine, behind the abdominal cavity. Treatment for these is exactly the same and includes removal of the testicle and of the long chain of lymph nodes extending all the way up to the kidney, where the testicle originally came from in its early development. If any lymph nodes are found to be involved with cancer, radiation is added to the surgery. If the cancer has spread further, chemotherapy is also used effectively. The five year survival for embryonal cancer and teratocarcinoma treated by removal of the lymph nodes and radiation, even when the lymph nodes are involved, is about 50 percent.

Choriocarcinoma is the least common but most serious of the cancers of the testicle because it tends to spread very early through the blood stream and frequently has reached the lungs before the original tumor is even discovered. If the lungs are not involved, the lymph nodes are removed, but when it has spread to the lungs, chemotherapy is the treatment of choice.

twenty-one

Cancer of the Cervix, Uterus, and Ovary

The female reproductive system is made up of the ovaries, the fallopian tubes, the uterus, the vagina, and the external genitalia or vulva (See Figure 21.1). The uterus itself has two parts, the body of the uterus with its special lining (endometrium), and the cervix of the uterus which opens into the vagina. Although cancer can originate in any of these organs, cancer of the ovary, endometrium, and cervix are the most common.

CANCER OF THE OVARY

The ovary is a complex organ made up of many different types of cells which can give rise to a variety of cancers. Knowledge of the exact cell type, which can only be obtained by an operation and biopsy, is important for determining the best treatment. Different cancers range from very low levels of malignancy which rarely spread elsewhere and have five year survival rates as high as 80–90 percent, to those which are much more malignant, tend to spread early, and where the outlook is not nearly as good. About 20,000 women develop cancer of the ovary each year with the peak being between the ages of forty and sixty. There are a few uncommon cancers of the ovary which can appear in young women and even girls. The cause of this disease is not known. It has no relationship to race or socio-economic status.

Signs

Cancer of the ovary is one of the tumors that often grows to be quite large before causing distress and is very difficult to detect early. The earliest signs are usually a sensation of pressure or fullness in the lower part of the abdomen and occasionally the realization that clothing feels tight in that area. There may be pain in the lower abdomen and occasionally there are vague digestive symptoms such as feelings

246

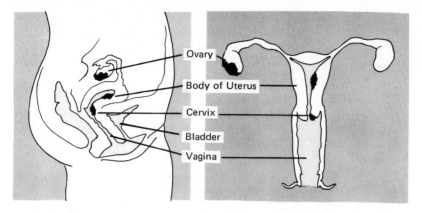

Figure 21.1 Location of the common cancer of the female genital system.

of fullness, nausea, or a change to irregular bowel habits. A later sign may be the accumulation of fluid in the abdomen or in the chest, the latter causing shortness of breath.

The routine pap smear does *not* help identify women who may have cancer of the ovary. The disease is first suspected by your doctor on pelvic examination. This may be a routine examination in which he notes enlargement of one or both ovaries, or it may be an examination to investigate any of the above signs. Abdominal fluid can often be removed with a needle through the top of the vagina or through the abdominal wall and examined for cancer cells. An enlarged ovary, however, is usually enough to start in motion studies that eventually lead to a biopsy and removal of the tumor. Several tumors that begin elsewhere can spread *to* the ovary. These include breast, stomach, and bowel. The breast is examined for any suspicious lumps, and the stomach and bowel are studied by x-ray. The ureter is frequently examined by x-ray (IVP) to see if it has been blocked off or pushed aside by a growing tumor. Finally, the lungs are usually examined by a chest x-ray, and the liver by a liver scan to look for spread to these two organs.

Is it Cancer of the Ovary?

Final proof requires surgery. The location of the ovary, inside the lower abdomen, makes a full-scale operation necessary just to get a biopsy. Therefore a biopsy, final evaluation of the extent of the disease, and the first step of its treatment are all carried out at the same time.

The initial treatment of cancer of the ovary is surgery. This tumor tends to spread locally, first to the neighboring structures, including

Treatment

the other ovary, the tubes, and the uterus, and later to other organs in the abdomen. The optimal operation is to remove both ovaries, the tubes, and the uterus, in order to remove as much tumor as possible. During the operation the surgeon can determine any spread of the tumor in the pelvis and abdominal cavity. This information will help determine later treatment.

It is possible to remove just the involved ovary if the tumor is of low grade malignancy and has not spread elsewhere. Cancer of the ovary has a strong tendency to spread to other parts of the pelvis and abdomen. Indeed, it frequently has done so by the time it is first discovered, in which case additional treatment with chemotherapy is usually given following recovery from surgery.

Because cancer of the ovary is hard to detect early, it is frequently quite advanced when treatment is begun. The overall results for all stages are not very good, with a five year survival rate of about 20 percent. When the tumor is discovered early and is still localized to the ovary, this increases to about 60 percent. With the availability of new drugs, particularly Adriamycin and Cis Platinum, the response rate of cancer of the ovary that has spread is greater than 50 percent.

In recurrence or advanced stages, cancer of the ovary tends to involve other organs in the abdomen, particularly the bowel. Obstruction of the bowel may cause vomiting and is treated by radiation, chemotherapy, or even surgery to bypass the obstructed area. Radiation can be given if the maximum safe dose was not received earlier. Chemotherapy gives relief to about half of the women who receive it. Another distressing sign of recurrence of cancer of the ovary is swelling of the abdomen from collecting fluid. Fluid may also collect in the chest, causing shortness of breath. The chest and the abdomen may be tapped to remove this fluid with a needle. The injection of drugs or radioisotopes into the abdomen or chest cavity can prevent or slow down accumulation of this fluid. A new operation transfers the fluid back into the circulating blood by means of a small tube buried under the skin.

CANCER OF THE BODY OF THE UTERUS

Signs

The single most important sign of cancer of the uterus is abnormal bleeding. Because this tumor is more common in older women, *any* vaginal bleeding or blood-tinged discharge after menopause should be brought to a doctor's attention promptly. At menopause, the same disease may cause unusually heavy periods, or bleeding between the periods. In this age group there are other causes of abnormal bleeding which have nothing to do with cancer, but the possibility of malignancy should not be overlooked. Other signs, such as pain in the lower abdomen or the back, are late signs and are usually preceded by abnormal bleeding. Cancer of the body of the uterus can occur in premenopausal woman although it is much less common.

Prolonged use of female hormones, particularly estrogen, either for contraception or during and after the menopause, may contribute to the development of this disease.

The diagnosis begins with a careful pelvic examination to determine the size of the uterus. Sometimes it is possible to obtain a diagnosis at that time by washing out the inside of the uterus with water to recover cancer cells, or using a suction device to get a small biopsy from the lining of the uterus. The final diagnosis can only be made by pelvic examination under anesthesia and "dilatation and curettage" (D & C) of the uterus. In this procedure the cervix is stretched or dilated with a series of metal instruments after which it is possible to scrape out (curettage) a large amount of the lining of the uterus for examination for cancer cells. Although this procedure takes only a few minutes it requires general anesthesia.

Is it Cancer of the Uterus?

If a biopsy obtained by D & C shows cancer in the lining of the uterus, several additional studies may be done to find out if the disease has spread. These include cystoscopy to see if there is spread to the bladder, sigmoidoscopy to see if there is spread to the colon, and an IVP to see if ureters have been pushed aside by the tumor. Since cancer of the uterus does not spread to these other organs very early, these studies may be omitted if the uterus is found to be small on examination.

The usual treatment for uterine cancer is surgery and radiation. When radiation is given before surgery, it is usually both external and internal. External radiation, given over two or more weeks, usually on an outpatient basis, is to the entire pelvis and the lymph nodes where this tumor often spreads. Internal radiation is delivered by cesium pellets that are inserted into the uterus and into the end of the vagina around the cervix. This is done under general anesthesia in the operating room through the vagina, although no real surgery is involved. The pellets are held in place by packing the vagina with a gauze plug. It is necessary to remain on your back in bed to avoid having the pellets move out of position. In the operating room a catheter is placed in your bladder so that your urine can be collected and you will not have to get up to go to the bathroom. You may also be placed on a special diet which will make it unnecessary for you to move your bowels while the cesium is in place, again to avoid any unnecessary movement. Since the pellets must stay in place two or three days, their position is checked by x-ray. During treatment you will be in a single room so no other patient is exposed. Visitors are

Treatment

kept to a minimum and asked to stand several feet from the bed. Nurses, who must care for many people undergoing radiation treatment, maintain a safe distance when they can, and do their work as quickly as possible without staying in your room too long. These precautions are for the safety of your friends and those taking care of you, but can make this time a fairly lonely experience. It helps to bring some reading materials or have a television set available to occupy your time. After the radium has been removed you are perfectly normal again and present no hazard to anyone. You can resume a normal social life, and can see your family and friends as much as you want. The operation, usually done four to six weeks later when the normal tissues have recovered, consists of removing the uterus, tubes, and ovaries.

Many centers now prefer to do the surgery first, in order to remove the uterus, tubes, and ovaries, and to check the lymph nodes and look for distant spread. If there is no spread and the tumor does not invade deeply into the wall of the uterus, additional radiation treatment may not be necessary. If radiation is needed after surgery, it is given the same way as before surgery.

The results of treatment of cancer of the body of the uterus are very good. The survival rate for all women is 70 percent. This relatively good outlook is due to the fact that so many of these tumors are discovered early, usually because of bleeding, before they have spread beyond the lining of the uterus. Eighty percent of all cancers of the body of the uterus are still in this early stage when they are first treated and most of them can be cured.

If it is going to recur at all, this tumor usually does so within two or three years. This means that a woman who has no evidence of recurrence by five years is unlikely to have one after that. The most common place for this cancer to recur is at the top of the vagina. The use of radiation therapy along with surgery decreases the likelihood of this but cannot eliminate it altogether. Women who have not previously had radiation are good candidates for radiation treatment for recurrence. Other places where this cancer may spread include the lungs, the liver, ovary, bowel, and the bones. These tumors are treated with female hormones (progesterone) which frequently slows down their growth. If this treatment fails, other chemotherapy or radiation may be used.

CANCER OF THE CERVIX The cervix is the portion of the uterus that extends into the top of the vagina. The cancer that develops there usually comes from the cells that cover the surface of the cervix. The development of cancer of the cervix is a very slow process in which the normal cells first become slightly abnormal or premalignant and then gradually, over three to twenty years, become truly malignant, evolving into a cancer that invades the underlying muscle of the cervix and is capable of spreading outward to other organs nearby. The slow rate of progression from normal to premalignant to malignant has made this cancer one of the easiest to detect and prevent, and even to treat at an early stage with a very high level of success. There are about 20,000 cases of cancer of the cervix each year. This number is decreasing as this cancer is more frequently being found when the woman still has only premalignant changes and can receive treatment before she develops "invasive" cancer. Cancer of the cervix can occur at any age from twenty-five to seventy. It is different from cancer of the body of the uterus in that it is frequently seen in premenopausal women, while cancer of the body of the uterus is more common during or after menopause.

The cause of cancer of the cervix is not known, but several factors suggest that it may be related to venereal infection. It is rare in women who have never had intercourse, and more common in those who have early and frequent intercourse, particularly with several different partners. It is more frequent in women of lower socio-economic groups. It is relatively infrequent in Jewish women. Venereal infection with one particular virus (Herpes II) has been found frequently in women with cancer of the cervix, but recently evidence indicates that this is probably just coincidence and that this virus does not cause the disease. There is no established relationship between contraceptive pills and the development of cancer of the cervix. However, women with abnormal Pap smears should definitely choose some other form of contraception.

Cancer of the cervix has benefited from early detection more than any other tumor. The pap smear, which is capable of detecting abnormal cells during the premalignant phase of this disease, has made this possible. (See Figure 21.2). This is done as part of the routine pelvic examination by scraping the cervix gently and putting the cells that are collected on a microscope slide for examination. Every woman over the age of 18 who has become sexually active should have a pap smear done once a year. For greater accuracy you should not douche for a couple of days before having a pap smear and it should not be done during your menstrual period.

Early Detection

The pap smear is reported back as one of five classifications:

Class I: The cells are completely normal.

Class II: Some abnormal cells but no evidence of cancerous changes. This smear should be repeated in three to six months.

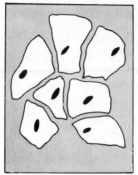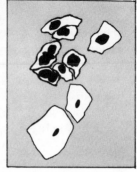

Normal   Early Cancer

Figure 21.2 Identification of cancer of the cervix by Pap smear. Changes can be recognized in cells that are scraped from the cervix long before a true cancer develops.

Class III: Some cells are suspicious or show "dysplasia" but do not show definite evidence of cancer. These changes may be due to inflammation of the cervix which will respond to simple treatment. If repeated pap smears continue to be suspicious a biopsy is often suggested.

Class IV: The cells are strongly suggestive of cancer. The pap smear is usually repeated immediately and further studies, including colposcopy and biopsy, are done at the same time. These often show non-invasive cancer (carcinoma in situ).

Class V: Cells are unmistakably cancer. A biopsy is always taken to confirm the diagnosis.

Every woman whose Pap smear is not normal (Class I) should have her cervix examined by colposcopy with biopsies taken of any suspicious areas. This is an outpatient procedure and is not uncomfortable.

Signs   The most common sign of cancer of the cervix, like that of cancer of the body of the uterus, is abnormal bleeding. In this case, however, the bleeding is more apt to follow mechanical irritation such as intercourse or douching. Any abnormal bleeding or discharge between menstrual periods should be investigated. Pain in the lower portion of the abdomen or the pelvis is usually a late sign and is rarely the first indication of this disease.

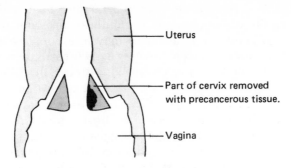

Figure 21.3 Cone biopsy of the cervix showing tissue removed.

The steps taken to make a diagnosis of cancer of the cervix include a pelvic examination, where an obvious abnormality of the cervix may be seen, the finding of cancer cells in the pap smear, colposcopy, and biopsy. They can all be done in the office. Colposcopy is examination of the cervix with a magnifying instrument which allows the doctor to inspect the abnormal areas more carefully. This instrument is not painful since no part of it goes inside you. Biopsies can be taken at the same time, using a small pinching instrument which is either painless or felt as a mild cramp. A larger biopsy (conization) in which a cone of tissue from the cervix is removed, requires anesthesia (See Figure 21.3).

Once the diagnosis of cancer of the cervix has been made, the next step is to determine the extent. This requires a more thorough pelvic examination, done in the hospital under general anesthesia for complete relaxation of the muscles of the abdomen and the pelvis. Cancer of the cervix tends to spread locally to the neighboring tissues, including the sides of the pelvis, the top of the vagina, the remainder of the uterus, and forward to the bladder or back to the rectum. The colon and rectum are examined by sigmoidoscopy and barium enema, and the bladder and ureters are examined by cystoscopy and an x-ray study of the ureters (IVP). Occasionally a lymphangiogram may be done to see if there is evidence of spread to the lymph nodes near the uterus.

Treatment for cancer of the cervix is surgery or radiation, depending on the stage of the disease. The very earliest stage of cancer of the cervix requiring treatment is cancer in situ ("in place"), in which the tumor is confined to the surface cells of the cervix and does not invade the muscle beneath them. This stage is usually treated by hysterectomy if the woman is no longer of child-bearing age, if her family is complete, or if childbearing is not important to her. In younger women the ovaries may be left in place. If a woman wishes to have more children, this very early form of the disease may be treated by a cone biopsy of the cervix with careful follow-up by repeat Pap smears and colposcopies to guard against any recurrence.

All other stages of cancer of the cervix, where there is invasion into the muscle, extension up into the uterus or down into the vagina, or into any of the neighboring tissues or organs are usually treated by external and internal radiation. In more advanced or recurrent disease, surgery may be necessary. Involvement of the bladder or rectum are occasionally treated by very radical surgery. If the cancer has spread back to the rectum or forward to the bladder, one or both of these organs may be removed along with the uterus, tubes, and ovaries. If the rectum is removed, it must be replaced by a colostomy (see Chapter 17 on Cancer of the Colon). Similarly, if the bladder is removed it must be replaced by an opening on the abdominal wall for collecting urine. (See Chapter 20 on Cancer of the Bladder). The need for such radical surgery is always recognized before the operation and should be discussed thoroughly with your doctor. This type of operation is reserved for women who are in good general condition and whose tumor has spread to organs *near* the uterus, but has *not* spread to other places. The chance of completely curing the disease must justify the extensive surgery.

Complications of radiation for carcinomas of the cervix or body of the uterus include radiation injury to the bladder and rectum, development of a communication (fistula) between the bladder and vagina, or rectum and vagina, damage to the bones of the pelvis with subsequent fractures, and unhealing sores or radiation burns of the upper vagina. With modern equipment and techniques these complications are rare.

Complications of surgery include damage to the ureters where they pass close to the uterus on their way to the bladder, leakage of urine from the ureters, development of an opening between bladder and vagina, or rectum and vagina, and non-healing of surgical wounds from infection.

The results of treatment of cancer of the cervix are excellent, primarily because it is often treated before it has a chance to become dangerous. Early detection by Pap smear and the slow progression of this disease make it possible to treat it very early, with almost 100 percent success. Further steps to eradicate this disease clearly depend on extending annual Pap smears to all women.

twenty-two

Cancer of the Head and Neck

The head and neck include many important organs crowded together in a relatively small space, which can give rise to a variety of tumors. This chapter will be confined to the more common ones, including lip, mouth, tongue, larynx (voice box) and the thyroid gland (See Figure 22.1).

About 45,000 people develop cancer of the head and neck in the United States each year, including 9,000 who develop cancer of the thyroid. With the exception of cancer of the thyroid, these tumors have many things in common. They are all rare under the age of forty, and reach their peak incidence at the age of sixty. Eighty to ninety percent of all cancers of the head and neck occur in men, and many of them are related to personal habits. Although the exact cause is not known, they are much more common in people who use large amounts of tobacco or alcohol.

CANCER OF THE LIP AND TONGUE

Smoking is associated primarily with cancer of the lip and the tongue. Unlike cancer of the lung which is associated with cigarette smoking, these two cancers occur more frequently in men who smoke pipes or cigars. The use of chewing tobacco or snuff also shows up here in that men who store their quid inside their lip or cheek are more apt to develop tumors in that same location. An uncommon form of late syphilis or the use of large amounts of alcohol are both associated with cancer of the tongue and of the throat. Inadequate care of the teeth and poor oral hygiene are frequently associated with cancer of the mouth. Finally, cancer of the lip almost invariably occurs on the lower lip and is much more common in men who work outdoors and have prolonged exposure to sunlight. People who have developed one cancer in the head and neck area are much more likely

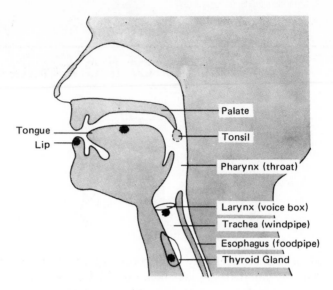

Figure 22.1 Locations of the common cancer of the head and neck.

to develop a second tumor somewhere else in the same area later on. These secondary tumors are presumably due to the same causes as the original which lends support to the likelihood that these habits are indeed responsible for the disease.

Cancers of the head and neck are predictable in their behavior. They tend to spread first to the lymph nodes high in the neck, nearest to the cancer, and then to the other lymph nodes lower in the neck. Spread to the lymph nodes of the neck is relatively slow and late in cancer of the lip, but earlier and more common in cancer of the tongue, mouth, or the throat. Only late in the disease do these tumors spread to other parts of the body, usually the lung.

Where they can be observed, particularly in the mouth, many begin as pre-malignant areas of white plaque (leukoplakia), or red patches (erythroplakia). The white plaques are not cancer but are pre-cancerous since a significant percent will eventually become malignant. These areas may be thin films that are greyish-white or thickened, raised plaques of tissue that are harder and drier than the normal surface. Erythroplakia, on the other hand, is a more advanced stage of change which corresponds to carcinoma in situ in other parts of the body (such as cancer of the cervix of the uterus). These areas are usually sharply outlined red patches in which the cells have undergone definite changes in the direction of cancer.

Cancers of the lip, tongue, or inside of the mouth usually develop as sores or ulcers that do not heal. These may be raised, firm areas with cauliflower-like surfaces, they may be small punched-out craters with hard edges, or they may be areas of hardness or thickening that can be felt by the tip of the tongue. The important thing about these sores is that they are not sore; they are usually almost painless. This is in contrast to the usual canker sore or other minor infection in the mouth in which the discomfort is completely out of proportion to the small size of the injury. Cancers of the back of the mouth or the throat are much harder to feel and may show up as difficulty swallowing, a disturbance of hearing or pain in the ear (some nerves from the ear connect with those of the throat), pain on swallowing, or swelling or lumps in the neck. Cancer of the larynx or voice box usually shows up very early as hoarseness and only much later as swelling or lumps in the neck or difficulty breathing. Lumps in the neck usually indicate spread to lymph nodes, regardless of where the original tumor is.

If you notice anything unusual inside your mouth the first thing to do is feel around with your finger and look in the mirror, or have someone else look for you. Everyone experiences hoarseness and sores in the mouth from time to time, but any such abnormality that lasts for more than two weeks should be called to the attention of your doctor or dentist. His examination should include inspection of your mouth and throat with a good light, feeling inside your mouth with his finger, and feeling your neck for any lumps that may be enlarged lymph nodes.

Any suspicious area should be biopsied. This can usually be done in the office under local anesthesia. If the suspicious area is in the throat or in the voice box, the biopsy can only be done as part of a more thorough examination (direct laryngoscopy) in which the area is examined through a hollow lighted tube under general anesthesia and the biopsy obtained at the time. This may require being in the hospital for a day or two. Cancer of the inside of the mouth requires x-ray studies to see if it has spread to the bone of the jaw or the roof of the mouth. A chest x-ray is taken to see if the tumor has spread to the lungs.

Most cancers of the head and neck are treated by surgery or radiation and for some there is actually a choice between these two forms of treatment. For this reason, it is very important for you to discuss the suggested treatment and alternatives for your own particular cancer with your doctors. If surgery has been recommended there is every reason to ask for a consultation with a radiation therapist or, if radiation therapy has been recommended, to ask for a consultation with a surgeon. In some hospitals people with cancers of the head or neck are now seen together by both specialists so the best treatment can be advised. This should be a more common practice.

In general, radiation or surgery may be used for small tumors —less than ¾ of an inch in diameter—that are easy to get at and where the amount of tissue removed will not result in any disability or serious scarring. Surgery under these circumstances is quick and causes very little discomfort or loss of time from work. Most cancers of the lip can be completely removed with very good cosmetic results. Surgery is frequently the best or only treatment when the tumor involves the underlying bone, such as the jaw in cancer of the gum or the floor of the mouth, because the bone frequently fails to heal after radiation.

Radiation, or radiation and surgery, are used for larger tumors where the amount of tissue that would have to be removed by surgery alone would result in serious disfigurement or loss of function. Under these circumstances, radiation therapy definitely gives better functional and cosmetic results with much less scarring. For tumors that are not easy to get at, such as the back of the tongue or the throat, radiation is often the only reasonable treatment. In some cases, radiation therapy has the advantage of surgical backup if the tumor is not controlled by the original radiation.

Cancer of the forward or mobile part of the tongue can be treated with radiation or surgery or a combination of both. Small tumors can often be removed surgically without limiting motion of the tongue to interfere with good speech. Larger tumors are usually treated with radiation and surgery. Tumors of the back of the tongue are much harder to treat, by either surgery or radiation. Occasionally large tumors of the tongue or mouth are treated with chemotherapy before either surgery or radiation to try to reduce the size of the tumor so that it can be completely removed or destroyed.

The type of radiation therapy used for cancers of the head and neck is usually external radiation, but occasionally internal radiation, using radium needles, is given for cancer of the tongue or the floor of the mouth. The major disadvantage of radiation is that it takes several weeks and may be associated with considerable soreness of the mouth and difficulty swallowing during much of that time. A long-term side effect of radiation of the head or neck area may be permanent dryness of the mouth.

Two special forms of surgery are occasionally used for some tumors of the head and neck. Laser surgery uses the intense heat of a laser beam which can be focused on a tiny area. Cryosurgery is just the opposite and uses the extreme cold of liquid nitrogen to destroy small areas of tumor by freezing.

<table>
<tr><td>

Cancer of the larynx has its own special considerations for treatment. Early cancers which are small and, at the most, involve only a small portion of one of the two vocal chords can frequently be treated by surgery or radiation. Serious consideration should be given to this choice of treatment. The only disability resulting from this surgery is slight but permanent hoarseness of the voice. Larger tumors are best treated by surgery, or radiation and surgery, if there is a possibility of curing them and still preserving the voice. Finally comes the still larger tumor which is also very curable by surgery, but at the great expense of complete loss of the voice. In this operation (laryngectomy), the voice box is completely removed and the windpipe (trachea) is brought to the outside as a hole low in the neck. Breathing is through this new hole (tracheostomy) and no longer through the normal route of the nose and mouth.

</td><td>

CANCER OF THE LARYNX

</td></tr>
</table>

About a third of all people with cancer of the larynx, or about 3,000 each year, require total laryngectomy. Psychologically, this is a very serious operation but the results in terms of curing the disease more than justify it. A person who has a laryngectomy (a laryngectomee) must share his disability and subsequent rehabilitation with his entire family. Positive attitudes and good support are very helpful. It is particularly helpful to see for yourself that the disability can be overcome. A visit from a fully rehabilitated laryngectomee, who has learned to use his new voice well, should take place *before* you have your operation. The fact is that most laryngectomees returned to their normal occupations and lives, having acquired a very acceptable form of vocal communication, and you should see this for yourself. Before surgery you should also receive detailed instructions of the various things that must be done after your operation. These include the vital functions of breathing, eating and talking.

Laryngectomy

Breathing: The Tracheostomy. For several weeks and often permanently, the tracheostomy will be kept open by means of a metal tube or airway. The proper cleansing of this is of vital importance since the inside can become blocked with dried secretions. Most laryngectomy tubes consist of two tubes, an outer sleeve which is tied in place most of the time, and an inner sleeve which can be removed easily for cleansing. You will be shown how to do this while you are in the hospital, and before you go home you will be shown how to remove both tubes and replace them. After several weeks, when the tracheostomy is well healed, many people can get along well without any tube.

With a tracheostomy, your ability to cough is greatly reduced because you cannot close off your throat to build up pressure. Later you will be shown how to produce a reasonable cough, but the first few days you must rely on suctioning, where a small rubber tube is inserted into the trachea to stimulate you to cough and to remove the secretions by suction. You will be taught to do this yourself, too.

Some other precautions must be observed. It is obviously dangerous to go swimming since your vent for breathing is well below the usual level of your mouth and nose. Similarly, care must be taken to avoid getting much water in the tracheostomy when you are showering. Rubber shields have been made for this purpose or you can protect the tracheostomy with your hand. In daily life most people feel safer protecting their tracheostomies with some kind of a shield of porous cloth that will keep foreign objects out. Beyond that, the tracheostomy can be easily and tastefully concealed with appropriate clothing or jewelry. The air that you breathe must be artificially moisturized, a function normally carried out by the inside of the nose. Some find it necessary to moisten the protective cloth, particularly in the winter, and everyone who has a tracheostomy should maintain a high level of humidity in his home.

Eating. The other piece of support equipment that you may have after your operation is a feeding tube (nasogastric or NG tube). This is a soft plastic tube that was inserted down into your stomach by way of your nose and foodpipe when you were asleep. This is to allow you to receive food without having to swallow very much while your throat is healing. Liquid meals are injected into the tube, another skill that you will acquire for yourself. The feeding tube is usually needed only for a few days.

Speech. The most serious longterm disability to overcome following laryngectomy is regaining your speech. Until you do so, the only way you can communicate more than very simple ideas is by writing notes. Developing esophageal speech requires time and patience but is accomplished successfully by more than 75 percent of all people who have a laryngectomy. This works by swallowing air to accumulate a bubble in the stomach and esophagus, and then burping the air back out slowly to make a continuous noise in the throat. The words are formed by shaping the mouth and tongue as one would in ordinary speech. Excellent teachers are available and you should begin your training before leaving the hospital. A few people combine esophageal speech with the use of a mechanical device, and still fewer must rely solely on mechanical speech. The device most frequently used is a small battery-powered buzzer that is held in the hand

and applied to the side of the neck. The vibrations of the buzzer are transmitted through the mouth and shaped into sounds and words by moving the lips and tongue in the usual way. Although the voice produced by this is mechanical and monotonous, and not nearly as good as well-developed esophageal speech, it provides perfectly acceptable communication.

Results of treatment of cancer of the larynx, even by total laryngectomy, are excellent. In order to help people who must face this disability, a large number of Lost Chord Clubs or New Voice Clubs have been formed. Information concerning the nearest club can be obtained from the International Association of Laryngectomees, American Cancer Society, 777 Third Ave., New York, NY 10017.

Most tumors of the head and neck spread in a predictable fashion to the nearby lymph nodes. If the tumor has already spread to these nodes by the time it is first seen, it is usually advisable to remove them by an operation called a neck dissection. This may be done at the same time the original tumor is removed if the tumor is small, and it is certain that it can be completely removed. A neck dissection may also be done following successful radiation therapy to a tumor of the mouth. On the other hand, there is usually no point in removing the lymph nodes in the neck if the original tumor has not been eliminated, either by surgery or radiation.

A neck dissection is done prophylactically, when there is a high likelihood that lymph nodes are involved even though they are not yet enlarged. An alternative is to treat the neck with radiation and watch carefully for nodes to appear, doing a neck dissection only if it becomes necessary. With some tumors, such as cancer of the lip, this is perfectly acceptable since this tumor tends to spread rather slowly.

Removal of Lymph Nodes

The results of treatment of the more common tumors of the head and neck are shown in Table 22.1. Although many of these tumors can be cured, the treatment required may be radical and disfiguring, particularly if surgery offers the best chance of cure. Difficult as the decision is, the disease justifies the treatment because uncontrolled growth of head and neck tumors may be even more disfiguring and distressing than the treatment, and are eventually fatal.

Results of Treatment

Many of the tumors that recur do so in the neck without ever spreading to other parts of the body. When they do go elsewhere, it is usually to the lungs. Recurrence of cancer of the head or neck can be treated by additional surgery, radiation therapy, or chemotherapy, but usually cannot be permanently cured unless they are limited to lymph

Follow-Up and Recurrence

Table 22.1. Results of Treatment of Cancers of the Head and Neck

Location	Treatment	5 Year Survival Rate (%)* without spread to nodes	with spread to nodes
Lip	Surgery or Radiation	80–90	50
Tongue	Surgery or Radiation	40–70	25–30
Floor of Mouth	Surgery or Radiation	60	30
Back of Tongue and Throat	Radiation	25	10
Larynx	Surgery or Radiation	60–95	60

* More exact figures within the ranges shown depend on the location and size of the tumor, and the grade of malignancy.

nodes high in the neck that have not received previous treatment. If a high dose of radiation was used in the initial treatment it usually cannot be repeated. Moreover, surgery in areas that have been heavily radiated has an increased risk because of poor healing. Chemotherapy can occasionally reduce the size of the tumor and provide relief from discomfort.

Late complications of these tumors include respiratory obstruction and inability to swallow. Both of these can be relieved temporarily by surgical procedures but they usually do not extend life. Further treatment should be discussed carefully with your family and your doctor, considering all of the alternatives, before making a choice. It is important to weigh what can be accomplished against the disfigurement and disability that may be involved.

CANCER OF THE THYROID

Cancer of the thyroid has little in common with other tumors of the head and neck and is included here only because of its location. The thyroid gland is a little larger than a walnut which has been split in half, with one half at each side of the windpipe low in the neck. The function of this gland is to regulate metabolism and energy. Failure of the thyroid gland to function properly (hypothyroidism) causes sleepiness, apathy and mental dullness, weight gain, intolerance of cold, and weakness. Abnormal increased thyroid function (hyperthyroidism) causes irritability, increased activity, weight loss in spite of a large appetite, intolerance of heat, rapid pulse rate, and sweating. The gland is made up of several types of cells that can cause different tumors, the most common of which are papillary carcinoma and follicular carcinoma.

While the cause of most cancers of the thyroid is not known, one very important association is recognized. Radiation, particularly early in life, increases the incidence of cancer of the thyroid about thirty times over the normal population. It was common practice in the United States in the 1920s and up through the early 1940s to treat a variety of childhood illnesses with x-ray. These included enlargement of the thymus gland, tonsillitis, and enlarged lymph nodes in the neck. As many as ten percent of these young people developed cancer of the thyroid when they grew up, often thirty or more years after the x-ray treatment. This form of treatment was discontinued as soon as the risk was recognized and now, thirty-five years later, we are beginning to see fewer people with thyroid cancer who previously received x-ray treatments. However, we still do not know when this risk will be completely over. If you know that you received x-ray treatments as a child or teenager, you should call it to the attention of your physician so he can examine your thyroid at regular intervals.

Cancer of the thyroid usually appears as a painless swelling or asymmetry low in the neck, noticed while looking in the mirror or by other people. It is often picked up on routine physical examination. Less frequently, when the tumor extends beyond the thyroid gland, it may cause hoarseness or difficulty swallowing.

Signs

Since there are many noncancerous tumors that cause enlargement of the thyroid gland, several studies are done to determine the likelihood of malignancy. These include careful examination of the neck, examination of the vocal chords with a small mirror to see if they both move properly, an x-ray study of the neck to determine that there is no difficulty swallowing, and a thyroid scan to evaluate the tumor itself. The normal thyroid gland has a large appetite for iodine and most of the iodine that enters the body quickly finds its way to the thyroid. If a small amount of radioactive iodine (I^{131}) is given, the size and shape of the gland can be recorded by a special instrument and shows up as an outline of black dots on a photographic film. Cancer of the thyroid does not take up the radioactive iodine as well as normal thyroid and therefore shows up as a light area against the darker background. A large thyroid nodule can be biopsied with a needle but more frequently the biopsy is done as part of an operation to remove part or all of the thyroid gland.

Is it Cancer of the Thyroid?

The usual treatment for cancer of the thyroid is to remove all of the gland because many of these tumors are present on both sides, even though they first appear on one side. The lymph nodes are usually removed only if they appear to be involved. The most common type of thyroid cancer, papillary carcinoma, tends to spread very slowly

Treatment

and only to the nearby nodes. The nodes can be removed years later if they become involved without compromising the chances for cure, which for this tumor are over 90 percent. Papillary carcinoma is a very slowly progressive tumor and a person may live twenty years or longer, even with known spread.

The next most common cancer of the thyroid, follicular carcinoma, also spreads to the neighboring nodes but also can spread directly to the lungs. It is treated very much in the same way but the overall chances of cure are slightly lower. Other more rare forms of thyroid cancer are more aggressive, and harder to cure.

Removal of the thyroid gland is a delicate operation because of several important structures that are close by. On each side, a small nerve passes by the thyroid gland on its way to the voice box (larynx). Damage to either of these nerves results in permanent hoarseness. Similarly, immediately behind the thyroid gland are four small glands measuring about 1/4 inch in diameter, the parathyroids. These control the use of calcium by the body. Two or even three of these four glands may be removed without difficulty, but loss of all of them results in numbness, muscle cramps, tingling in the fingers and around the mouth and other distressing symptoms. When present these symptoms can be relieved by taking large amounts of calcium in the form of milk and calcium tablets. Unless these structures are directly involved with the tumor they should be spared when the thyroid gland is removed.

Following removal of the thyroid gland it is necessary to take a thyroid hormone preparation by mouth. The dose is regulated to provide a high level of energy and metabolism but not to the point of giving the distress of hyperthyroidism mentioned previously. This high normal dose also tends to suppress the growth of any remaining thyroid tissue, including residual tumor.

Tumors that recur after surgery or have spread elsewhere can sometimes be treated with radioactive iodine, the same material which was used to help find the tumor in the first place. When it is being used for treatment, a much larger dose of radioactive iodine is given than when it is used for diagnosis.

twenty-three

Skin Cancer, Melanoma, and Sarcoma

There are three important cancers of the skin, each originating from a different type of cell. *Basal cell* carcinoma comes from round cells that are deep in the skin while *squamous cell* carcinoma comes from the flatter cells that are near the surface. These two tumors look very much alike and both are usually of such low-grade malignancy that they are not considered truly malignant cancers. Indeed, it has been estimated that 50 percent of the population will develop at least one of these common skin cancers during a lifetime of seventy years. If treated early and properly, these two tumors are very rarely fatal. *Melanoma* originates in the pigmented cells of the skin, the cells which determine one's normal skin coloring and which multiply and increase in darkness in the process of tanning from exposure to the sun. Melanoma is much less common than basal cell or squamous cell carcinoma, but is also a much more serious disease.

These three skin cancers have one important factor in common; they are all thought to be caused by excessive exposure to sunlight. The two common skin cancers are rare in blacks, but melanoma is more common, particularly in African countries where it tends to occur on the soles of the feet, suggesting that chronic injury to the skin may be a factor. It is much less common in blacks in the United States. Skin cancers are not contagious. They cannot be transmitted by direct contact, through towels or swimming pools.

COMMON SKIN CANCERS

Basal cell and squamous cell are two very common skin cancers which occur more frequently in older people, with basal cell carcinoma occurring about four times as often as squamous cell. They are definitely related to long exposure to the sun and are occupational hazards for farmers, ranchers, sailors, outdoor sportsman, and even sun worshipers. They are more common in parts of the world where sunlight is intense, and are seen most frequently in people who burn easily, those with fair skin, light eyes, and light hair. They are much more frequent on the exposed parts of the body, with about 90 percent appearing on the face, neck, hands, and arms. In addition to exposure to sunlight, both of these tumors occasionally occur as hereditary diseases or previously non-malignant skin conditions, particularly senile keratosis, which is often seen on the face and back of the hands of the elderly as white scaly plaques. In addition, squamous cell carcinoma can occur in areas previously exposed to high doses of x-ray, or to chemicals such as coal tar products and arsenic, chronic unhealed or poorly healed wounds such as burn scars, or long term infections of bone (osteomyelitis).

Is it Skin Cancer? Both of these common skin cancers vary in appearance and frequently can be told apart only by microscopic examination of a biopsy. They usually appear as thickened or ulcerated areas on the face or hands, or as plaques of thickening beneath the skin with the surface appearing to be intact and normal. They may be flat or raised, scaly or ulcerated, but they do not heal and go away. The biopsy needed for diagnosis is usually taken from the edge of the tumor, to include a tiny piece of normal skin. This can be done either with a small round cutting instrument (punch biopsy) or with a scalpel. The biopsy is done under local anesthesia and is usually too small to require a stitch to close the wound.

Treatment These tumors tend to spread locally, invading the underlying tissues, rather than spreading to lymph nodes or other parts of the body. Basal cell tumors virtually never go to lymph nodes or beyond, while squamous cell carcinomas do so only occasionally. For this reason, the treatment is entirely directed towards the original tumor. Neighboring lymph nodes, usually in the neck, armpit, or groin, depending on where the original tumor is, are not removed unless they are obviously involved. Since these tumors are easily seen they are usually treated early. Surgical removal or radiation are equally effective. For small tumors, where only a small scar will remain, frequently in a facial line, surgery is preferred over radiation which requires daily visits for one to three weeks.

For larger tumors, where more extensive surgery would be disfiguring, radiation is frequently preferable. In more advanced tumors, particularly where the tumor involves the bones of the face, radiation is not curative and quite extensive surgery may be necessary. Fortunately, such large skin tumors are rare. They usually have been present for ten or more years and frequently had previous treatment when they were smaller. Extensive and disfiguring surgery to the face is very hard to accept. It requires careful consideration and planning by the patient and the surgeon. It should always be planned in cooperation with a plastic surgeon who is skilled at facial reconstruction in order to minimize the defect. These tumors are very rarely fatal and more than 95 percent of the common skin cancers are completely cured when they are first treated. Of those that recur, most can still be cured by additional surgery or radiation therapy.

Because radiation and surgery are equally effective in treating many skin cancers, a real choice is available. To a large extent, this is influenced by the location and size of the tumor and the availability of treatment in your community. You should not hesitate to discuss both forms of treatment with your doctor to be sure that you understand this choice.

People who have been treated for skin cancer should be examined periodically to look for possible recurrences. New skin cancers are common in people whose skin has already shown this tendency to develop tumors. Squamous cell cancer of the skin does occasionally spread to other parts of the body, including the lung, liver, bone, or brain. These rare occurrences are treated with chemotherapy.

MELANOMA

Melanoma (malignant melanoma) has a much more complicated relationship to exposure sunlight. Like the more common skin cancers, melanoma is more frequent on exposed parts of the body, such as the head, neck and trunk of men and the head, neck and legs of women. Melanoma is increasing in frequency. Its incidence has doubled in the past ten years and the frequency on the neck, trunk and legs has increased six times since 1940. There are now approximately 10,000 new cases of malignant melanoma in the United States each year. Melanoma is most frequently seen in the elderly but also occurs in young adults. It is very rare in children and is not related to pregnancy.

Melanoma differs from the more common skin cancers in one respect. In spite of the fact that all of them appear to be related to exposure to sunlight, melanoma is more common in people who do not have chronic long-term exposure. It is not an occupational hazard of those who work outdoors, but rather of those who work indoors and only occasionally are exposed to the sun (i.e. teachers, office workers, and other white collar workers). Because it is seen in people who are fair skinned and tend to burn easily, it is thought to be related to occasional severe sunburn rather than chronic exposure. The increasing incidence of melanoma is thought to be due to the fact that more people are exposing more of themselves to the sun than in the past.

Signs Two-thirds of all malignant melanomas begin with already existing moles. Since the average individual has fifteen to twenty moles on his body, the real question is "When should I begin to worry?". The main thing to look for is a change in a previously existing mole or the appearance of a new mole. The change may be in the size of the mole, the color, the appearance of ulceration or scaling, crusting, itching, bleeding on minor injury, or increasing elevation above the surface of the skin. Melanomas are highly variable and do not present any single typical picture. In shape they may be large or tiny, with sharp borders or very indistinct ones. They may be flat, slightly elevated, or mushroom-like growths that are elevated well above the skin surface. They may range in appearance from tan and brown to red or purple-black or deep black. They may even be *white*, since some melanomas lose the pigment that characterized this type of cell.

Is it
Melanoma? Final diagnosis is made by biopsy. This can usually be done under local anesthesia. A dark tumor of the skin should *always* be biopsied and should *never* by treated by burning with an electric needle, freezing, or any other form of destruction that does not remove the entire tumor intact for examination by the pathologist. A biopsy shows that it is (or is not) melanoma and how deeply it extends into the skin, both of which are important in determining eventual treatment.

Treatment Melanomas are very capricious and unpredictable tumors that tend to spread in the small lymphatic vessels in the skin, to the nearby lymph nodes, and also to distant parts of the body. This spread may take place very late or it may take place when the original tumor is very small or occasionally when it cannot even be found at all. Melanoma is treated by removing the tumor and a large area of surrounding skin. The margins should be two to three inches on all sides of the tumor except when it is on the face where smaller margins are acceptable. Even when the entire tumor is removed during a biopsy, removal of additional skin, including the scar, should be carried out in a second operation to insure adequate margins.

Removal of a large piece of skin frequently requires the use of a skin graft taken from some other part of the body, usually the thigh, to cover the defect. A very thin "shaving" of skin is used for this purpose. The skin grows back to its full thickness in the place that it was taken from, leaving no scar at all. Unlike the more common skin cancers, radiation has no place in the treatment of melanomas while it is still in the skin and has not spread.

Melanoma spreads to nearby lymph nodes. When the nodes are obviously involved, they are usually removed, if there is no evidence of spread to other parts of the body. Smaller and more superficial melanomas, which do not penetrate deeply into the skin, rarely spread to the lymph nodes, making removal of the nodes unnecessary. Conversely, larger and thicker melanomas which penetrate more deeply into the skin are more apt to have spread to the neighboring nodes, even if the nodes are not noticeably enlarged. There is some controversy at the present time about whether lymph nodes that are not obviously involved should be removed or not. Many surgeons feel that if the tumor is sufficiently deep and likely to have spread to lymph nodes, usually in the axilla or the groin, these nodes should be removed. If the tumor is located where it could spread to more than two sets of nodes, such as the middle of the back, many surgeons feel that removal of all of these lymph nodes is not justifiable. Similarly, if the tumor is found to have already spread to the lungs or other distant parts of the body, there is little point in removing the lymph nodes.

Adjuvant chemotherapy is being tried, in addition to surgery, to improve the results with some less favorable melanomas, particularly those on the trunk, those that have recurred locally, or when lymph nodes are involved. Melanoma can spread to almost any other part of the body, including the skin, the lung, liver, and brain. Moreover, distant spread can take place without any involvement of the neighboring lymph nodes. Distant spread is treated with chemotherapy with good remissions about 25 percent of the time. The drugs most frequently used include imidazole carboxamide, BCNU, methyl-CCNU, and phenylalanine mustard.

The overall five year survival rate for treated melanoma is 60 percent, ranging from 90–100 percent for the very superficial tumors, to 40 percent for tumors that penetrate through the skin into the fatty tissue underneath. Involvement of the regional lymph nodes by tumor is also important. If the nodes are free of tumor, the five year survival rate is 60–70 percent, while if the nodes are involved it is only 20 percent. Melanomas on the head and neck have a better outlook than those on the trunk and, for any given tumor, women have a slightly better outlook than men.

After treatment for melanoma, you should be followed for recurrence for life. If it is going to appear, a recurrence usually does so within five years. However, melanoma is one of the few tumors that can recur ten, fifteen, or even twenty years after removal of the original tumor.

The relationship between exposure to sunlight and the occurrence of both of the common skin cancers and melanoma suggest that we should avoid unnecessary exposure to the sun. For those who do not tan, excessive exposure is clearly dangerous. For those who do tan, gradually increasing exposures, to promote good tanning and avoid burning, is the only safe route. The wise use of effective sun screens will permit those of us who are sun worshipers to continue our practices without too much danger.

THE SARCOMAS

When I found the lump under my arm my wife went into a panic. Even my doctor went pale when he saw it. I was told that it could be malignant or benign — whatever it was, it had to come out.

Sarcomas are cancers of the structural and connective tissues of the body. These include bone (osteosarcoma), cartilage (chondrosarcoma), fibrous connective tissue (fibrosarcoma), fat (liposarcoma), muscle (myosarcoma), and blood vessels (angiosarcoma). While most can appear at any age, osteosarcoma is more common in young people between ten and twenty-five, and chondrosarcoma is more common between thirty and sixty. As a group, sarcomas are rare tumors, with about 7,000 new cases in the United States each year. The cause is not known. They are definitely *not* related to common injuries, although athletic injuries in children often bring about discovery of the tumor. The single exception is the more-than-coincidental occurrence of sarcomas in the scars of serious burns. In experimental animals, both chemicals and viruses cause sarcomas.

Signs

Sarcomas appear as an enlarging, non-tender swelling or mass which is usually painless. Sarcomas of the bone most frequently occur just above the knee, or in the upper arm, while sarcomas of cartilage are common in the pelvis, the ribs, and the spine, as well as in the arm and the leg. Of the other sarcomas, 40 percent occur in the leg, 20 percent in the arm, 20 percent in the trunk, 10 percent in the head and neck, and about 10 percent in the back wall of the abdominal cavity. Some of these are so well hidden by overlying normal tissue that they may become quite large before being noticed.

Is it Sarcoma?

The diagnosis of sarcoma is usually not difficult to make. X-ray and ultrasound studies show changes in bone or cartilage. They also show abnormal masses in softer tissues. A bone scan, following the injection of an isotope that is picked up by the tumor, helps detect sarcomas of bone. X-ray of blood vessels (arteriogram or angiogram) show whether these vessels are pushed aside or whether the tumor has an abnormal blood supply which is often characteristic. Chemical changes in the blood are often found in sarcomas of bone (elevation of the calcium and the enzyme alkaline phosphatase). A chest x-ray is very important in evaluating sarcomas because as a group they tend to spread rather early and usually to the lungs. Sarcomas are quite different from each other in their behavior, and therefore require different forms of treatment. For this reason the biopsy is usually done as a separate procedure before any treatment is planned. Depending on where the tumor is the biopsy may be done under local or general anesthesia. It is usually done as an open biopsy to get an adequate piece of tumor rather than as a needle biopsy.

If the sarcoma has not spread, the first treatment is usually surgery. **Treatment** The extent of the operation depends on the type of sarcoma and its location. Because many sarcomas occur in the arm or the leg, treatment for cure may require very radical surgery, including amputation. Contemplation of such a loss is a tremendous shock to anyone, and is not decreased by the fact that the person is often a child. For many years the cruel alternative was quite simply "your limb or your life".

More recently a few cancer centers are modifying the treatment of some sarcomas by combining less radical surgery with radiation therapy. The operations are still extensive, and bone involvement may require replacement with artificial bone or even an artificial joint, but the limb is saved, although its function may be less than normal. Radiation required to help control these tumors is extensive and may be given before or after the surgery. Many sarcomas spread early by the blood stream and, even when there is no evidence of spread, eventually show up again, usually in the lungs. For this reason removal of the original tumor is not considered to be enough treatment for some sarcomas. Trials of adjuvant chemotherapy are also being carried out to try to eliminate cells that may have spread before the tumor was discovered. The notable exception is sarcoma of cartilage which grows slowly and spreads much later.

When a sarcoma recurs or has spread to the lungs, the treatment is usually chemotherapy. Adriamycin, frequently in combination with other drugs, has a response rate of about 50 percent. Surprisingly, surgery also has a role in the treatment of some sarcomas that have spread. If there is only one or at most a few tumor nodules in the lungs and they are confined to one lung, they can be removed without removing much normal lung tissue. While this aggressive surgical approach is rarely curative it can offer a comfortable life, sometimes for years.

Treatment of sarcomas in children is one of the bright and encouraging areas in cancer treatment. One type of sarcoma of muscle in children (rhabdomyosarcoma) can be cured more than 50 percent of the time by a combination of surgery, radiation, and chemotherapy, if it has not spread. Similarly, sarcoma of bone, which was almost always fatal ten years ago, may also be successfully treated with radical surgery combined with radiation and chemotherapy. If the tumor has not spread the two year survival is about 40 percent and over half of these children may be cured. The picture in adults is not as good. Sarcoma of the bone in adults has only a 20 percent five year survival rate while the others range from 20 percent to 90 percent five year survival, depending on the type of sarcoma. The very gratifying results of the treatment of sarcoma in children have stimulated intense study of combined forms of treatment for these tumors in adults.

twenty-four

Leukemia and Lymphoma

Leukemia is a disease of the white blood cells and the bone marrow. The bone marrow is white fatty material located in the cavities of most of the large bones in the body. It is the factory where blood cells are made. The cells originate from early or primitive stem cells which develop into the various families of blood cells, normally to be released into the circulating blood as mature blood cells. These families include the red cells which carry oxygen to the tissues, platelets which help the blood to clot and prevent bleeding, and white cells which fight infections. The white cells are further divided into three groups, lymphocytes which are responsible for the immune response, granulocytes which eat up bacteria that cause infections, and monocytes which eat up any dirt or foreign material that may get into the body.

The immature cells in the bone marrow are called blasts. In leukemia, the immature blasts of white cells grow out of control. First they crowd out normal bone marrow cells and later they spill over into the circulation. In children this process is labelled "acute" because it usually comes on very suddenly and progresses rapidly. The interval between the very first signs of illness and making the diagnosis of leukemia is often less than three weeks. The same disease in adults may be "chronic" because it is slower to progress.

I never did feel sick, just weak and tired. Leukemia is a lot of little miseries, no real pain. But even they can get to you once in a while.

You would think that a disease like acute leukemia that can react so violently and suddenly must be a painful disease. It really isn't. It's the procedures that go along with it for treatment that are a nuisance.

Leukemia is not like it is in the movies. You don't go around looking like you're deathly ill or in constant pain all the time. I could do most of the things I wanted

273

to do. The real problem is that I just didn't have much energy. I missed a lot of school. Since I've gotten better I've been able to do everything I've wanted to. I've gone camping and traveled and I've gone back to my normal life.

ACUTE LEUKEMIA OF CHILDHOOD

The most common leukemia in children, acute lymphocytic leukemia or ALL, makes up about 80 percent of all childhood leukemias. Acute granulocytic leukemia, also known as acute myelocytic leukemia or AML, accounts for most of the other cases. This name comes from the fact that the primitive blast cells that become granulocytes are called myeloblasts.

Childhood leukemia is rare before age one and most frequent between three and six. The cause is not known, but radiation, drugs that injure the bone marrow, viruses, and genetic factors have all been suggested. The increased incidence of leukemia among Japanese who received heavy radiation from the atomic bomb blasts, and American children who were exposed to fallout from the testing of nuclear weapons indicates that radiation contributes to this disease. We now feel that unwarranted exposure of women to diagnostic x-rays during pregnancy may increase the possible risk to the unborn child.

Virus-like particles have been seen in leukemia cells but have rarely been isolated. Genetic information that may come from such viruses has not been found in any human leukemia. Most important, there is no evidence that leukemia is spread from one person to another, either within families or within communities.

Genetic factors play an unusual but demonstrable role in this disease. The incidence of leukemia in the average population is about four in every 100,000 children. However, leukemia is relatively common among children who have hereditary diseases where chromosomes break easily. The most common of these is mongolism or Down's Syndrome, where approximately one percent of the affected children eventually develop leukemia. In families where one child has leukemia the chances of another child developing the disease are one in 720. In identical twins this increases to one in five.

Signs

The signs of leukemia are directly related to the crowding out of normal bone marrow elements by leukemic cells. Interference with production of red cells causes anemia which shows up as paleness of the skin, tiredness, listlessness, and shortness of breath. Lack of production of platelets causes bleeding of the gums, nose bleeds, easy bruising, small hemorrhages of the skin which cause red spots known as petechia, blood in the urine, rectal bleeding, or bleeding into any internal organ. Lack of production of normal white cells that fight infection is associated with sore throats, sores in the mouth, pneumonia, and urinary infections usually with an elevated temperature. Pressure from the leukemic cells may cause aching pains over the bones, particularly those of the arms, legs, or the spine, where the large bone marrow cavities are located.

The ninth grade was a bad year for me. I went skiing during one of our vacations and I got more bruises than I thought I should and they stayed around a long time. After that I began getting red dots on my legs. I thought it was a bad case of acne but they stayed under my skin and that didn't make much sense. Finally I was getting very tired so that when I walked home from school I would have to stop and rest several times. It finally got to the point where I had to stop half way up a flight of stairs. That's when we found out.

The diagnosis of leukemia is made by finding abnormal, immature blast cells in the circulating blood obtained by sticking the finger. This is confirmed when microscopic examination of the bone marrow shows abnormal blasts crowding out normal cells. Bone marrow is obtained by inserting a needle into the bone or removing a small piece of bone. This is usually done on the hipbone under a local anesthesia. **Is It Leukemia?**

The goals in treatment of acute leukemia are to produce and maintain a complete remission for as long as possible. The disease is said to be in complete *remission* when no abnormal leukemic cells can be found in the circulating blood or in the bone marrow, and the bone marrow has resumed all its normal functions. The child in complete remission feels and acts perfectly well. **Treatment**

The first remission usually requires two to four weeks of treatment in the hospital, after which the child can go home and continue treatment as an outpatient while taking many of his medications at home. Readmission to the hospital is usually required only for infections, bleeding, or recurrence. The treatment itself falls into three phases. First, remission is induced with drugs, usually including Vincristine and Prednisone and one or two other agents. In ALL, complete remission can be achieved in about 95 percent of children. The second or *consolidation* phase consists of giving special treatment to the head and spine because leukemic cells tend to hide there and cannot be reached by the usual drugs. To get to leukemic cells that may be in the brain or spinal cord, a drug (usually methotrexate) is injected directly into the spinal canal by means of a needle. This is very similar to giving a spinal tap or LP. An alternative is to give radiation to the head and spine. Before this treatment was used, half of the children who went into remission developed recurrence of their disease in the brain or in the spine within eighteen months. This figure is now less than seven percent.

The goal of the third phase is to maintain remission for as long as possible. Several drugs are used. These often include methotrexate given weekly, 6-mercaptopurine taken by mouth daily, and one or more other drugs. These are continued for at least three years.

In addition to treatment that directly attacks the disease, several supportive measures may be used. Various types of blood cells can be transfused to replace those not being formed in adequate numbers by the bone marrow: red cells for anemia, platelets for bleeding, and white cells for infection. If the white cell counts gets too low, the child may be placed in a protective room in the hospital to try to avoid infections until his bone marrow recovers its ability to make white cells. Infections that appear are treated with antibiotics.

When large numbers of leukemic cells are killed, uric acid from the waste products of the destroyed leukemic cells may accumulate in the kidneys and form stones. Allopurinol is a drug that is used to prevent this.

Acute myelocytic leukemia—AML—is treated in much the same way but with a different set of drugs. In addition, some children with AML are being treated by bone marrow transplantation. In this procedure, healthy bone marrow from a close relative is injected into the bone marrow spaces of the child with leukemia. The actual transfer of the bone marrow is carried out under sterile conditions in the operating room with the donor and the patient asleep. In order to make room for the healthy marrow to replace it, the leukemic bone marrow is first destroyed by radiation or chemotherapy. This also destroys most of the remaining normal bone marrow of the patient, leaving the door wide open for infections until the new marrow has a chance to establish itself. During this period every precaution is taken to avoid infection, including keeping the child in a sterile room in the hospital for several weeks until the new bone marrow is well established and functioning properly. Failure of the new bone marrow to grow is obviously a serious complication. Another complication is "graft vs. host disease" in which cells produced by the new bone marrow attack some of the patient's own cells. The risk of this happening is reduced by using a close relative as a donor and by our ability to actually match the cells and select a donor whose cells are most nearly identical to the patient's.

Complications of Treatment. The risks of the treatment of leukemia involve those of the drugs given in high doses to obtain and maintain remission. The common side effects are described elsewhere but these same drugs may also impose additional problems for the child. These include the possibility of sterility, some interference with growth and development, and the possibility, by no means proven by our experience to date, of developing another tumor later in life.

Children receiving chemotherapy for leukemia should take Tylenol rather than aspirin or aspirin containing compounds, to avoid the risk of bleeding, and should avoid any vaccinations while they are under induction or maintenance treatment. Exposure to any contagious disease such as chickenpox, measles, or mumps should be reported immediately to your physician. Other things that should be reported include a temperature greater than 102°, abnormal bleeding anywhere, severe headaches, blurring of vision, weakness, difficulty walking, stiff neck, yellowness of the skin, mouth sores, or unusual nausea or vomiting.

Results of Treatment. The treatment of ALL represents one of the triumphs of modern cancer therapy. Previously this disease was uniformly fatal in a matter of weeks or months. Now more than 95 percent of children with ALL can be brought into complete remission and more than 50 percent can expect to remain in remission for more than five years. At what stage one can speak of cure is not clear yet since recurrence has been known to occur after five or even ten years. However, it is quite likely that a significant number of these children will be permanently cured.

Signs of recurrence or relapse in leukemia are the same as the original symptoms. Bone marrow changes may be found several weeks before they show up in the blood so they are often checked as part of the routine followup exams. Relapse can be treated by inducing a second or even third or fourth remission, occasionally with the same drugs that were used the first time, but often with a different set. Second or later remissions can be long lasting.

The results of treatment of AML have not shown this improvement and only about 20 percent of these children can be maintained in remission for five years.

Leukemia in adults is very similar to the childhood disease with the exception that, in addition to the acute form seen in children, there are two chronic forms in adults which are much more slowly progressive.

LEUKEMIA IN ADULTS

The predominant leukemia of childhood is acute lymphocytic leukemia where the involved cell is a member of the lymphocyte family. After the age of 15, this disease is replaced by acute myelogenous leukemia, or AML, also occasionally called acute non-lymphocytic leukemia or ANLL. This disease can occur any time between the ages of fifteen and seventy-five. The symptoms are exactly the same as acute leukemia in childhood.

Acute Leukemia

Treatment for adult acute leukemia is chemotherapy, the most commonly used drugs being cytosine arabinocide and thioguanine. Other drugs include 6-mercaptopurine, methotrexate, cytoxan, prednisone, and vincristine. Complete remissions can be induced 50–70 percent of the time. The overall outlook, however, for prolonged remissions in adults with AML is not nearly as good as in childhood leukemia, with an average survival of about 1 year after remission. Other supportive forms of treatment include replacement of normal blood cells that are crowded out by the leukemia cells in the bone marrow.

Chronic Granulocytic Leukemia

The abnormal cells in granulocytic leukemia is the granulocyte produced in the bone marrow, one of the most important cells for fighting infections. This disease occurs most commonly between the ages of thirty and sixty. The first signs depend on which one of the three cell components of the blood is damaged most severely. The diagnosis is occasionally made by chance, in the absence of any symptoms, when a blood study shows abnormal cells or the spleen is found to be enlarged on routine examination.

The diagnosis is made by examining samples of the blood and bone marrow by microscope, both of which show a large number of granulocytes. A unique aspect of the these abnormal white cells is that on close inspection they can almost always be shown to have an abnormal chromosome, known as the Philadelphia chromosome after the city where it was first discovered. This chromosome is only found in the abnormal granulocytes and other bone marrow cells. It is not found in other normal cells in the same person, nor is it found in any cells in family members. For this reason, the abnormal chromosome is considered to be acquired with the disease and not inherited. Beyond that, the exact relationship of the abnormal chromosome to the cause of the disease is not known.

Treatment of chronic myelogenous leukemia is chemotherapy, the most commonly used drug being Busulfan. With this and other drugs, it is almost always possible to induce complete remission to where only a few abnormal granulocytes remain in the bone marrow. Remission, however, cannot be maintained indefinitely and the average survival is about three years.

Chronic Lymphocytic Leukemia

The last of the adult leukemias, chronic lymphocyte leukemia, is a disease of still older people in their fifties, sixties, and seventies. This disease can be very slow in coming on, showing up as enlargement of lymph nodes or the spleen, but with no other symptoms. Often there is no anemia or abnormal bleeding and this disease is frequently discovered on routine examination. In some people it is more active, causing fatigue, weakness, and abnormal bleeding. Again, the diagnosis is made by examining the blood and bone marrow by microscope.

Treatment of this disease depends on how active it is. When it is mild, treatment may be withheld until some symptoms appear, often as long as several years. When the disease is active or progresses to the point where treatment is needed, chemotherapy helps to reduce the size of the lymph nodes and the spleen, and to reduce the number of abnormal lymphocytes in the blood. The course of this disease is more variable than the other leukemias. While the average survival is about five years, people with very slowly progressing disease may live fifteen years or longer.

Another disease in the adult leukemia family is multiple myeloma, in which there is an overproduction of a form of lymphocyte known as a plasma cell. This is the cell that is responsible for the production of antibody, one of the major factors in fighting infections. In myeloma there is an over-production of plasma cells in the bone marrow throughout the body (hence the name *multiple* myeloma). As in the other leukemias, the myeloma cells crowd out the normal bone marrow resulting in anemia from lack of red cells, abnormal bleeding from lack of platelets, and frequent infections from lack of normal white cells. In addition, the myeloma cells can attack the bone itself. This results in pain in the bones, particularly in the back, high levels of calcium in the blood from bone destruction, and kidney stones if the kidneys cannot keep up with the increased load of calcium they must get rid of. In addition, myeloma cells often dump large amounts of abnormal proteins into the blood, instead of normal antibody to fight infections. This places a further burden on the kidneys and often leads to kidney failure.

The diagnosis of myeloma is made by examination of the bone marrow, by x-rays of the bones, and by examination of the blood and urine for the abnormal protein produced by the myeloma cells. The extent of the disease can be estimated by x-ray studies of all of the bones and measurement of the amount of abnormal protein in the blood and urine. The degree of replacement of normal bone marrow by myeloma can be estimated by measuring the remaining normal marrow functions in terms of anemia and numbers of platelet and normal white cells. Kidney function is measured accurately to see if the kidneys have been injured by the disease.

Treatment of myeloma includes chemotherapy backed up with radiation to areas where bone pain is severe. Infections must be treated vigorously with antibiotics because many natural defenses are damaged in this disease. Continued physical activity, often requiring orthopedic braces, is important to slow down the progress of bone

Multiple
Myeloma

destruction. Drinking large quantities of fluids helps to avoid kidney problems by flushing out the excess calcium released by the bones and the abnormal protein produced by the myeloma.

If the disease is discovered early and is not very extensive, good treatment may provide several years of comfortable life. If the disease is already widespread when first treated, survival may be only one or two years.

LYMPHOMAS

In addition to a variety of leukemias, adults have another family of similar diseases of the lymphatic system, known as lymphomas. The lymphatic system includes the spleen and a network of glands (lymph nodes) and small vessels distributed throughout the body (See Figure 24.1). One type of white blood cells (lymphocytes) are manufactured in the lymph nodes and the spleen, and enter the circulation through this network. These are important cells for fighting infections. The fluid part of the blood seeps out of blood vessels into the tissues where it bathes and nourishes the cells of the body. The lymphatic system, with its extensive network of tiny tubules, collects this fluid (lymph) and returns it to the main circulation of the bloodstream.

Lymphomas are a group of diseases in which there is over-production of the cells found in lymph nodes and the spleen. One form of lymphoma, Hodgkin's disease, was first described as early as 1832 by an English doctor, Thomas Hodgkin. Today all lymphomas are classified as either Hodgkin's disease or non-Hodgkin's lymphomas, and these two large groups have several subdivisions. It is beyond the scope of this book to go into all the complexities of this family of diseases. The main difference is that in general Hodgkin's disease responds somewhat better to treatment, and has a better overall outlook than non-Hodgkin's lymphomas, perhaps because it tends to remain localized longer in one area.

About 15,000 people develop lymphomas each year. About half have Hodgkin's and the other half non-Hodgkin's lymphomas. Hodgkin's disease is rare in children and occurs most frequently between the ages of twenty and forty-five, while the other lymphomas tend to occur later in life. The lymphomas affect men slightly more frequently than women. While the cause of most cases is not known, the incidence is greater in people who received large amounts of radiation, such as the Japanese survivors of the atomic bomb blast in World War II. Although several lymphomas in experimental animals are caused by viruses, it has not been proven in humans.

Signs

The lymphomas usually show up as one or more enlarged lymph nodes, or glands, most commonly in the neck or the armpit, less

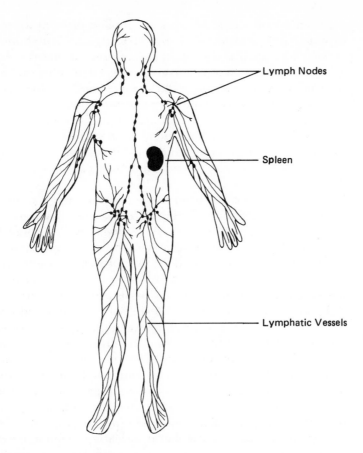

Figure 24.1 The lymphatic system.

commonly in the groin or elsewhere. The lumps are firm and pain-less. Some lymphomas, particularly Hodgkin's disease, may be found on a routine chest x-ray as enlargement of the lymph nodes in the central part of the chest (the mediastinum). Less frequently, a persis-tent fever of unknown cause, sweating at night, itching, weight loss, or weakness may be the first clue to these diseases.

More advanced disease can involve many organs including the liver, lungs, digestive tract, kidneys, and bones. The lymph nodes and spleen are the source of white blood cells that fight infection (lym-phocytes). Lymphomas, particularly Hodgkin's disease, tend to crowd out normal lymphocytes and replace them with abnormal ones. This can gradually lower one's resistance to infections.

In all likelihood, lymphomas start in a single lymph node and spread from there. Hodgkin's disease is characterized by a fairly methodical spread from one lymph node to others in the nearby areas, such as from the neck to the armpit or to the inside of the chest, without large skip areas. The non-Hodgkin's lymphomas tend to spread in a much less predictable fashion, so that the disease may appear in the neck and in the groin, and even in lymph nodes inside the chest or abdomen almost at the same time. The diagnosis is made by a biopsy of any of the enlarged lymph nodes. The biopsy is examined carefully by the pathologist for the presence of Reed-Sternberg cells which will distinguish between Hodgkin's disease and non-Hodgkin's lymphoma, and for cellular patterns which have important implications for treatment and overall outlook.

Staging Once the diagnosis has been made the next step is to determine as accurately as possible the extent of the disease. Physical examination includes all parts of the body where lymph nodes can ordinarily be felt (particularly the neck, armpits, and groin) and examination of the abdomen by hand to see if the liver or spleen are enlarged. A chest x-ray will show enlargement of lymph nodes in that area. Lymph nodes deep in the abdomen and pelvis can be examined by an x-ray technique (lymphangiogram). A special dye is injected into the network of lymphatics in the web between the first and second toes on each foot. Although this is a long way from the target area, the dye makes its way up through lymphatic channels of the leg and about a day later can be seen outlining the lymph nodes in the pelvis and deep in the abdomen. X-rays of the skeleton, particularly if there is tenderness, can show if there is bone involvement. Similarly, biopsy of the bone marrow, usually from the hip, can determine if the tumor has spread to the marrow. Fever, sweating, itching, or weight loss suggest that the disease may involve internal organs, particularly the liver.

As with many other tumors, the extent or stage of the disease is important in the choice of treatment and the expected results. In Stage I, there is involvement of a single group of lymph nodes, confined to one area of the body such as the neck or the armpit. In Stage II, two lymph node areas are involved but they must be adjacent to each other and both must be in the upper half or both in the lower half of the body, the dividing line being the diaphragm that separates the chest from the abdomen. In Stage III, lymph node regions on both sides of the diaphragm are involved (such as neck and groin), and the spleen may be diseased. Stage IV means diffuse involvement outside of the lymph node areas and often includes the liver and bone marrow.

To increase the accuracy of the staging and help choose the best form of treatment, a staging operation is often done to look for spread to lymph nodes and other organs inside the abdomen where they cannot be evaluated by physical examination. This staging operation is most often used for Hodgkin's Disease. As part of this procedure, biopsies of the liver are obtained as well as of lymph nodes from several areas. The spleen is also removed. Some radiation therapists prefer to treat the lymph nodes in the abdomen even when they are not known to be involved. When treatment is going to be given to that area anyway, there is not much need for a staging operation, except to remove the spleen.

Lymphomas are treated by radiation and chemotherapy. If the disease is confined to one area of the body, it is usually treated only with radiation, treating not only the area of known disease but also the adjacent areas. For a tumor in the neck this would include the neck, both armpits, and the middle of the chest. At the other end of the spectrum, the main form of treatment for Stage IV disease is chemotherapy with several drugs. The most commonly used combination in this country carries the nickname of MOPP and consists of mustargen (nitrogen mustard), oncovin (vincristine), procarbazine, and prednisone. These drugs are given in fourteen-day cycles, separated by fourteen-day rest periods, and are usually continued for six or more cycles. Many other drugs and combinations are also used. While the main treatment for Stages II and III is also radiation, chemotherapy is often added for particular types of tumors or if there is involvement outside of the lymph node areas. The treatment of Hodgkin's and non-Hodgkin's lymphomas differ in many details for different stages and even for different types of tumors within each of these major groups.

Treatment

The results of treatment of Hodgkin's disease represents one of the triumphs of cancer research. Previously uniformly fatal, now more than 50 percent of *all* people with Hodgkin's disease, regardless of stage, are free of disease ten to fifteen years later and presumed to be cured. Stages I and II can be cured about 90 percent of the time. Treatment of Stage IV disease with MOPP results in about 80 percent complete remission, and five and even ten years later, half the people are still free of disease. While the results of treatment of non-Hodgkin's lymphoma have improved, they are not as good, with an average five year survival for all stages of about 30 percent.

twenty-five
Brain Tumors

The brain can be thought of as a very complex electronic switchboard or computer capable of acquiring, sorting, integrating, storing, and eventually feeding back vast amounts of information. It is composed of different tissues that include the electronic wires themselves (neurons) and several supporting tissues, most of which are able to develop tumors. Brain tumors are different from most cancers in that they never spread to other parts of the body. Some are very slow growing and simply push the surrounding normal brain tissue aside, often over a period of years, without ever invading the normal tissue. These are considered to be benign brain tumors. More malignant brain tumors may grow rapidly and invade the normal surrounding brain tissue. Both benign and malignant brain tumors share one thing in common. They do not have much room to expand. The skull is a solid container which is completely filled by the normal brain. Any new growth that takes even a small amount of space does so at the expense of the normal brain, causing compression and pressure inside the head. Even a small slowly growing tumor which would give no trouble elsewhere usually has to be removed from the brain, either because it is located in a critical area where it interferes with some normal function, or because it is causing pressure on the entire brain.

About 85 percent of brain tumors are in adults, usually between the ages of fifty and sixty. There are also some brain tumors which occur only in children. About 11,000 new brain tumors occur in the United States each year. Their cause is not known but they are definitely *not* related to head injuries. A few rare hereditary diseases are associated with brain tumors. In experimental animals, both chemicals and viruses are able to cause brain tumors. Workers in some parts of the rubber industry have been found to have an incidence as much as eight times that of the average population, suggesting a chemical cause for some of these tumors.

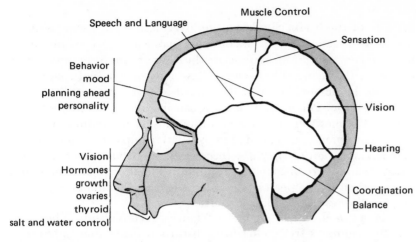

Figure 25.1 Functions of various areas of the brain that may be impaired by brain tumors. The symptoms that result are often related to the exact location of the tumor.

Along with tumors that originate in the brain, we must consider a much larger number of tumors that spread to the brain from elsewhere. These metastatic tumors *to the brain* are much more common than tumors *of the brain*. Although these are not true brain tumors, they may give the same signs. Steps required to evaluate them are the same and occasionally they are removed surgically. All adults suspected of having a brain tumor are studied carefully to look for a primary tumor somewhere else that may have spread to the brain. The most common ones are cancer of the lung, the breast, kidney, thyroid gland, and melanoma. About 50 percent of people who die of melanoma have brain involvement, as do 30 percent of those dying of cancer of the lung.

I feel like a different person—some days I'm myself and some days I'm not. I can't control or even understand the changes, which is very confusing for my *children. I even react differently to the same situations from one day to the next.* I blame my treatment. It is better to blame the treatment—to protect yourself.

Signs

Brain tumors have two ways of causing signs: alteration or loss of some specific function of the brain due to the presence of the tumor in a specialized area, and pressure on the entire brain from increased pressure inside the skull. Many of the various functions of the brain have precise locations, so that a tumor in one area will interfere only with the function of that area (see Figure 25.1). These localized signs may include loss of sensation or muscle function in a particular part of the body such as the right arm or leg. Because the "wires cross over", these signs on the right side would result from a tumor on the *left* side of the brain. Similarly, the loss might be of recognition of words or the capacity to speak, of vision in one or both eyes, or partial loss from both eyes. More subtle are the signs of tumors in the areas of the brain that control behavior. These may be gradual changes in behavior or personality which are hard to recognize until they are quite extreme. Personality changes can include irritability, moodiness, lack of motivation or concentration, absentmindedness or sleepiness. The changes can erode family relationships or cause poor job performance before they are recognized for what they really are. These changes are often harder on family members, particularly the spouse, than on the person who has the tumor. We do not like to see our loved ones become less lovable.

A more dramatic sign is a seizure or convulsion. This, too, usually originates from a localized disturbance and then spreads to involve most of the brain. In this case the disturbance is an electrical one with abnormal electrical shock waves starting up in the brain tissue in or near the tumor and then spreading to the normal brain tissue elsewhere. There are two main groups of seizures. A major seizure, or grand mal, is a violent muscular reaction associated with complete loss of consciousness. The person usually falls to the ground and stiffens with a series of jerking movements. Because there is some tendency towards unconscious breath holding during the seizure, the skin may become white or even bluish. The jerking motions gradually decrease over a few minutes but the person remains in a deep sleep for an hour or more afterward. Although a major seizure can be very frightening to witness, it is usually harmless and the person having it has little or no recollection afterwards. You should not try to restrain an individual who is having a seizure in any way. About all that can be done is to protect her from injuring herself against furniture or other hard objects. Glasses should be removed and tight clothing loosened. The head should be turned to the side in the sleeping phase to prevent the relaxed tongue from interfering with breathing. Nothing should be given by mouth during the seizure or afterward until the person is fully conscious and able to talk and swallow.

The minor seizure, or focal seizure, is less dramatic and may even go unnoticed. This is more of a behavioral seizure and may consist of a glassy stare for several minutes, inability to answer questions or inappropriate answers, some form of inappropriate behavior such as getting up to walk around aimlessly or plucking at the clothing, making chewing motions, or appearing to be drunk. Again, this abnormal behavior usually lasts only a few minutes. It is not followed by a period of sleep but there is usually no memory of anything that took place during the period of the seizure. Following this, the person may be confused for a few minutes or may be alert immediately. Again, no attempt should be made to restrain the person during the seizure but she should be protected from walking into objects that could cause injury. If the person appears angry or aggressive you should not try to reason with her or restrain her.

Signs of pressure on the brain include headache, nausea, vomiting, dizziness, and unsteadiness on the feet. Late signs of greater pressure may include dullness of intellect, sleepiness, and blurring of vision. The headache is usually worse upon awakening in the morning and may even cause one to wake up. It tends to appear off and on throughout the day and is usually a generalized throbbing headache. It is a "touchy" headache, made worse by coughing, straining, or sudden motions of the head. When nausea or vomiting are present, they usually appear at the same time as the headache. Beyond headache, which can usually be controlled with medication, brain tumors are rarely associated with severe pain. For many, however, awareness that the brain is not functioning properly is pain enough.

The various functions of the brain and the remainder of the central nervous system are so beautifully organized that it is often possible to get a great deal of information just from the history and physical examination. Essentially, these examinations determine which nerves are functioning properly and which are not. Examination involves testing of sensation, including vision and hearing, muscular ability, and reflexes over much of the body. Each of these can be mapped and related directly to its place in the brain. Increased pressure in the brain can be recognized by shining a light into the pupil of the eye and looking at the nerve and small blood vessels that enter the back of the eye directly from the brain. Occasionally tumors located at the base of the brain, at or near the pituitary gland, may cause hormonal disorders of a wide variety, including disturbances of growth, thyroid gland function, ovarian function and menses, the turnover of water and salt, and resistance to stress.

Is It a Brain Tumor?

The next step in examining the brain is to see if it is producing abnormal electrical waves. As mentioned initially, the brain can be considered a complex electronic computer. It has a normal pattern of electrical waves that it creates itself. These can be monitored by placing small wires on several places on the scalp and measuring the electrical changes taking place inside the head (electroencephalogram, or EEG). This painless study can reveal abnormal wave patterns which may give clues as to the presence and even location of a brain tumor.

More precise location of a brain tumor is obtained by injecting a radioactive isotope into the arm, using an isotope that is selectively picked up and concentrated by the brain tumor, but not by the normal brain tissue. This "brain scan" is painless and simply requires lying still while a camera goes back and forth beside the head recording the radiation given off by the isotope. The amount of radiation used for this study is small and constitutes no risk.

X-rays of the skull may show destruction of bone. A more refined technique, computerized tomography, or CT scan, is able to provide pictures representing cross-sectional views of the brain to look for any displacement of brain structures from their normal locations. By injecting an x-ray dye into the blood vessels that go to the brain (angiogram), usually under sedation or even anesthesia, it is possible to take x-ray pictures of the blood vessels on and within the brain to see if they are being pushed aside. The same pictures often can locate a tumor by its abnormal blood supply. Finally, the brain has four small cavities inside it filled with fluid, which communicate with the coverings over the spinal cord in the middle of the back. By putting a small needle in the back, it is possible to drain off some of this fluid and allow air to replace it (pneumoencephalogram). When the cavities within the brain are filled with air, they stand out sharply on x-ray pictures, so their position, shape, and communication with each other can be checked. This procedure is usually done under anesthesia. Biopsy of a brain tumor, required for the final diagnosis, is usually obtained at the time of surgery to remove the tumor rather than as a separate procedure. Not all of these tests are required for any one brain tumor.

Treatment   The best treatment for most brain tumors is surgery, removing the entire tumor or as much of it as possible. Some brain tumors are so well separated from the normal brain tissue that they can be removed completely with little chance of recurrence. Others grow slowly and may be operated on several times over a period of years, whenever the signs of the original tumor come back. Still others are unlikely to be cured by surgery alone and require additional treatment with radiation or chemotherapy. These are the tumors that extend into the normal brain like the roots of a tree and the margins between tumor and normal tissue cannot be seen (See Table 25.1).

Brain operations are done under general anesthesia and require removing a portion of the skull. The head must be completely shaved before the operation to avoid infection. The bone is replaced at the end of the operation and once the hair has grown back there is no obvious defect. Even the scar is invisible. The brain is a very delicate structure which can be injured easily. Many brain operations are now done with the aid of an operating microscope to see the delicate structures better and increase the safety. Some tumors are difficult to get at and the task for the neurosurgeon is to remove as

Table 25.1. Brain Tumors

Tumor	Age	Growth	Treatment	Outlook
Astrocytoma cerebellar	Children & Adults	slow	Surgery, may be repeated	Good, years or permanent cure.
Low grade astrocytoma	Children & Adults	slow	Surgery & radiation	Good if totally removed.
Glioblastoma multiform	Adults	rapid	Surgery, radiation, & chemotherapy	Poor, less than 1 year.
Brain stem glioma	Children & Adults	rapid	Radiation	Usually fatal.
Ependymoma	Children	slow–rapid	Surgery, radiation, & chemotherapy	Grade I–89% 3 years; Grade IV–10% 3 years.
Medulloblastoma	Children	slow	Surgery, radiation, & chemotherapy	20 percent–five year survival; many recur.
Meningioma	Children & Adults	slow	Surgery	Good, permanent cure.
Pituitary tumors	Adults	slow	Surgery, radiation	Good, permanent cure.

much of the tumor as possible without harming the normal brain. A person who has a brain operation may be quite sleepy for several days because of the swelling of the brain that takes place. Swelling and bruising can also be seen in the soft tissues of the face if the operation was on the front of the head. People who have had brain operations are frequently kept half-sitting in bed to decrease this swelling. All of these changes disappear within a few days.

When the tumor cannot be completely removed, surgery is frequently followed by radiation. This, too, has side effects, including hair loss and swelling of the brain. Radiation treatments are spaced out and a drug is frequently given (decadron) to decrease the swelling. Hair loss, in preparation for surgery, as a result of radiation, or both, is upsetting and should be planned for. It can come on very suddenly in radiation treatment. A wide variety of wigs are available that can be matched up before the hair is lost. An inexpensive way for a man to get one is to buy a woman's wig and cut it to his own style. Many men find that growing a moustache or beard helps to compensate for loss of their normal hair. Radiation occasionally causes loss of eyebrows and eyelashes, but these usually grow back.

If a single area of the brain is involved with a tumor that has spread from elsewhere, and there is no evidence of spread to other organs, surgery is sometimes done to remove this tumor. If studies show that the tumor has spread to several areas of the brain, surgery is not recommended and radiation or chemotherapy are used, depending on the type and sensitivity of the original cancer.

Results   Many people are able to resume all of their normal activities and go back to work following the treatment for a brain tumor while others may have permanent defects from the tumor or the surgery required. The overall results depend very much on the type of tumor. Some are completely cured by surgery alone while others are rarely cured even by the combined efforts of surgery, radiation, and chemotherapy.

Recurrence of a brain tumor often gives the same signs as the original. The major problem is pressure from the tumor within the skull. Decadron and other drugs which combat swelling in the brain frequently are useful at this stage. Death from a brain tumor is usually painless and quiet, with increasing sleep, and unconsciousness as the various functions of the brain stop.

(Please see the index for terms that are defined in the text.)

ADENOMA. A benign tumor of glandular tissue.

ADJUVANT TREATMENT. Additional treatment, usually of a different kind (for example, chemotherapy after surgery), to try to increase the chances of permanent cure.

ANASTOMOSIS. Surgical joining together of two hollow structures to establish continuity, as in the bowel after removal of a diseased portion.

ANEMIA. Inadequate number of red blood cells due to bleeding, iron deficiency, infection, damage to bone marrow, or replacement of bone marrow by leukemia.

ANTIBIOTIC. A substance produced by living organisms such as bacteria or molds, which can destroy other bacteria. Some antibiotics have anticancer activity.

ARTERY. A vessel which carries oxygen-rich blood from the heart to the tissues.

AXILLA. The armpit.

BACTERIA. A term for a group of living organisms, larger than viruses, which may be seen only through a microscope, and are the cause of most infections.

BENIGN. Not malignant or cancerous, harmless.

BIOPSY. A small sample of tissue taken with a sharp instrument for evaluation under a microscope to determine if cancer cells are present.

BLADDER. Sac that holds the body's liquid waste before it is eliminated (gall bladder, urinary bladder).

BLAST CELL. Immature blood cell, usually found only in the bone marrow.

BONE MARROW. The spongy material which fills the cavities of the bones, in which many of the blood cells are produced.

BLOOD COUNT. An examination of the blood to count the number of white and red blood cells and platelets.

COPING. The psychological mechanisms for dealing with problems.

CANCER. A general term for more than one hundred diseases, all of which have an uncontrolled growth of cells. The resulting mass, or tumor, can invade and destroy surrounding normal tissues. Cells from the cancer can spread through the blood or lymph system to start new ones, in other parts of the body (see metastasis).

CARCINOGEN. Any substance that causes cancer.

CARCINOMA. A form of cancer which arises in the tissues that cover or line such organs of the body as skin, intestines, uterus, lung, breast, and others (see epithelium).

CARCINOMA IN SITU. An early stage in the growth of cancer when it is still confined to the tissue in which it started.

CBC. A complete blood count.

CELL. The living units from which animals and plants are built. In the center of each cell, there is a denser portion called the nucleus which controls the cell's metabolism and reproduction. It also contains the chromosomes, which carry the genetic information, the genes. The material outside of the nucleus is called the cytoplasm.

CHROMOSOME. A structural unit of heredity, which is present in each cell nucleus, contains numerous genes for hereditary traits. Human cells have forty-six chromosomes, each made up of thousands of genes.

CLINICAL. Pertaining to the study and treatment of disease in human beings by direct observation, as distinguished from laboratory research.

CNS. central nervous system, referring to the brain and spinal cord.

COBALT THERAPY. A form of radiation treatment.

COMBINATION THERAPY. The use of two or more modes of treatment: surgery, radiation, and chemotherapy, in combinations to treat cancer.

CRYOSURGERY. Freezing of tissue using liquid nitrogen or dry ice, to eliminate abnormal cells on the cervix or vocal cords.

CYST. An abnormal sac which contains a liquid or semi-solid material; may be benign or malignant.

CYTOLOGY. The science which deals with the study of living cells. Cells which have been sloughed off, or scraped off, from such organs of the body as uterus, lungs, bladder, or stomach are examined under the microscope for early signs of abnormality. The Pap test used for early detection of cervical cancer is an example of this method. Also referred to as exfoliative cytology.

DIAGNOSIS. Identifying a disease by its signs, symptoms, course, and laboratory findings.

DYSPLASIA. Very early changes in cell structure that may be premalignant.

ELECTRON BEAM THERAPY. A form of radiation treatment used mainly for tumors near the surface of the body.

EPIDEMIOLOGY. The study of incidence, distribution, environmental causes, and control of disease in a population.

EPITHELIUM. The type of tissue which lines skin surface and some of the hollow internal organs, and comprises the body's extensive glandular apparatus. Carcinoma is derived from epithelial tissue, in contrast to sarcoma, which is derived from supporting tissues.

ESOPHAGUS. The food passage from the mouth to the stomach; the foodpipe or gullet.

ESTROGEN. A female hormone produced mostly by the ovaries which is essential to reproduction. It is involved in the menstrual cycle, and produces female secondary sex characteristics, such as breast development.

ETIOLOGY. Cause, as applied to cause of disease.

EXCISION. Surgical removal of a diseased part of the body, including cancerous growths.

GENES. The hereditary units of life which control the cell's transfer of a trait or process.

GENETICS. The field of study concerned with heredity.

G.I. TRACT. Abbreviation for gastrointestinal (digestive) tract.

GUAIAC TEST. A chemical test used to detect hidden blood in the stool. A simple method allows stool specimens to be placed on special guaiac-treated paper slides. These slides are then treated and checked by a doctor or lab technician. The test is well-suited to screening programs for colon-rectal cancer because the specimen can be prepared at home.

HEMATOCRIT. A measure of the number of red blood cells; they are decreased in anemia.

HEMATOLOGY. The study of the blood and blood-forming organs.

HEMOGLOBIN. A measure of the number of red blood cells; they are decreased in anemia.

HORMONES. Chemicals that help regulate the body mechanisms, including growth, metabolism, and reproduction.

HYPERPLASIA. Increase in number of cells of a tissue or organ, but not necessarily related in any way to cancer.

HYPOPHYSECTOMY. Removal of the pituitary gland, most frequently for recurrence of breast cancer.

IMMUNE REACTION. A reaction of normal tissues to foreign substances. These foreign substances can be chemicals, particles, microorganisms, or cells. The reactions can be mediated through antibodies, or through the direct action of lymphocytes.

IMMUNOLOGY. Branch of science dealing with the body's resistance mechanism against disease or the invasion of a foreign substance.

IMMUNOTHERAPY. Treatment of cancer by stimulating the body's own immune defense mechanism against the disease (not of proven value).

INFECTION. Invasion of the body by disease-producing organisms.

INJECTIONS. Introduction of drugs into the body by a hollow needle. Injections may be given intramuscularly (into a muscle), intravenously (into a vein), or subcutaneously (just under the skin).

INTRAVENOUS. Given into a vein, as with intravenous medication or feeding.

INVASION. The escape of tumor from its site of origin with resulting spread into surrounding tissues.

IRRIGATE. To wash out.

JAUNDICE. Yellowing of the skin and the whites of the eyes from backing up of products of blood breakdown. Caused by rapid breakdown of red blood cells, liver disease, or blockage of the common bile duct.

LARYNX. The organ of sound production, the voice box which contains the vocal cords. Laryngectomy is removal of the larynx.

LESION. Any abnormality of body tissue, due to an illness, injury, or defect at birth.

LINEAR ACCELERATOR. A type of equipment used for radiation therapy.

LIPOMA. A benign tumor derived from fat tissue.

LUMBAR PUNCTURE. (Abbreviated L.P.) Same as spinal tap. A technique for removing small amounts of the fluid which bathes the brain and spinal cord. A narrow needle is inserted in the middle of the back under local anesthesia. In leukemia, this fluid is tested for the presence of blast cells, as well as other elements.

LYMPH. A clear fluid which circulates throughout the body, containing white blood cells (called lymphocytes), antibodies, and nourishing substances.

LYMPH GLAND. Tissue which is made up of lymphocytes and connective tissue, and produces lymph and lymphocytes (also called lymph nodes). These lymph glands, or nodes, normally act as filters of impurities in the body.

LYMPH SYSTEM. The circulatory network of vessels, spaces, and nodes carrying lymph, the almost colorless fluid that bathes the body's cells. The system is important in the body's defense against infection.

MALIGNANT. Cancerous; a growth of cancer cells.

METASTASES. The spread of cancer from one part of the body to another, usually by the lymph and blood systems. Cells in the new cancer are like those in the original tumor.

MITOSIS. The process of cell reproduction by which new cells are formed.

MUCOUS MEMBRANE. The specialized surface layers of certain body cavities and internal tubes (such as mouth, nose, gastrointestinal tract, and female genital tract) consisting of epithelial lining plus underlying supporting tissue.

MUTATION. A change in the genetic information of a cell that alters its behavior and is transferred to the new cells that result from cell division. A mutation may be induced (as by radiation) or it may be spontaneous, occurring naturally with no known cause.

NEOPLASM. Any new abnormal growth of cells or tissues. It may be benign or malignant, but is customarily used to describe a cancerous tumor.

NUCLEAR MEDICINE. The study dealing with the administration of radioactive materials in the diagnosis of disease and treatment of certain cancers.

ONCOLOGY. The study and treatment of cancer as a special branch of medicine.

ORGAN. Several tissues grouped together to perform one or more functions in the body.

OSTOMY. A surgical procedure that creates a stoma, or artificial opening. A stoma of the intestinal and urinary tracts permits the elimination of wastes through the abdominal wall. A stoma of the respiratory tract permits the passage of air through the neck. An ostomate is someone who has had this form of surgery.

PALLIATIVE TREATMENT. Providing relief from symptoms of a disease but not directly curing the disease; alleviating pain. Palliation.

PALPATION. A detection procedure using the hands to examine organs without the aid of instruments.

PANCREAS. A large gland behind the stomach that secretes digestive fluids and the hormone insulin.

PAP SMEAR. (Papanicolaou smear or Pap Test). A screening test for cancer of the cervix. Cells are obtained from the surface of the cervix and studied under a microscope.

PAPILLOMA. A tumor which generally arises in skin or in epithelial cells of internal organs, and characteristically rises above surrounding surface.

PATHOLOGY. The branch of medicine involved in making diagnoses from the examination of tissues.

PHARMACOLOGY. The study of drugs, their absorption, distribution throughout the body, and excretion.

PHARYNX. The area between the mouth and esophagus, the throat.

PLASMA. The liquid portion of the blood in which the cells are suspended. Contains many proteins and minerals necessary for normal body functioning.

PLATELETS. Small circular or oval disks present in blood which are necessary for blood to clot. Produced in the bone marrow. A platelet count refers to the number of platelets in the blood.

POLYP. An overgrowth of tissue projecting into a cavity of the body, as in the lining of the colon, the nasal passage, or the surface of vocal cords.

POSTMORTEM EXAMINATION. An autopsy. Examination of the body of the deceased in order to determine or study the cause of death.

PREMALIGNANT. A term applied to certain early cell changes, which possess the potential to become malignant. This may take many years.

PRESSURE SORE (or bed-sore). Breakdown of the skin in people who are unable to change position frequently, usually over prominent bones such as the hips, lower back, or heels.

PROCTO. Short for proctosigmoidoscopy, an examination of the first ten inches of the rectum and colon with a hollow, lighted tube.

PROGNOSIS. A prediction regarding the outcome of a disease.

PROSTHESIS. An artificial replacement for a missing body part, for example, breast, leg, arm, eye.

PROTEIN. A naturally occurring compound in meat, eggs, milk, and some grains, which is essential to growth and repair of all living cells. The main component of all animal tissues.

PROTOCOL. Standardized procedures followed by physicians so that results of treatment of different patients can be compared.

QUACKERY. The practice of using untested or unproven methods of treatment for a disease. A quack is someone who gives such treatment.

RADIATION. Energy waves or particles given off by a source. Visible light is a form of low energy radiation.

RADIATION THERAPY. Treatment using high energy radiation from x-ray, cobalt, radium, and other sources for the destruction of cancer.

RADIOACTIVITY. Spontaneous release of radiation energy by some chemicals. Used to detect or treat cancer. Careless use can cause cancer.

RADIOLOGIST. A physician with special experience using radiant energy, usually x-ray, in the diagnosis of disease. Not to be confused with radiation therapist who treats cancer with radiation.

RECURRENCE. Reappearance of a tumor either locally, where the original tumor was, or distally, in some other part of the body (metastasis).

REHABILITATION. The restoration of a sick or injured person to self-sufficiency in daily living and to gainful employment at his highest attainable skill.

RELAPSE. Return of a disease after its apparent improvement.

REMISSION. Complete or partial disappearance of the signs and symptoms of a disease, or the period during which a disease is under control.

SARCOMA. A form of cancer that arises in the connective tissues, including bone and cartilage, fat, fibrous tissue, and muscle.

SIDE-EFFECT. Extra or secondary effect of treatment. The feeling of well-being associated with morphine or cortisone, and nausea or loss of hair associated with some chemotherapy drugs, are examples of pleasant and unpleasant side effects.

SIGNS. The effects of an illness as seen and observed by an outsider. Signs and symptoms are close enough in meaning that they are used interchangeably in this book.

SPINAL TAP. See Lumbar Puncture.

SPLEEN. An organ in the abdomen that is responsible for removing old or damaged red blood cells from the circulation, and for producing some kinds of white blood cells.

SUPPORTIVE THERAPY. All treatment for general support, but not directly attacking the disease.

STAGING. Determining the extent of growth of a cancer so that proper treatment can be given and a prognosis offered.

STOMA. An artificial opening on the surface of the body.

SYMPTOM. The effects of an illness as felt by the patient.

THERAPEUTIC. Pertaining to treatment.

THERAPIST. A person with special skills in treating illness or disability.

THERAPY. The treatment of disease.

THERMOGRAPHY. A technique for measuring the surface temperature of parts of the body to detect underlying disease. It is used along with mammography and palpation for discovering breast cancer in its earliest stage.

THROMBOCYTOPENIA. Refers to a decreased number of platelets in the blood.

TISSUE. A collection of similar cells. There are four basic tissues in the body: epithelial, connective, muscle, and nerve.

TOMOGRAM. An x-ray technique to detect small tumors, usually in the lung.

TOXICITY. A word frequently used to describe the undesirable side effect caused by a drug.

TUMOR. An abnormal mass of tissue or growth. Although some tumors are harmless (benign), the terms "tumor" and "cancer" are used interchangeably in this book, to mean cancerous or malignant.

VEIN. A blood vessel carrying blood from the tissues towards the heart and lungs.

VIRUS. A tiny parasite which invades cells and alters their chemistry so that the cells are compelled to produce more virus particles. Viruses cause many diseases, including some experimental cancers. No human cancer has been proven to be caused by a virus.

VITAMIN. Chemical substances which are essential for the maintenance of normal growth and body function. These substances are sufficiently abundant in most normal diets.

WHITE BLOOD COUNT (WBC). Refers to the number of leukocytes or white blood cells.

X-RAY. Penetrating radiations of the same general nature as light, but invisible, with an extremely short wave length, used to help diagnose and treat cancer.

Chemotherapy *(Cont.)*
    for cure, 155–56
    decisions regarding use, 30
    drugs used in, 160–62
    effectiveness, 106–7, 156–57, 167–69
    hormone treatment, 165–67, 168,
        212–13, 243, 244
    for leukemia, 276, 277–78
    for lymphoma, 283
    and metastases, 134, 135–36
    for sarcomas, 271–72
    side effects, 11, 99, 159, 163–65, 167,
        183, 185, 186
    for stomach cancer, 233
    unproven drugs, 138–43
Chewing tobacco, 255
Children:
    attitudes towards hospitals and doctors,
        82, 102–4
    cancer in, 97–111, 271–72, 274–77
    death of, 107–9
    as emotional support, 35
    grief of, 93–96
    knowledge of cancer, 44–46, 97–98
    legal responsibility for, 106
    reactions to cancer, 43, 46–47
Chondrosarcoma, 270
Choriocarcinoma, 133, 135, 156, 245
Clinical Center, of National Institutes of
    Health, 114
Clinical trials, participation in, 68–69
Colon, examination of, 129
Colon cancer, 121, 134
    complications, 219
    diagnosis, 216–18
    early detection, 216–17
    metastases, 218, 222–23
    recurrence, 222–23
    risk factors, 214–16
    signs, 216–17
    treatment, 218–22
Colostomy, 219–22, 254
Committee for Freedom of Choice in
    Cancer Treatment, 139
Communication, 48, 52, 90, 92, 100
    doctor-patient, 24, 25–27
    lack of, 31–33
Competition, as defense mechanism, 77
Computerized tomography (CT), 127–28,
    288
Confidence, in doctors, 24, 60, 58, 100
Consciousness, during dying, 84
Constipation, 186, 193
Contraception, 251
Control, loss of, 9, 82, 193
Coping mechanisms, 20–24
Cortisones, 167
Cost, of treatment, 112–14
Cough, 125

Counseling services:
    for cancer patients, 38–40, 93, 114
    for family, 101–2, 114
Cremation, 87
Cryosurgery, 258–59
CT scan. *See* Computerized tomography
Cure, definition, 14
Cure rate, of cancer, 6–7, 25, 110, 136,
    137, 224
Cystectomy, 241

Death:
    acceptance of, 23, 73, 76, 78–79
    attitudes towards, 83, 93–96
    of children, 107–9
    fear of, 16–17, 38, 73, 94
    meaning of, 96
    place of, 81–83, 85–86, 107–8
    procedures following, 85–87
    process of, 83–85
    right to, 79–81
    talking about, 16–17, 77, 93
Deferral, as coping mechanism, 20, 22
Denial, 5–6, 20, 42, 47, 52, 76–77, 100
Dependency, 24, 48–49, 71, 193
Depression, 9, 42, 51, 90, 77–78
Diagnosis:
    of bladder cancer, 240
    of brain tumor, 287–88
    of breast cancer, 201–3
    of cervix cancer, 25–53
    of colon cancer, 216–18
    of head and neck cancers, 257
    of kidney cancer, 238
    knowledge of, 27–28, 61
    of leukemia, 275, 278, 279
    of melanoma, 268
    of prostate cancer, 242–43
    of sarcoma, 270–71
    of skin cancer, 266
    techniques, 125–33, 144–45
    of thyroid cancer, 263
    of uterus cancer, 248–49
Diarrhea, 178, 186, 215, 244
Dilation and curettage, 249
Diet:
    as cause of colon cancer, 214
    during radiation treatment, 178, 179,
        180, 185, 186
    elemental, 187–88
Digestive tract, examination of, 129
Digestive tract cancer, 182–83, 230–36
    treatment side effects, 159, 163, 178
Disfigurement, from surgery, 145,
    205–6, 266
Distraction, as coping mechanism, 20, 22
Doctors:
    attitudes of, 25, 60–61, 74, 99

Intellect, impairment of, 107

Radiation sickness, 180
Radiation therapy, 65, 113, 137, 170–80, 183
  for bladder cancer, 241
  for breast cancer, 210
  for colon cancer, 222–23
  for digestive cancer, 232
  for head and neck cancers, 257–58
  internal, 172, 249, 258
  for kidney cancer, 238
  long term effects, 106–7
  for lung cancer, 229
  for lymphoma, 283
  side effects, 177–80, 185, 186
  for skin cancer, 266–67
Rectal examination, 129, 217–18, 242
Rectum cancer, 214–23
Recurrence, 133, 137
  of brain tumor, 290
  of breast cancer, 210, 211–13
  of colon cancer, 222–23
  control, 157–58
  fear of, 13–15, 48, 103
  of head and neck cancers, 261–62
  of kidney cancer, 239
  of leukemia, 275, 277
  of lung cancer, 228–29
  of melanoma, 269
  of ovary cancer, 248
  of skin cancer, 267
  of uterus cancer, 250
Rehabilitation:
  following laryngectomy, 259–61
  following mastectomy, 209–11
Rehabilitation Act, 119
Rejection, 33, 38, 51, 76, 103, 209
Relationships:
  doctor-family, 52–53
  doctor-patient, 24, 30, 35–36, 58–62, 93, 142–43
Religious beliefs, 8, 17, 35, 66, 78, 106
Remission, of leukemia, 275–76, 277, 278
Reproductive organs, 179
Retinoblastoma, 156
Phabdomyosarcoma, 271
Right to die, 79–81
Role changes, 42–44

Salivary gland cancer, 135
Sarcoma, 109, 135, 137, 145, 156, 169, 172, 270–72
School attendance, 105–6
Seizures, 286–87
Self-acceptance, 18
Self-administration, of medication, 70, 193
Self-assertion, 24–27
Self-awareness, 18
Self-confidence, 208

Self-esteem, loss of, 8–9, 204
Self-image, 205
Self-pity, 12, 78
Seminoma, 244
Sensation, loss of, 5, 285
Sexual activity, 49–52, 164, 178, 207–9, 243
Sexual attractiveness, 51, 206, 211
Sexual development, effect of therapy on, 106–7
Shock, 5, 42, 76
Side effects:
  of chemotherapy, 11, 99, 159, 163–65, 167, 183, 185, 186
  of narcotics, 193
  of radiation treatment, 172, 177–80, 183
  of surgery, 219
Signs of cancer, 226, 262–63, 268, 274–75, 280–82, 285–86
Skin cancer, 121, 136, 137, 171, 265–72
Skin reactions to treatment, 163, 177–78
Smoking as cause of cancer, 8, 225–26, 227, 230, 239, 255
Sore throat, 186
Sores, 126, 178, 257
Speech, following laryngectomy, 260–61
Spinal cord cancer, 5
Squamous cell carcinoma, 121, 265–67
Sterility, 50, 276
Stomach cancer, 136, 169, 232–34
Suicide, 9
Sunlight, cause of skin cancer, 265–66, 267–68, 269–70
Support systems, 31–40, 47–52, 53–55, 93, 99–104
Surgeons, choice of, 57–59
Surgery, 11, 26–27, 29–30, 68, 134, 135–36, 144–53, 258
  complications, 151–52, 254
  preparations for, 146–48
  postoperative period, 149–51
  procedures, 148–49
  second opinions, 59–60
  types of, 57–58
Survival time, 210, 222, 238–39, 241, 250, 272, 280
  doctor's estimate of, 74–76, 137
Swallowing, difficulty in, 4, 84, 126, 179, 183, 231, 232, 262

Taste, loss of, 179, 185–86
Tension, reduction of, 20
Teratocarcinoma, 245
Testicle cancer, 137, 156, 171, 244–45
Thyroid cancer, 137, 262–63
Time, limited, 19, 26–27
Tongue cancer, 255–58
Tracheostomy, 259–60